# AIDS,
# HEALTH,
# and
# MENTAL HEALTH

## A Primary Sourcebook

# AIDS, HEALTH, and MENTAL HEALTH

A Primary Sourcebook

*Judith Landau-Stanton*
*Colleen D. Clements*

*with Associates:*
**Robert E. Cole**
**Ann Z. Griepp**
**Alexander F. Tartaglia**

*with:*
**Jackie Nudd**
**Elisabet Espaillat-Piña**
**M. Duncan Stanton**

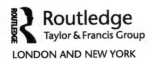

Routledge
Taylor & Francis Group

LONDON AND NEW YORK

First published 1993 by Brunner/Mazel, Inc.

Published 2018 by Routledge
2 Park Square, Milton Park, Abingdon, Oxon OX14 4RN
52 Vanderbilt Avenue, New York, NY 10017

First issued in paperback 2018

*Routledge is an imprint of the Taylor & Francis Group,
an informa business*

Library of Congress Cataloging-in-Publication Data
Landau-Stanton, Judith.
    Aids, health, and mental health : a primary sourcebook / by Judith
Landau-Stanton and Colleen D. Clements.
        p.   cm.
    Includes bibliographical references and index.
    ISBN 0-87630-688-1
    1. AIDS (Disease)   2. AIDS (Disease)—Social aspects.   3. AIDS
(Disease)—Psychological aspects.   I. Clements, Colleen D.
II. Title.
RA644.A25L364   1993
362.1'9697'92—dc20                                    92-30578
                                                            CIP

ISBN 13: 978-1-138-86923-3 (pbk)
ISBN 13: 978-0-87630-688-8 (hbk)

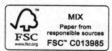

MIX
Paper from
responsible sources
FSC
www.fsc.org   FSC™ C013985

Printed in the United Kingdom
by Henry Ling Limited

## DEDICATION

To the extended family: My father, David Landau, my first inspiration in the field of social medicine and all the fathers and mothers who took his place; my mentors in psychiatry, Vera Bührmann, Lynn Gillis and Dick Cheetham; my husband, Duke Stanton, who unstintingly shares his creativity, ideas and wisdom, and is a constant source of encouragement and love; my children, Johan, David, Raoul, and Cathy, who have unselfishly allowed me the joy of authorship and motherhood; and the many generations of my family and friends, and the families of all the patients who made this book possible.

And for Rudy whose sacrifice came first . . .

JLS


For Norman, again.

CDC

# Contents

# Contents

PART I: APPLIED SYSTEMS THINKING IN HIV/AIDS PREVENTION

PART II: BIOPSYCHOSOCIAL INTERVENTION:
CLINICAL MANAGEMENT

# Contributors

**Judith Landau-Stanton, M.B., Ch.B., D.P.M.**
Psychiatrist; Professor of Psychiatry and Family Medicine; Director of the AIDS Training Program; Family Therapy Training and Clinical Services in the Division of Family Programs of the Department of Psychiatry, University of Rochester School of Medicine and Dentistry, Rochester, New York.

**Colleen D. Clements, Ph.D.**
Clinical Associate Professor of Psychiatry; Associate Director of the AIDS Training Program of the Division of Family Programs and Faculty of the Psychiatry and Law Program of the Department of Psychiatry, University of Rochester School of Medicine and Dentistry, Rochester, New York.

**Robert E. Cole, Ph.D.**
Clinical Associate Professor of Psychiatry (Psychology); Director of Research and Evaluation of the AIDS Training Program of the Division of Family Programs of the Department of Psychiatry, University of Rochester School of Medicine and Dentistry, Rochester, New York.

**Ann Z. Griepp, M.D.**
Assistant Professor of Psychiatry, Coordinator of HIV Psychiatric Services of Department of Psychiatry, and trainer, AIDS Training Program, Division of Family Programs, Department of Psychiatry, University of Rochester School of Medicine and Dentistry, Rochester, New York.

**Alexander F. Tartaglia, D. Min.**

Director of Chaplaincy Services and Training at Strong Memorial Hospital and Pastoral Advisor; Trainer, AIDS Training Program of the Division of Family Programs of the Department of Psychiatry, University of Rochester School of Medicine and Dentistry, Rochester, New York.

**Jackie Nudd**

Former Executive Director of AIDS Rochester, Inc.; Community Consultant with the AIDS Training Project of the Division of Family Programs, Department of Psychiatry, University of Rochester School of Medicine and Dentistry, Rochester, New York.

**Elisabet Espaillat-Piña**

AIDS Community Educator, Puerto Rican Youth Development, Rochester, New York; Senior Health Educator–Part-time, AIDS Training Program of the Division of Family Programs, Department of Psychiatry, University of Rochester School of Medicine and Dentistry, Rochester, New York.

**M. Duncan Stanton, Ph.D.**

Professor of Psychiatry (Psychology); Director of the Division of Family Programs of the Department of Psychiatry, University of Rochester School of Medicine and Dentistry, Rochester, New York.

# Preface

Health care professionals are familiar with dealing with chronic illness and loss. Most of us have worked with cancer patients and their families, and all of us have lost friends and family members. The authors are no different. One of us (JLS) had experienced many losses, both personal and professional:

"Many of my patients had taught me to deal with death. My first lesson was given me by a surgical patient dying of an untreatable malignancy, despite all our best efforts. He collected his family members around him and invited me to join them. He then shared with us all, in a loving and dignified way, his personal preparations for death. He told us that he was ready to die. He had made all his financial arrangements, and was at peace with his Maker. He helped us plan his funeral. He shared with his wife and children his plans for their future. He told them which members of their extended family he most valued and wanted to have involved in the raising of his children. He parted with his wife in a moving and real way that taught me how precious a relationship can be.

"But nothing in my past had prepared me for the loss of Rudy, a staff member, in 1982. He died after a long, mysterious illness that was not diagnosed until the very end. What did his death stand for? Even statistically, he was not counted. The kids on the adolescent program I directed were distraught. He was their favorite counselor; none of them cared that he was gay. He changed before our eyes. Once an extremely good-looking young man, he became wasted to the point of emaciation. His skin became covered with blotchy red lesions. He became difficult to recognize. Then we heard that he had been hospitalized with an undiagnosed malady, that he had pneumonia and might not survive. Within six months of his first symptoms, my staff member was dead.

"Had I not personally lost this friend, the AIDS Training Program might not have been developed. When the then director of mental health for Monroe County, Andreas Pederson, Ph.D., forwarded a request for proposal (RFP) to me, I decided to apply. The National Institute of Mental Health (NIMH) was offering grants for the training of health care professionals in the prevention of AIDS, and our first AIDS Training Project was born."

Before the spread of HIV disease, the daughter of one of the authors (CDC) was working in a genetics lab and went down to the mail room to pick up a package that had come in for one of the geneticists. As she picked it up, blood oozed out of it and spilled on her clothes. She experienced fear and concern, but was relieved to learn it was blood taken from a racehorse for HLA typing. Long before universal precautions, the lab head had always stressed the danger of blood products or any human biological material. His lab would not have sent something through the mails in an unsafe container that could break during transit.

After HIV disease had become known, one of the members of the AIDS Training Program was accidentally stuck with a needle used to draw a patient's blood. She was very concerned. Reassurance that the patient didn't fit the profile for HIV positivity did not relieve her fear; she knew that without a direct test for the virus there was no way to predict whether a patient carried the virus for AIDS. Only testing at six-month intervals could realistically alleviate her concerns.

Because so many health care professionals and other members of society had forgotten the precarious victories against human pathogens and the always-present threat of infectious diseases, the fears about HIV disease reach abnormal proportions since they lack a context to normalize them. In our risk-conscious society, even small risks become exaggerated, while unreal risks become accepted as catastrophic. The population is constantly told of doomsday scenarios: Global Warming, Nuclear Accident Meltdown, Meteor Impact, Ozone Depletion, Alar, Dioxin, Landfill Overload, New Madrid Earthquakes, Radon, Microwave—the list is almost endless. Also, in order to prevent the spread of HIV, public service messages emphasize the deadly risk to everyone, creating AIDS-fear. In this context, normal fears and concerns can rapidly become pathological and irrational, making efforts at realistic prevention difficult.

This volume is the story of our personal and professional struggles with HIV infection and its prevention. We attempt to normalize and mainstream HIV disease so that we can look at it as we have looked at other dreaded diseases: tuberculosis, polio, pancreatic or ovarian cancer, Huntington's, malaria, Creutzfeldt-Jakob, or Ebola fever. Another goal is to normalize therapy with HIV patients, so that the major emotional responses that accompany HIV diagnosis and course of illness can be fruitfully handled by health care professionals, patients, and families. Our approach incorporates the application of systems theory as a tool for therapy and a means of better understanding HIV disease. We also try to give a normal historical sense of HIV disease and a systemic view of ethical and policy questions.

This book reflects the experiences of our AIDS Training Programs and the gift we received of sharing the life stories of many AIDS patients. Early in our work in AIDS training, we produced a video montage that, in short clips, gave a broad and personal view of the major questions and experiences of HIV disease. AIDS patients, or Persons-With-AIDS, allowed us to use video clips of themselves for the montage. We remember with gratefulness the two gay men, Kevin and Paul, who consented to be part of that montage or whose families did. We remember the Puerto Rican married couple, Carmen and Pedro, who contracted HIV from intravenous drug use and shared their story on the video. All four are now dead, although we can still watch their life stories on the tape. We want to thank them all and their families for sharing their lives, and we want to say goodbye to them. The book is in essence the training program designed, taught, and evaluated by our AIDS Training Program.

Part I on *Applied Systems Principles in AIDS Prevention* should provide, the map and tools for dealing with HIV disease in a systemic way. Chapter 1 gives an overview of the current ways of thinking about HIV disease and some of the results of those patterns of thinking. Chapter 2 describes three patients with AIDS and begins seeing them not only as biological systems, but as individuals with needs and plans for their lives and as members of an interactive family and community, who live in and are influenced by the world around them. Chapter 3 looks at individuals at risk for HIV disease, both in terms of individual behavior patterns that may be dangerous, and in terms of membership in groups where the prevalence of the virus creates the critical mass for exposure to HIV that can constitute a public health epidemic and an ongoing risk for those groups. In addition to the biological exposure risk and the individual psychological risks for contracting HIV, it also describes social, economic, and cultural factors that place individuals and their groups at high risk.

Chapter 4 then looks at health care professionals as one of the groups at special risk for contracting HIV. Here, too, it looks at this question in a systemic way, including the physical exposure risk, the individual psychological risks of denial and burnout, and the family and extended network risks that health care professionals also need to pay attention to. Chapter 5 gives the health care professional a method for staying up-to-date about this new and developing disease. It places HIV disease in its historical context and then provides a quick summary of our increasing knowledge of HIV disease. It also takes one year in the ongoing HIV story and outlines the important developments and new information from that year. Finally, it gives steps that the health care professional can take to keep abreast of this disease and develop the resources necessary to achieve that goal.

Part II on *Biopsychosocial Intervention: Clinical Management* looks at the clinical and policy issues in HIV disease that mental health care professionals and other health professionals will encounter, and suggests therapeutic techniques for dealing with HIV disease. Chapter 6 is a medical summary of our diagnostic and treatment knowledge and techniques, geared for the non-AIDS specialist. It discusses HIV testing and counseling, and outlines common opportunistic and primary diseases in order to give health care professionals an understanding of the biological and psychological issues their patients may be grappling with. Chapter 7 discusses the neuropsychiatric and general psychiatric aspects of HIV disease. These opportunistic infections and primary diseases are perhaps the most difficult to manage. AIDS dementia takes its toll not just on the patient who begins to feel that his personhood is slipping away. It also is difficult for the patient's family, social network, and health care providers. This chapter provides tools for dealing with such difficult issues and attempts to normalize the neuropsychiatric problems of HIV.

Chapter 8 introduces the Rochester Model of family systems therapy, using cases to illustrate techniques, including: contacting, engaging and overcoming resistance; initial session strategies; working with traditional and nontraditional family systems; accessing the professional support system; dealing with apparent cut-offs, grief, and loss. Chapter 9 explores the community aspects of HIV disease prevention and management, providing practical techniques for spiritual, religious, and culturally sensitive intervention. It describes the ways in which community resources can be mobilized for the treatment and prevention of HIV disease. Finally, Chapter 10 develops a theory of ethics called Systems Ethics and applies it to AIDS clinical cases and policy decisions. The advantages of this theory are described, along with its particular relevance to HIV disease.

## ACKNOWLEDGMENTS

Of course, a book of this nature is the culmination of the contributions of a number of colleagues. Since the associates (Cole, Griepp, and Tartaglia) listed on the title page, in addition to contributing case material and discussion to the book, participated in the writing of specific chapters, we have listed them as authors on those chapters. The contributors (Espaillat-Piña, Nudd, & Stanton) are also listed on appropriate chapters.

We would also specifically like to mention all our colleagues who have worked on the design and/or implementation of the NIMH AIDS Training Project, who have helped with the book, and whose expertise is reflected in it. These include: Richard Reichman, M.D.; Michael Keefer, M.D.; William Valenti, M.D.; Kenneth Dorner, R.N., BSN; John Lambert, M.D.; Gloria Horsley, R.N., MFCC; Shelley Miller, M.S.; Rev. Enrique Rivera; Paul Graman, M.D.; Elisabet Espaillat-Piña; Rev. Gregory Coles; Robert Tocco, CAC, M.S.; Robert Allan, M.A.; Sybil Baldwin, ACSW, CSW; Lorelei Heliotis, M.S., R.N., C.S.; Stella Diamanti-Kostias, M.D.; Frederick

Steier, Ph.D.; Michael Tarcinale, Ph.D., R.N.; Lyman Wynne, M.D., Ph.D.; Eleanor Macklin, Ph.D.; and Jeffrey Kelly, Ph.D.

We wish to thank the University of Rochester School of Medicine's AIDS Center (directed by Richard Reichman, M.D.), the Department of Psychiatry, and the Office of Research and Project Administration for serving as unfailing resources. We also want to thank the community organizations that immeasurably enriched our work through sharing their commitment to, and knowledge of, the community: AIDS Rochester, Inc.; Puerto Rican Youth Development Organization; the Rochester Area AIDS Task Force; Daybreak Drug and Alcohol Treatment Center; Anthony Jordan Health Center and Baden Street Settlement, Inc.

We are also indebted to Monroe County clinics, hospitals, and health and mental health agencies (too numerous to mention) for their ongoing support in our efforts. A few of these have provided not only trainees but facilities and trainers: Hillside Children's Center, Park Ridge Chemical Dependency; St. Mary's Hospital; the Strong Memorial Hospital Education Committee; and the community network of the Family Therapy Workshops Consortium (Hillside Children's Center, Family Services of Rochester, and the University of Rochester Family Therapy Training Program).

We are also indebted to the National Institute of Mental Health, which provided the initial incentive and funding for our AIDS Training Program (Contract # 278-88-0008), and specifically to Dr. Melvyn Haas, who served as our project officer, for his encouragement, inspiration, and support. He continues to be available with ready wit and wisdom, and this book would not have been written without him.

We are grateful for ongoing funding and support from the New York State AIDS Institute (# C-008512), and (# C-009669), and to Steven Onderdonk, our project officer there, as well as to Albany Medical Center AIDS Program for their funding and support through the Human Resources and Services Administration New York/Virgin Islands Education and Training Center (ETC).

In addition, we would like to thank Richard Reichman, M.D., M. Duncan Stanton, Ph.D., Susan McDaniel, Ph.D., Michael Keefer, M.D., Pieter le Roux, D. Litt. et Phil., Pavel Bem, M.D., and Michele Stratton, M.S., for their helpful comments on an earlier version of the manuscript. Also, our heartfelt thanks to Carole Dill, Erin McReynolds, Carol Wilber, and Pat Atkins for their support, and to Carole Dill for her indefatigable typing.

Our own families have contributed in no small way by sacrificing their time with us to ensure that this work was able to reach completion. Thank you to each and every one.

We also wish to reaffirm our gratitude to the AIDS patients and their families who have made such an important contribution to all of us. Without them, this book could not have been written. We mourn the deaths of some of those who have contributed their stories and are no longer with us. Their names are now on the AIDS Quilt put together by the Names Project and too large now to be shown in its entirety. We've used one of those quilt panels as the cover of our manual, brochures, and booklets, and will always remember the real names.

These names and identifying information have been changed to protect their confidentiality, although all of them have been publicly active in AIDS prevention education. Thank you Amy, Brian, Belinda, Bill, Carmen, Emily, Gino, Julian, Helene, Kevin, Latisha, Maria, Mary, Max, Paul, Pedro, Roberto, Sal, Tim, Todd, Walter. . . .

*Judith Landau-Stanton*
*Colleen D. Clements*

# PART I

## Applied Systems Principles in AIDS Prevention

# CHAPTER 1

# Correcting AIDS Metaphors and Myths with a Systems Approach

## AIDS AND SYSTEMS THEORY

"In preventing AIDS," said C. Everett Koop when he was the United States Surgeon General, "the moralist and the scientist could walk hand in hand."[1] A pediatric surgeon, Koop came to his systems way of thinking about AIDS from his years of clinical experience working with very sick children and their families. He saw first-hand the interconnectedness of life experiences, ranging from the small silk sutures he used to reconnect a newborn's congenitally deformed esophagus (esophageal atresias)[1] to the family's role in supporting the child's recovery and development, to the social systems that hold members in a relational compact of compassion and care. When he looked at AIDS, he saw the larger system:

> "The politics of AIDS poses a threat not only to the health of some Americans but also to our constitutional safeguards of basic rights, to our ethics of care and compassion, to the very fabric of American society. Within the politics of AIDS lay one enduring, central conflict: AIDS pitted the politics of the gay revolution of the seventies against the politics of the Reagan revolution of the eighties." (p. 197)

Koop's clinical systemic view highlights the usefulness of systems theory, which gives the foundation for the moralist and scientist to build an integrated approach to AIDS. Something very exciting happened in the world of ideas this century. It has gone by many names: Family Systems Theory,[2] General System Theory,[3] Hierarchy Theory,[4] Chaos Theory,[5] Community Ecology,[6] Ecosystems Ecology,[6] Wholistic Theory.[7] Whatever the name, systems theory has become the modern methodology, used by biologists (ecosystems research, population dynamics), physicists and biomathematicians (chaos dynamics and "Attractors"), medical researchers (homeostasis, chaos systems in cardiac arrhythmias), and therapists (family therapy, co-dependency counseling). Because it is a synthesis, it can help answer questions in the humanities.[8] This new tool can help us fully understand the interrelated problems generated by the HIV (Human Immunodeficiency Virus) infectious disease process[9] and its syndromic classification, AIDS. Our educational and clinical models, which will be described in this book, apply the systems method in both educational and clinical intervention with AIDS. This approach gives breadth to the explanation and understanding of the HIV infectious disease process that is not possible with more traditional methods.

This chapter will explore the nature of the HIV infectious disease process and illustrate how the informational foundation for interventions can be developed. It will also summarize the practical usefulness of systems theory for AIDS educators, clinicians, counselors, therapists, and policy makers. We will begin this exploration by addressing issues of perception: How AIDS has been seen or construed, and how it has increasingly secured a place in society's consciousness. The vehicles for these perceptions are the metaphors and myths that have gotten in the way of a positive approach to this disease and to the care of people who have contracted it.

## THE METAPHORS OF AIDS

When HIV disease first caught the attention of the health care system, conflicting medical metaphors arose. Even when disguised as acronyms, such as "GRID" (Gay-Related Immune Deficiency), these metaphors were still present. Though closely related, these metaphors are slightly different from the way of hiding the reality of AIDS, which Shilts describes as "AIDSpeak,"[10] or from the myths and misconceptions about HIV disease. The metaphors are broad analogies that frame the way professionals and the public think about AIDS without examining their deeper meaning.

Our University of Rochester AIDS Program experienced these metaphors and their rippling effects at all levels of the social system, including in: (a) front-line work in setting up community agencies, (b) specialized clinical treatment of AIDS patients, (c) academic research on medical and psychiatric problems, (d) therapy with AIDS patients and their families, and (e) ethical and policy questions raised by this disease. It became clear early on that a narrow and isolating picture of AIDS could give rise to troublesome metaphors that failed to capture the complete picture of AIDS. In fact, these metaphors could serve to disconnect the clinical, medical, research, family, community, pastoral, and social value systems from each other, causing adverse effects through all parts of the system. The metaphors were often silently accepted by society and, as a multidisciplinary team of AIDS educators and clinicians, we felt it was important to bring them "out of the closet" and develop more accurate metaphors.

Part of the problem was the name of the disease itself. After 10 years of experience with this disease, we still do not have an adequate name for it. The term AIDS refers to a syndrome and can be too narrow and misleading. The Centers for Disease Control's (CDC's) "HIV infection" does not convey the severity of the illness or its propensity to attack the nervous system directly. Ostrow's [9] "HIV infectious disease process" is medically correct but is too awkward. Perhaps the most telling and all-embracing metaphor about AIDS is the lack of a good name for it. For the sake of convenience, we have abbreviated Ostrow's term to HIV disease, which will be used throughout the book.

At least nine metaphors have been applied to AIDS, as follows:

## 1. AIDS as a Homosexual Illness

GRID (Gay-Related Immune Deficiency) and the Gay Plague were early versions of this metaphor. The more scientific appearing GRID carried less hidden moral condemnation than Gay Plague, but both described the phenomenon as exclusively a gay man's illness, something attached to homosexuality. This early identification of the disease with homosexuality created long-lasting effects. Because of it, American researchers initially missed the signs of the disease in intravenous drug users, in recipients of transfusions, in hemophiliacs, in babies and children, and in women. For years, its occurrence in these populations, even when recognized, was downplayed.

Because of acceptance of this metaphor, only one of the major ways of transmitting Human Immunodeficiency Virus (HIV) was emphasized, sexual behavior among homosexuals. Blood transmission was not sufficiently stressed, resulting in the infection of about 12,000 blood recipients before blood banks finally instituted screening.[10] Meanwhile, HIV infection continued to spread through intravenous (i.v.) drug users and injection drug users (IDUs) in the urban centers and among the minority poor. Until very recently, significant programs of education and prevention were not developed, arriving too late for many. While European researchers were paying close attention to the disease in Africa, among a primarily heterosexual population, American researchers were focused on the gay community.

The American focus highlighted the gay community's realistic experiences of homophobia and its movement for Gay Civil Rights as the central issues. But a result of the gay rights emphasis was the difficulty encountered in attempts to close bathhouses in San Francisco and New York City for health reasons, when political goals superseded a very serious risk to health and life. In 1982, Gaetan Dugas (the initial carrier in the study documenting the spread of HIV) was still going to bathhouses, while gay community leaders continued to oppose critics of multiple sex partners and the bathhouse lifestyle. In 1983, a meeting of gay leaders and bathhouse owners came to no resolution, and the owners suggested there was a mere one in 3,127,443 chance of contracting AIDS in bathhouses. San Francisco's Public Health Director opposed closing the baths or requiring posted warnings to alert tourists during the Gay Freedom Day Parade. A compromise among gay community leaders and the Milk Club and Toklas Club, supporting some restrictions on the baths, collapsed just before a press conference called by the Public Health Director to announce restrictions.[10]

By October 9, 1984, when the Director did close the baths at another press conference, the San Francisco AIDS Foundation still objected, based on civil rights reasons and the fact that there were already AIDS education posters in the bathhouses. Only the Milk Club, at considerable personal cost (ostracism) to members, supported the closings. And by that time, about two-thirds of the gay men who eventually tested HIV positive (HIV+) were already infected. The San Francisco gay community's choice to see this problem as a gay rights issue, rather than a gay health issue, allowed the easy spread of the virus through the mechanism of bathhouses. This politicizing of a disease occurred even though a 1980 gay physicians' conference had pointed with increased concern to the behaviors that even then had led to an 8,000 percent rise in enteric diseases (intestinal infection) and a 93 percent infection rate for Cytomegalovirus (CMV) and Epstein-Barr (E-B) pathogens, as well as a 66 percent infection with Hepatitis B and rising venereal disease rates.[10]

This metaphor of AIDS as a homosexual illness connected the disease with the movement to gain homosexual rights, making AIDS a political football. Although present-day AIDS education programs no longer refer to AIDS as a gay disease, the residual effects of this metaphor are important to understand since the approach to the disease is still guided by the metaphor.

## 2. AIDS as HTLV-III/LAV: The Prize for Competitive Research and Economic Gain in Medical Science

The dispute between French and American researchers over discovery of the virus and the marketing rights for the test produced another metaphor. The French researcher, Luc Montagnier, working from a better-informed theory, gave the Pasteur Institute preeminence by his discovery of the virus. Montagnier wished to call it lymphadenopathy-associated virus (LAV) because he felt that this virus was not a human T-lymphocyte virus (HTLV) type. He correctly believed that it was more closely related to a family of animal viruses, the retroviruses that caused visna, caprine arthritis encephalitis (CAE), and equine infectious anemia (EIA), all of which are lentiviruses (slow viruses). These (slow) retroviruses may cause both immune deficiency and severe neurologic disorders.

The American researcher, Robert Gallo, having received research samples from the Pasteur Institute, also claimed to have discovered the virus. He wished to call it HTLV-III since he felt it was a member of the group of viruses that he had discovered could cause leukemia in man and other animals. His insistence on linking what finally became known as Human Immunodeficiency Virus (HIV) to the HTLV-I and -II classification sent investigators off on the wrong track and also deemphasized any neurological symptoms of the disease. For a time, the virus used a hyphenated name, HTLV-III/LAV, before an international agreement was reached by political process, and the virus finally became known as HIV. Gallo is now involved in an investigation to determine if he inappropriately claimed joint discovery of the AIDS virus.

The mind-set engendered by this metaphor tended to keep many physicians unaware of the lentiviruses when thinking about this disease (even though Gallo has done significant work on the genetic and morphologic homology— evolutionary and structural similarity— of the lentiviruses such as HIV, Visna, CAE, and EIA[11]). In public discussion the virus is usually presented as a retrovirus, without its linkage to the lentiviruses, which limits our understanding of HIV disease. This metaphor of HTLV-III/LAV also delayed the recognition of the significance of the primary neurological aspects of the disease.

### 3. AIDS as Defined as Severe Opportunistic Infection and Active Illness

Finally, of course, the disease became known as Acquired Immunodeficiency Syndrome, or AIDS. Persons whose immune systems are compromised by HIV disease are more susceptible to other infections and illnesses not caused directly by HIV. In other words, organisms that do not generally affect people (or if they do, the illness is circumscribed) frequently affect HIV + people severely. These illnesses seen as an accompaniment to HIV disease are called opportunistic infections and have been used as the diagnostic criteria of AIDS.

Physicians in the United States developed a list of opportunistic infections and physical manifestations that qualified for making the diagnosis of AIDS. These diagnostic criteria were derived from a study of the American gay population and were, therefore, very specific to this population. Pneumonia caused by pneumocystis carinii (PCP) was the principle defining disease for AIDS, along with Kaposi's sarcoma (a form of cancer). Due to accidents of geography and subpopulation, these were the early criteria that most clearly defined the full-blown disease for American researchers. This gave rise to the metaphor of AIDS as opportunistic infection and active illness. Defining AIDS in terms of opportunistic infection and active illness is a diagnostic manual classification approach, rather than a full etiological (causal) and natural history of the disease approach. It is not a systemic, dynamic way of looking at the disease, but rather an end-stage diagnostic perspective that limits the view of AIDS as a progressive spectrum.

This metaphor resulted in a diagnostic dichotomy. When the virus was discovered and individuals could be tested for HIV infection, there were now two groups, one diagnosed as having AIDS and one diagnosed as being HIV positive. As a result, a number of misperceptions sprang up among the public and those tested for the virus. Some thought that being HIV+ did not mean the disease was present, since it was not AIDS. In Magic Johnson's announcement that he had tested HIV positive during an insurance examination, he stressed that he did not have AIDS, but was only HIV+. This dichotomy continues to be confusing to the public. Patients who were dying from primary AIDS dementia were still not diagnosed as having AIDS, since they did not have an AIDS-defining illness. In addition, individuals from other countries, with a different set of opportunistic infections and physical manifestations, were not immediately classified as AIDS cases. AIDS-related complex (ARC) was then introduced as a third separate diagnosis, further confusing the natural history of the illness. There were three discrete boxes, rather than an illness process. This has remained the epidemiological classification, although the Centers for Disease Control (CDC) are currently modifying the AIDS definition according to criteria derived from the impact of the virus on the immune system. (A CD4 cell count below 200 cubic mm. (cu mm) will probably be considered as AIDS-defining.)

Currently, the focus remains on full-blown AIDS in the numbers reported by the CDC and World Health Organization (WHO). But, because HIV is a lentivirus (a "slow virus" taking some years to manifest itself), the complete spectrum of infection is important and the numbers of end-stage cases of HIV disease (AIDS) are not the significant statistics for epidemiology or public health. Rates of HIV seropositivity or, better still, the presence of virus, rather than seroconversion (the development of antibodies to HIV), are the statistics that are really needed. The metaphor of AIDS as opportunistic infection and active illness has played a role in obstructing the gathering of this information. It has also impeded the viewing of the disease as a progressive and unpredictable spectrum in which people may be severely ill at one time and relatively well at another.

Two of the images employed by our group to help people understand the unpredictable progress of the disease were the CDC's iceberg imagery (HIV seropositivity at its base, ARC in the middle, and AIDS at the tip) and an airplane (HIV seropositivity at the rear, ARC in the middle, and AIDS at the front). We asked people to imagine seeing different portions of the iceberg at different times, or people moving forward and backwards in the plane, in order to have them understand that HIV disease may present differently at different stages.

## 4. AIDS as a Unique and Newly Created Disease

Because AIDS was first discovered in the early '80s in the United States, and there was no earlier record of it, it was assumed to be a new disease, a sudden epidemic unlike anything before in medical history. This produced another metaphor—that of a new and unique strange disease. The image of newness and strangeness precipitated feelings of fear and panic. It was compatible with a Sodom and Gomorrah belief that AIDS suddenly struck from the sky as God's punishment. It generated feelings of helplessness in medical care professionals. It disconnected the disease from the comfortable body of knowledge about diseases, and from a medical approach to its prevention and treatment.

The combination of newness, strangeness, impotence, and fear contributed to the separation of AIDS patients from other patients. This de-medicalization of AIDS—its not being managed like other epidemics—has had consequences both for public health and for the care of the individual AIDS patient. But the scientific reality of HIV disease does not support such a metaphor. The *Lancet* reported the presence of HIV in a British sailor who died from an undiagnosed ailment in 1959.[12] HIV disease is not so new and some hypothesize that it has existed in contained pockets of humans in the tropics for thousands of years. HIV disease is not unique; Ebola fever shares many similarities. Joshua Lederberg predicts a host of emergent viruses that will give medical science challenges, some currently identified, some still to be discovered as hidden zoonotic (carried by animal) viruses (such as Seoul virus, Junin virus, and Hantaan virus).[13]

There are other "slow virus" diseases that are fatal, untestable except at autopsy and animal culture, and potentially transmitted through medical procedures. Creutzfeldt-Jakob (CJD) is an example of a recently understood disease that fits this category, although its specific cause (pathogen) has not been identified. Since 1974, it has been known that CJD can be transmitted through many medical and surgical procedures (for example transplants, electrode implants, human dura mater grafts, Applanation Tonometry during eye examination, otologic (inner ear) grafts, power drills and saws, and inoculation of Human Growth Hormone to treat children for dwarfism.)[14,15,16] Bovine Spongiform Encephalopathy (BSE), popularly called "Mad Cow Disease" in Great Britain where it is making the safety of British beef suspect, is an animal form of CJD. Pet food made from cows infected with BSE has transmitted the disease to cats, and its implications for public health are very troublesome.[17] It is now known that HTLV-I also can be transmitted through blood transfusions.

As virology opens up new questions and understanding, HIV disease will probably become reincorporated into medical science as one of a number of emergent viruses. At that stage this metaphor will be replaced. For the present, a broader view of such viral diseases is needed in order to increase awareness of the general risks in medicine and to increase the sense of competency in health care professionals dealing with these risks.

## 5. AIDS as Sex

Because AIDS prevention first started in the gay community, most notably in San Francisco, sexual behavior became the prime target for AIDS education and prevention. Condoms were the symbol of this emphasis on "safe sex." HIV infection became linked in people's minds with sex, creating still another metaphor. It is only recently that drugs have emerged as another image for AIDS transmission, although Shilts' book again documents the early spread of HIV in the drug-using community parallel with its spread in the gay community. He suggests that the first documented carrier of HIV was a drug-abusing San Francisco prostitute with three children who all had AIDS.[10] While she tested positive, and was probably infected as early as 1976, she continued to work as a prostitute until her death in 1987. Her infection probably occurred because of her history of substance-abuse. The first European death, and later documentation of HIV infection, was that of a Danish surgeon, who probably contracted HIV during surgical procedures in a missionary hospital in Zaire. She died December 12, 1977.[10]

Despite diverse sources of spread, the metaphor of sex and sexual behavior became locked in as the principal image for AIDS. This introduced all the psychological, social, and cultural complexities of human sexuality. Previous experience with the epidemiology of syphilis has not been sufficiently applied to the development of education and prevention interventions for HIV infection. Society still clings to the notion that education on behavioral risks and safe sex will be sufficiently effective in the prevention of the slow spread of HIV infection.[18] Condoms, and now bleach kits for sterilizing drug users' works, are assumed to have an extremely high rate of effectiveness if used. A high rate of compliance is presumed among populations where compliance is known to be a major problem.

Perhaps the most important negative consequence of the AIDS-sex metaphor is the exclusive linkage of AIDS and sex. Our knowledge about our sexuality, its sensitivity, intimacy, or privacy, and the psychodynamic intricacies of our sexuality all become problems in AIDS education and prevention. The more general problem, however, is the effect such a linkage will have on healthy human sexuality. There are already indications that Puritan agendas (and a devaluing of the body and its functions) are being stimulated by public discussion of HIV infection. Conversely, there is danger that the all-important intimacy of sexuality could be lost. We feel it is important to avoid both these consequences.

The reports of changing social attitudes toward multiple sexual partners, as well as the fear among singles about sexual behavior, may reflect actual changes in social values about sexual pleasure, or a new ideal about what should constitute sexual behavior. Elementary and secondary health education curricula are a renewed battleground between premarital abstinence and premarital sexual enjoyment. Monogamy (long-term monogamous relationships) is presented as the ideal safe-sex behavior, and even if the intention is safety rather than judgment, the practical effect is to devalue non-monogamous relationships. Commentators talk about the end of the Sexual Revolution. This implies a return to more restrictive social codes about sex, less openness in discussion, and stronger taboos.

The other pole is to confront individuals with the explicit realities and graphic public expression of sexual behaviors. Such an approach can be in direct conflict with their personal wish for privacy or with the restrictions of their cultural value systems. For example, some Native American cultures designate individuals who may talk to each other about sex and those who may not. There are rules of communication making some family members available for such conversations and some not, depending on kinship. By challenging these traditions or values, AIDS education and treatment would be inviting unnecessary difficulty. Teaching condom use is a concrete example of this dilemma. Sensitivity to people's perceptions about their use or even about their open distribution, is necessary for successful education and prevention.

## 6. AIDS as Self-Inflicted Illness

The concept of self-inflicted, or behaviorally-caused, disease is becoming more prominent in American medicine. For example, smoking, obesity and other nutritional disorders, sedentary life style, and substance abuse are progressively being regarded as "well-deserved" and "avoidable." The demand for a "healthy life style" is increasing in the medical care system. There are even discussions in the literature of restricting the availability of medical care for those whose diseases are "caused" by an unhealthy life style. [19,20]

When self-inflicted illness concepts are combined with the very negative perception of such behaviors as illegal drug use, nicotine use, alcoholism, homosexuality, and promiscuity, there is the risk of negative judgment and punitive treatment of the patient by the health care system. There is also the risk that medical resources, already curtailed by political cost-containment choices, will be further rationed for such behavior, and that access to treatment facilities will be limited.

The self-inflicted illness metaphor is destructive. It undermines the essential empathy and compassion that health care professionals must bring to their interactions with patients and clients. This problem is compounded because AIDS information frequently stresses that *behaviors* put individuals at risk for contracting HIV. But if personal behaviors, rather than exposure to the virus, are stressed as the risk factor, it is very easy to attribute personal responsibility and blame to those infected with HIV. This self-inflicted (self-chosen) illness metaphor can lead to the unacceptable progression of the following ideas:

self-chosen risk behavior
↓
self-accountability
↓
self-blame
↓
self-deserved illness
↓
moral instead of medical treatment
↓
non-deserving of medical or social resources

When the behaviors are already viewed by the culture or society as immoral or bad, empathy and compassion are diminished. Health care professionals are not immune to this bias. There is need to call attention to the flaws of this metaphor and the risk of emphasizing personal risk behavior over viral infection.

## 7. AIDS as a Malthusian Solution to Overpopulation

One of the little-discussed effects of the current emphasis on environmentalism (the '90s may be the decade of pop ecology) has been the valuing of green spaces and the devaluing of human populations that adversely impact on these "natural" habitats. The political Green Party in Europe and the philosophic school of Deep Ecology both call for a considerable reduction in the current level of human population. Genuine overpopulation problems in third-world countries, particularly Africa and India, also contribute to the willingness to see a Malthusian solution to population pressure. In addition to famine, disease is one such powerful mechanism. Thus, the newly emerged disease, AIDS, can be viewed by some as having a beneficial outcome.

Some view the African AIDS crisis with alarm. At an international AIDS conference in Naples, Italy, in 1987, a warning was raised that Africa would be a "hecatomb." Others, such as the past leader of Earth First, David

Foreman, wrote in the group's publication: "AIDS is not a malediction, but the welcome and natural remedy to reduce the population on the planet . . ." University of Cape Town anthropologist Virginia van der Vliet notes that there is reason to question how motivated some South Africans are to deal with AIDS: "There are clearly some who feel that AIDS is God's answer to both South Africa's political and population problems."[21] When studies estimate that more than half of South Africa's population over age 15 will be infected by HIV by the year 2000; when 3 percent of all South African blacks, 5 percent of those attending prenatal clinics, 14 percent of mine workers, and 17 percent of males at STD clinics are infected now, this is not a fantasy of population control. Nor are the statistics limited to South Africa. In Zambia, 19 percent of blood donors and 27 percent of hospital staff are infected; in Kampala, Uganda, 70 percent of blood donors; in Nairobi, Kenya, 85 percent of prostitutes; in Zimbabwe, 7 percent of blood donors and 20–30 percent of the general population; and in Namibia, 66 percent of returning SWAPO members.[21]

The benign neglect of African populations will strike a familiar chord with the American gay community, the urban ghetto minorities, and the substance abusing population. When over two-thirds of New York City substance abusers seeking treatment at clinics are HIV infected and when that infection has simmered unattended since 1976, it is not difficult to conceive that certain populations are being written off. Populations with little perceived utility can be sacrificed by a cost-effective model of politics and medicine. An HIV + rate of one in 77 New York City women of child-bearing age anonymously screened at hospitals is a signpost for the eventual depletion in numbers of certain populations. When the African and American experiences are combined, there is a definite Malthusian flavor to certain AIDS policies and interventions.

This needs to be explored in a calm way, without the rhetoric or paranoia that can overtake activist groups and make them part of the problem rather than part of the solution. The metaphor's underlying link with certain environmentalist beliefs further complicates the task.

## 8. AIDS as Romantic Death

The HIV disease experience also shares something with the social and cultural response to tuberculosis in the 18th and 19th century. Dying with tuberculosis became highly romanticized and eroticized, the disease making the individual more heroic and sexually attractive in the public's mind. Death itself became romanticized and eroticized as evidenced in the cultural expressions of the era, such as Mimi's demise in the opera, La Bohème. With regard to HIV disease, this same phenomenon may be expressing itself in the popular culture of today. A positive side of this metaphor is that many individuals facing terminal illness from HIV disease have been recognized as achieving heroic stature. They have also been humanized, as in the movie *Long Time Companion*, where members of the homosexual community were portrayed as attractive, approachable, and worthwhile. The Names Project, which toured the country with an ever larger quilt made from pieces commemorating persons who had died from AIDS, has been able to touch the common and unifying human nature beneath the sexual identity differences. [22]

On the negative side of the metaphor, not all AIDS patients can attain such heroic stature or an idealized journey to death. The need to be seen as ordinary sufferers of a very devastating disease can get submerged in this romanticism and fantasy. Repressing the losses that HIV infection routinely causes or glossing over the ugly and destructive side of HIV's reality can create a fantasy that is alien to the patient's experience and impossible to come to terms with. Romanticizing dying with AIDS can also stand in the way of effective education and prevention. Coupling AIDS and romantic death has two other effects. It can remove hope and a will to live, influencing an individual to welcome death prematurely or to run toward death by active suicide, passive withdrawal, or refusal of medical treatment. Dying can be seen as the heroic and erotic thing to do, almost a requirement.

Finally, the potential linkage of AIDS, sex, and death into a pathological eroticism should not be overlooked. Our team struggled with this metaphor until our experience of videotaping several exceptional AIDS patients convinced us that it was both relevant and useful. These people continued to grow as human beings while dying from the disease. One patient, who died within weeks of being videotaped, was a remarkable person, but he was also romanticized by the video. A Puerto Rican couple, Carmen and Pedro (who will be discussed later), who were taped progressively through the course of their illness, showed how self-destructive choices can be turned around by the strength required to meet the challenge of illness. During a poignant session, Pedro, with rapidly deteriorating health, revealed that he had bought a coffin and taken photos of himself inside the coffin, waving goodbye. This concrete embracing of reality and death, as well as sharing it with those remaining alive, is striking and unusual. Health care professionals should consider both positive and negative aspects of this metaphor, and be prepared to look for, and reinforce, the positive and loving perspective whenever possible.

We have also learned to consider the dangerous effect of romanticizing death and unwittingly encouraging suicide or treatment refusal when there is a strong cost-containment agenda and pressure on the medical care system. [23,24] The potential that such romanticizing can be co-opted and misused for strictly economic goals is serious enough that it should be addressed.

## 9. AIDS as a Spotlight for Society's Problems

We find it useful to use specific images to express the metaphor of AIDS as a spotlight for society's problems. AIDS can be seen as a finger in the dike, enlarging the crack and exposing the weaknesses of the wall. It can be viewed as a searchlight that increases the visibility of problems in the health care and social systems, or as a spotlight that shows up specific problems. For example, the problem of keeping HIV test results and diagnosis confidential highlights the general problem of confidentiality.[25] Utilization, regulatory, and insurance reimbursement reviews; mandatory reporting of drug testing, blood alcohol levels, child abuse, and sexually transmissible diseases; as well as Duty to Warn precedents in case law, are all ongoing and significant limitations on confidentiality that have become routine in the health care system. The desire for anonymity or confidentiality of HIV test results conflicts with such common practices in the medical system. There are many other questions raised by HIV disease that perform this same function.

The metaphor of AIDS as a symptom of society's problems can provide a framework for dealing with larger, underlying problems within the medical system, the family, the community, and human society. It allows for bi-directionality, since resolution of these underlying larger problems can in turn assist in understanding and reaching workable solutions for HIV issues. This metaphor permits "joining" of HIV issues to general issues in a way that emphasizes commonality and prevents separation or alienation. This serves to integrate AIDS services and personnel, as well as the clients and patients, into the larger human community. The metaphor accomplishes this without either exaggerating the spread of HIV disease or resorting to doomsday scenarios, both potentially dangerous.[26]

Identifying and understanding the metaphors of AIDS prevalent in the community are essential to effective AIDS intervention and prevention. The construction of additional positive metaphors can also be a useful tool. The misconceptions produced by some metaphors need to be corrected, and a systems perspective can aid in the construction of metaphors that are more accurate and useful.

## AIDS MYTHS AND THEIR MANAGEMENT

Unarticulated and unexamined metaphors are one thing; myths are quite another. Although both have as their goal an explanation of human experience, metaphors are meant to be accurate images. AIDS metaphors should reflect the reality of AIDS and to the extent that they obscure, confuse, or distort, they are not useful or acceptable. Myths, however, may be mistaken beliefs given uncritical acceptance in support of existing or traditional practices and institutions. They may be propagated to conceal and deceive, or perpetuated for hidden psychological reasons. They may become integral to the popular culture. From the beginning, AIDS has had its share of this type of myth, myths that have been honest mistakes or that conceal prejudice against, or hatred of, certain groups. These are the myths that distort risks, mask other agendas, or reinforce popular biases. Shilts calls this "AIDSpeak."[10]

The myths of AIDS fall into three main categories: (1) Myths about risk, (2) Myths about prevention and treatment, and (3) Myths about human behavior.

## 1. Myths About Risk

The development of understanding of this newly emerged virus has been remarkably rapid considering the historical medical context of research and the combating of new diseases. Thanks to the Recombinant DNA technology that was so recently developed and the advances in molecular biology that have made biotechnology such an undreamed-of success, researchers have actually identified the viral source (or pathogen), described it, and proposed medical interventions at an accelerated rate. In 10 years, we have made truly extraordinary progress in understanding and treating HIV infection. This progress would not have been possible 30 years ago. So the emergence of this fatal disease occurred at a fortunate time in history. However, none of that has prevented fears and fallacies developing almost as rapidly as the research.

Because AIDS was discovered so recently and seemed to restrict its spread to certain clearly identified populations, the first error was to see it as a plague similar to bubonic plague. It was expected rapidly to wipe out continental populations, run its devastating course, and then wane after the destruction. Because the virus initially was not well-characterized, modes of transmission were frightening to contemplate. AIDS training still has to deal with some of the misconceptions that sprang up in this early period. Some of these are listed in Table 1-A.

But these overstated risk perceptions were not the only mistakes. Balancing them, and sometimes because of them, another set of common understated risk perceptions are listed in Table 1-B.

Both overstated and understated beliefs or myths about AIDS are still operative in public policy discussion and in the public's distrust of AIDS information. With the accumulation of experience and knowledge about HIV, some of the earlier myths have been abandoned, while some were seen as irrational even from the very beginning. For example, it has been reliably established that:

1. There was no mechanism for HIV infection when blood donation was done with disposable needles and gloved personnel, but there would have been a mechanism if blood were taken with reused needles and ungloved or with reused gloves. The risk was dependent on adequate infection control and was unnecessary and unacceptable, but the public's concerns needed to be accepted rather than ridiculed;
2. Experience with HIV infection indicated it was not easy to transmit

TABLE 1-A
Overstated Risks

HIV infection can be contracted by donating blood.

HIV infection can be transmitted through airborne contact.

HIV infection can be easily transmitted through touch.

HIV infection can certainly be transmitted through insect vectors.

HIV infection can certainly be transmitted through food handling.

HIV infection can certainly be transmitted through objects an infected person has touched.

HIV infection is very easy to catch.

HIV infection can very easily pass from patient to physician.

Individuals who are HIV+ must be quarantined.

HIV infection is rapidly spreading through every sector of society, equally.

TABLE 1-B
Understated Risks

HIV infection can never be transmitted through touching diapers, broken skin, etc. and there is never a need to wear gloves.

HIV infection has not been proven to be transmitted through sex, so sexual activity should not be limited or changed.

HIV infection concerns are unrealistic and a plot against homosexual rights and the gay community.

HIV infection precautions will lead to concentration camps for homosexuals.

Unexplained infection with HIV is actually caused by hidden sexual behaviors of the person infected, rather than by other unknown modes of transmission.

Universal precautions are demeaning and dehumanizing to patients.

Science completely knows and understands all the modes of transmission for HIV.

HIV infection does not discriminate in infectivity.

HIV infection is almost never a result of needle-sticks in health care workers.

HIV infection can never be transmitted through a bite.

Negative seropositivity means the individual does not carry HIV.

HIV does not cause AIDS.

this disease from one individual to another by indirect contact. Indeed, the epidemiology of HIV infection does not indicate that it is spreading evenly through all sectors of society, although the potential is there;

3. HIV is reasonably scientifically established as the etiology of most cases of Autoimmune Deficiency Syndrome—but not all AIDS-like illness,* although co-factors and perhaps immune system dynamics appear to accelerate the progression of the disease;[27,28]

4. Physicians are at risk for HIV infection and Universal Precautions are recommended; and

5. HIV infection is demonstrated to be a sexually transmissible disease, and blood banks recognize that HIV can be transmitted through blood transfusion.

New findings will continue to change our tentative conclusions about HIV infection, and this is uncomfortable for some, given the severity of the disease. Tests for seropositivity are not completely satisfactory, since individuals may have the virus without seroconverting for some time. The length of time is debatable, but it may exceed the six-month period previously assumed.[29] To be scientific, we also cannot assume that, at this early stage of experience with the disease, we are certain of every mode of transmission. Research indicates that HIV can be transmitted through oral sex, breastfeeding an HIV + baby, HIV + blood on broken skin, and caring for an HIV + baby without proper precautions, such as gloves when diapering. It is also unscientific to presume that an individual exposed to the virus in ways other than those recognized as high-risk, who also practices high-risk behavior, contracted the virus through the high-risk behavior route.

One of the effects of these Risk Myths on both the public and health care professionals is distrust of the experts. This is clearly the most negative consequence of these myths. This distrust can be corrected by adequate education and informed treatment. AIDS information needs to emphasize the probabilistic nature of scientific knowledge, as well as the evolving content of scientific knowledge, both of which are typical of good science. It needs to be abreast of the most recent research, and of the arguments and disagreements about HIV infection. The newest paths of research need to be placed alongside accumulating data that have stood the test of investigation. AIDS experts need to discuss the range of interpretation of data, from the "worst case" scenario to the "best case" scenario, and to advise both professionals and public to understand where a particular interpretation has been set. An institution may look at a best case interpretation while the individual who has just been placed at risk of infection may look at the worst case interpretation. Different agendas can drive interpretation of data. Knowing the full context can help everyone evaluate the data and the inter-

---

*Tom Spira, CDC. *Is there another agent that causes low CD$_4$ counts and AIDS?*

pretation more competently. Again, a systems perspective is useful in this task, providing the methodology for looking at the entire spectrum of such complex processes without becoming unnecessarily polarized.

Risk description and risk interpretation do not occur in a vacuum. The role of the Centers for Disease Control will not be the same as the role of the American Medical Association or the role of a school board. All these roles are legitimate, but they influence the interpretation of data on risk of HIV transmission. The role of an individual teacher in the school system and the role of the parents of a pre-school child will also vary. It is important to understand and try to integrate these varying interpretations of the same scientific data. The approach should be matched carefully to the context of the individual or organization, and an attempt should be made to broaden the understanding of the positions and roles of those involved.

There is also a question of presenting the most frightening (but not necessarily the most likely or accurate) interpretation, as opposed to the most neutral. It is not clear which is actually more effective in prevention, and there are some costs to the "Scare Tactic" method in risk presentation that need to be considered.[30,31,32,33] The scare might be effective, but it might result in paralysis of action, thus changing nothing. Or it might result in a fatalistic resignation and continuation of the same behaviors. It may produce the equivalent of hypochondria in health issues, resulting in modification of all behaviors (even low-risk and productive normal behaviors) and retreat into a constricted life style.

The scare might be ineffectual, a case of crying wolf too many times. Disbelief might then cause the rejection of all information and the reinforcement or acceleration of high-risk behavior. There can be an information burnout, as appears to have occurred in parts of the country with AIDS media information. Listeners will simply tune out because fear and their perception of a lack of progress with the disease are too high to tolerate over a long time. They may make no effort to change any of their behaviors and may deny the reality of HIV infection.

Both groups, those who are terrified or frozen and those who disbelieve, may become resistant to AIDS education and prevention. This has serious implications for both risk reduction and treatment.

## 2. Myths About Prevention and Treatment

In the early period of HIV infection, prevention was the central goal since treatment was supportive and limited. Advances have increased the treatment possibilities and extended the life span of AIDS patients, although in a qualified way. HIV + individuals have been able to remain healthy for longer periods of time before developing ARC or AIDS. As patients live longer, the profile of the disease is changing and neurological disorders are

**TABLE 1-C**
**Prevention and Treatment Myths**

Once an opportunistic infection appears, death is imminent.
Nontraditional healing can prevent AIDS patients from dying.
Suicide is the courageous way to control the process of dying with AIDS.
Scientists are not trying to work quickly enough on a cure for AIDS, caus-
ing unnecessary deaths.
Dying patients should be able to obtain any experimental drugs.
A positive mind-frame will prevent death from AIDS.
A healthy life style will prevent death from AIDS.
Health diets can prevent death from AIDS.
Condoms are the only solution to AIDS prevention.
Clean needles are the only solution to AIDS prevention.
Universal precautions will always prevent health care workers from con-
tracting AIDS.
Surgical gloves will never allow the passage of HIV.
Universal precautions are always feasible to use.
Ordinary gloves will protect Emergency Medical Technicians (EMTs)
against exposure to the AIDS virus.
Education of adolescents will reliably prevent high-risk behavior.
Substance abusers are not interested in protecting themselves from the
AIDS virus.
There is no documented transmission of HIV from a health care worker
to a patient.
The risk of dying with AIDS is over now that AZT and ddI are available
as treatment.
AIDS is now a chronic rather than fatal disease.
The health care system has the facilities to mass screen for HIV.
HIV + pregnant women always consider abortion.
"Safe sex" will definitely prevent AIDS.
There are adequate treatment or care facilities for those with AIDS
dementia.
Financing of HIV testing, medical treatment, and hospital care is adequate
to the need.
HIV + women always use effective birth control methods to prevent
pregnancy.
Research has been slow to understand and develop treatment for AIDS.

becoming more common. The myths about prevention and treatment reflect
the evolving nature of the disease. Some of these treatment myths are set
forth in Table 1-C.

HIV infection was originally quickly terminal, with little hope for survival. Focus was placed on "taking control of dying" and on acceptance of
death as a legitimate response. Suicide was considered an ethical option
by some. These responses can still be seen. For example, in New York State,
the gay community is still lobbying for passage of Living Will legislation,

and elsewhere the Hemlock Society and Society for the Right to Die have attracted considerable support, for both Living Will and physician-assisted suicide legislation. An alternate response to the acceptance and quickening of death is a search for hope and life outside medical science. Nontraditional healing, ranging from the crystals of New Age to old shaman practices, have been embraced. Mystical beliefs hold out some hope for individuals diagnosed with a fatal disease. A more conservative response is to pressure science to research herbal treatments such as the Chinese cucumber (Compound Q), to turn to experimental work in psychoneuroimmunology, or to campaign actively for relaxation of FDA research standards in order to make new potentially effective drugs available on a broad scale. The time seems short and desperation fuels many decisions.

There is also the political fear that government-funded science is slow to research and develop treatment. This fear is not well-founded, since the history of research on HIV infection is one of remarkably fast progress when compared to other new diseases of the past. However, the American research effort did suffer from systemic problems and initially was placed on the wrong path because of scientific assumptions that HIV was closely related to the HTLVs.

As experience with and knowledge about this disease have progressed along with research, the danger now seems the opposite of the earlier panic response, with myths of complacency replacing myths of crisis. "Safe sex" was not the best choice of words, and the belief that condom use alone will completely prevent transmission of HIV is unfortunate. The New York State AIDS Institute is now talking about "safer sex," a preferable phrase.[34] Similarly, some individuals feel that magical protection against their contracting the disease results from the sterilization of needles. Conversely, centers treating HIV + individuals also need to take care that the message to the community does not become: There is treatment, therefore the AIDS problem has been solved and there is no danger in high-risk behavior. AIDS education and counseling that stress the progress in treating AIDS as a chronic disease, while not mentioning that it remains fatal, will give a false sense of security.

The realities, not the myths, of infection control and the routes of iatrogenic transmission of HIV need to be stressed. As HIV + patients continue to live longer, there will be increasing contact with health care professionals. Also, with an increasing number of health care professionals being HIV + (approximately 5,000 in the U.S. in 1991), there will also be more contact between them and patients suffering from other illnesses. In terms of controlling iatrogenic transmission, the history of the battle to screen the blood supply is not encouraging [10] and the recent CDC conclusion that a patient was infected with HIV by her dentist (confirmed as clearly as science can confirm an effect, through DNA comparison) highlights the need for infection control of HIV. [35] Universal precautions are not always followed according to the book, and this needs to be documented accurately. It is not always possible, in emergency situations, to make use of such precautions. Institutions do not always have an adequate supply of barriers. Some barriers, such as surgical gloves, have a high rate of failure (virus passage)[36] or are ineffectual in some situations (glove tearing during orthopedic surgery, for example).

The response to prevention and treatment may also be altered by myths arising from cultural and social context. For example, the experience of professionals working with women who are HIV + is that effective birth control is sometimes not used with a primary partner, even if that partner is seropositive.[37] Health care providers frequently assume that HIV + women will consider abortion if pregnant. However, this is not usually the case. For example, if an HIV + substance-abusing woman living in an urban ghetto is given the risk figure of approximately 30 percent that her baby will contract AIDS, she may perceive this as relatively good odds, given the context of her life. To her, a 70 percent chance of a baby not having AIDS may be the best odds she's had in years. Her primary concern may very well be the likelihood of living long enough to take care of her child. For her, a 30 percent risk will not mean the same thing that it means to an HIV counselor or to a college student from the suburbs. Cultural myths need to be assessed by health care professionals and policy planners, and AIDS educators need to identify them.

Finally, the more chronic character of HIV infection opens a range of questions about the health care system, its financing, its distribution, and its ethical response to the needs of society as a whole versus its individual members. Health planners continue to assume that there is considerable "fat" in the health care system and that cost-containment is a realistic ongoing goal. Those economists who realize that this is also a myth still maintain the goal of cost-cutting, but then suggest that rationing is required and ethical, and that the development of new and truly useful technology be stopped.[38]

Activists for HIV treatment are now discovering the long-term cost-cutting agenda that has been in place in the medical care system for some time. Good quality care can easily become a social myth in this environment. For example, New York State hospitals reported last year that almost all were running significant deficits that impacted on quality of care, due to the regulatory and cost-containment measures the State had instituted over a period of time. New York has not felt the full brunt of the increased patient load due to HIV infection yet, but this irresistible force of patient need is rapidly approaching the immovable object of medical cost-containment, particularly in New York City.

An understanding of these larger systems dynamics is required for a good understanding of the treatment of HIV infection. Without it, the frustrations of trying to give medical care to AIDS patients will appear inexplicable and defeating. If the public is to be actively involved in policy decisions and policy planning, this understanding is also most important. It is crucial to try to avoid pitting one group's need against another's: transplant patients against AIDS patients, terminal AIDS patients against substance abusers wanting treatment, bypass surgery patients against Well Baby Clinics, HIV-negative obstetrics patients against HIV-positive obstetrics patients, patients over 65 against young adults. This competition is likely to increase, but it would be an ethical and medical tragedy if it did. The myth that there are such scarce resources that medical needs of individuals with HIV cannot be met without sacrificing medical needs of individuals without HIV should be held up for public examination.[39]

### 3. Myths About Human Behavior

Effective education and clinical care depend on a scientifically valid, sensitive and reasonably full understanding of human motivation and action, and of how various interventions can alter motivation and action. Change in knowledge, attitude, and behavior is the goal of such interventions, and this is a very complex undertaking. The many myths about effecting changes in human behavior, as well as about the nature of human behavior itself, make this difficult task even harder. Some myths regarding behavior are given in Table 1-D.

Attempting to demonstrate behavior change scientifically is a difficult task. It is easier to demonstrate accumulation of new knowledge, and it is often incorrectly assumed that such knowledge will inevitably lead to change in behavior. The problem is that it is not even clear that new knowledge necessarily leads to a change in motivation, and therefore behavior.[30,33,40] There are many ways that individuals can deal with new information, and these may not be the ways intended by education or training. Psychological mechanisms can produce unexpected results. Values and different ways of constructing priorities are also powerful confounders. It is incorrect to assume that substance abusers, for example, have a conscious death wish and are not very concerned about the risk of AIDS. But it is also incorrect to assume that health and optimal existence lead the list of their priorities. Their behavior, as documented by researchers, indicates a complex system of motivations and loyalties in which trade-offs are made that routinely put health and life at risk. It has been labeled self-destructive[41] and likened to slow suicide.[42] Health education in general suffers from the assumption that health (good physiological and psychological function) is a universal primary value and has high motivating force.

**TABLE 1-D**
**Myths of Human Behavior**

Knowing about risks prevents individuals from taking them.
Presenting the most terrifying versions of risk results in the most reduction of risks.
People believe what is presented to them as absolute knowledge.
People do not deny or repress information about risks.
The motivations for risk-taking are simple and well-understood.
Human behavior is malleable and easily changed.
It is impossible to change human behavior.
Sexual behavior can be effectively changed with presentation of didactic information.
The motivations for sexual behavior are simple and well understood.
Individuals are very much alike in motivation, risk assessment, and behavior change.
Equating sex with death, or risk of death, will change behavior.
Behavior modification, for a good end, is always ethical.
The goal of health is a primary motivating factor for all individuals.
Avoidance of risk is important to everyone.
Emotional responses can be easily changed.
If knowledge and attitudes are modified, behavior will always change.
The individual is in complete control of his/her behavior.
Systems or environments cannot structure individual action.
If only individuals, and not systems they work or live in, are targeted, behavior can be changed.
Changing lifestyles is easily accomplished.
Education and communication will solve all problems.

It is also difficult to evaluate risk-taking behavior. As a society, we have to find a balance between risk-taking and prudence or caution, and that balance varies in different contexts and cultures. Risk-taking is a normal function and a necessary one for optimal human functioning (or we would never cross a street).[43] Education that pushes the balance to extreme caution is likely to be dangerous if effective, and likely not to be effective because it runs counter to normal human response. Finding the balance is a sophisticated task and needs to be a major concern in any considered intervention with large groups of individuals.

There are also questions about how effectively behavior can be changed. Some assumptions about human nature are not validated by empirical research. There is a limit to the malleability of human beings on the basis of genetics and contextual constraints. When the targeted behaviors are sexual, the situation becomes very complicated. Knowledge and skills about sexual behavior are the tip of a very large iceberg and a thorough understanding of human sexuality in a systemic context is required.

In addition to these general considerations about the myths of human behavior and its modification, there are specific questions. The research in genetic counseling, for example, indicates that people distort, repress, and reject genetic information if it is threatening to them.[44] There is also a healthy skepticism towards experts and hidden agendas, and individuals want to test the validity of information before accepting it. Any dogmatic approach to information can backfire and result in rejection of all the information supplied. Trust is an important component of education and altering views, but it must be earned and it can be easily lost.

Scare tactics can also be dangerous to use. If too threatening, such information will be dealt with through a number of psychological mechanisms leading to denial or rejection. A famous media info-commercial about the impact of drug use on the brain, which uses a frying pan and eggs to illustrate its point, has been reworked by the public to submerge its message that brains get fried by drugs. The resulting joke ("This is your brain on drugs. This is your brain, two eggs and fries on drugs. This is your brain, two eggs, fries and orange juice on drugs") has blunted the message and listeners now laugh at the presentation of the commercial. In this way powerful scare messages may be converted into jokes and discounted. One version of scare tactic behavior modification is the equation of unsafe sex with death. Unfortunately, that may also equate any sex with death, an impossible message either to live with or to sustain a species.

The difference between education and propaganda should not be lightly dismissed. Propaganda can take many forms. These may include the publication or advertising of an overestimation of risks or a listing of atypical worst-case scenarios. Propaganda may emphasize the common wisdom of the "establishment" or rely on the power of emotional triggers alone. It may abuse group dynamics in order to achieve a hidden goal. True education, on the other hand, can give the individual tools that he or she can use for problem-solving. It respects the individual. Propaganda frequently brings premature closure to thinking about problems and solutions, becoming a barrier to further problem solving. In the case of HIV disease, an infection that is still being explored, premature closure is even more dangerous.

Health care providers need to assess the impact of their treatment and preventive education by rigorous evaluation of changes in knowledge, attitudes, and behavior. If this is not done, the health care provider may be convinced that the program is effective when the goals are not being met. Evaluation should be ongoing and thoroughly integrated with the program, so that the health care provider can be constantly aware of the need to alter or update the program.

Finally, sociological studies confirm that the individual's behavior can be altered only if the systems in which that individual works and lives support the change. If those systems are not supportive, and are not altered, the individual will, at best, experience frustration in his or her attempts to exhibit the new behavior and, at worst, not attempt to change. Conversely, if the individuals in the system are not open to change, the systems in which they work and live will not change either. In the case of HIV disease, these systems range from the family and community to work and institutional settings. It is helpful to understand how these systems function, both specifically and in terms of general systems theory, in order to effect change in prevention or treatment.

## CONCLUSION

We have illustrated the metaphors and myths of AIDS and how an understanding of the context in which they are embedded allows us to reject those that are not appropriate. The framework provided by systems theory can help avoid the pitfalls of inappropriate myths and metaphors surrounding HIV infection and be of invaluable assistance in constructing an accurate understanding of this disease. A true systems view incorporates the importance of both detailed specialization of knowledge and a broad synthesis of the multiple levels of explanation that constitute the whole system. Without an integrating view, detail can become confusing, even meaningless. Because HIV infection, the persons who have the virus, and the contexts within which they dwell need to be incorporated into shared human experience, systems theory is even more important when one is thinking about HIV infection. It is precisely the tool that can work.

## REFERENCES

1. Koop, C.E. (1991). *Koop: The Memoirs of America's Family Doctor.* New York: Random House.
2. Bateson, G. (1979). *Mind and Nature.* New York: Dutton.
3. Von Bertalanffy, L. (1968). *General System Theory: Foundations, Development, Application.* New York: George Braziller.
4. Pattee, H.H. (1973). *Hierarchy Theory: The Challenge of Complex Systems.* New York: Braziller.
5. Krasner, S. (1990). *The Ubiquity of Chaos.* Waldorf, MD: American Association for the Advancement of Science.
6. Kolasa, J., Pickett, S.T.A. (1989). Ecological systems and the concept of biological organization. *Proc. Nat. Acad. of Science U.S.A., 86:* 8837–8841.
7. Engel, G.L. (1980). The clinical application of the biopsychosocial model. *Journal of Medicine and Philosophy, 6*(2): 101–123.

8. Clements, C.D. (1989). Biology, man and culture: A unified science based on hierarchy levels. *Perspectives in Biology and Medicine, 33*(1): 70–85.

9. Ostrow, D.G., Atkinson III, J.H., Grant, I. (1990) Overview: The management of the HIV-positive patient with neuropsychiatric impairment. In D.G. Ostrow (Ed.), *Behavioral Aspects of AIDS* (pp. 171–186). New York: Plenum.

10. Shilts, R. (1987). *And the Band Played On: Politics, People, and the AIDS Epidemic.* New York: St. Martin's Press.

11. Gonda, M.A., Braun, M.J., Clements, J.E., Pyper, J.M., Wong- Stoal, F., Gallo, R.C., Gilden, R.V. (1986). Human T-cell lymphotropic virus type II shares sequence homology with a family of pathogenic lentoviruses. *Proceedings National Academy Science U.S.A. 83*: 4007–4011.

12. Williams, G., Stretton, T.B., Leonard, J.C. (1983). AIDS in 1959?. *Lancet, II*(8359): 1136.

13. Culliton, B.J. (1990). Emerging viruses, emerging threat. *Science, 247*: 279–280.

14. Weller, R.O. (1989). Editorial: Iatrogenic transmission of Creutzfeldt-Jakob disease. *Psycho. Med., 19*: 1–4.

15. Thadoni, V., Penar, P.L., Partington, J., Kalb, R., Janssen, R., Schomberger, L., Rabkin, C.S., Prichard, J.W. (1988). Creutzfeldt-Jakob disease probably acquired from a cadaveric dura mater graft. *Journal of Neurosurgery, 69*: 766–769.

16. Brown, P., Cathala, F., Raubertas, R.F., Gajdusek, D.C., Castaigne, P. (1987). The epidemiology of Creutzfeldt-Jakob disease: Conclusion of a 15-year investigation in France. *Neurology, 37*: 895–904.

17. Cherfas, J. (1990). Virus-like agent blamed for mad cow disease. *Science, 247*: 523.

18. Brandt, A.M. (1988). The syphilis epidemic and its relation to AIDS. *Science, 239*: 375–380.

19. Givens, T.G. (1986). A burning issue: Health and wealth up in smoke. *Archives of Internal Medicine, 146*: 1494–1495.

20. Sider, R.C., Clements, C.D. (1987). Medical caring for the smoker: Ethical responsibility works both ways. *Chest, 91*: 156–158.

21. Hyman, J. (Aug. 19, 1990). Ravages of AIDS cross all boundaries in South Africa. *Democrat & Chronicle*, p. 6A.

22. The Names Project, 2362 Market Street, P.O. Box 14573, San Francisco, California

23. Clements, C.D. (1987). The silence of ethics and economics of medicine. *The World and I, Nov. 1987*: 577–592.

24. Bloom, D.E., Carliner, G. (1988). The economic impact of AIDS in the United States. *Science, 239*(4840): 604–609.

25. Dickens, B.M. (1988). Legal rights and duties in the AIDS epidemic.*Science, 239*(4840): 580–586.

26. Fusmento, M. (1990). *The Myth of Heterosexual AIDS.* New York: Basic Books.

27. Lo, S., Tsai, S., Benish, J.R., Wai-Kuo Shih, J., Wear, D.J., Wong, D.M. (1991). Enhancement of HIV-I cytocidal effects in CD4 lymphocytes by the AIDS-associated mycoplasma. *Science, 251*: 1074–1076;

28. Lusso, P., Di Marzo, F., Enzol, B., Franchine, G., Jemma, C., De Rocco, S.E., Kalyana-Raman, V.S., Gallo, R.C. (1990). Expanded HIV-I cellular tro-

pism by phenotypic mixing with murine endogenous retrovirus. *Science,* 247: 848–852.

29. Imagawa, D.T., Moon, H.L., Wolinsky, S.M., Sano, K., Morales, F., Kwok, S., Sninsky, J.J., Nishanian, P.G., Giorgi, J., Fahey, J.L., Dudley, J., Visscher, B.R., Detils, R. (1989). Human Immunodeficiency Virus Type I infection in homosexual men who remain seronegative for long periods. *New England Journal of Medicine,* 320(22): 1458–1462.

30. Simon, K.J., Das, A. (1984). An application of the health belief model toward educational diagnosis for VD education. *Health Education Quarterly,* 11(4): 403–418.

31. Darrow, W.W., Siegel, K. (1990) Preventive health behaviors and STD. In K.K. Holmes, P. March, P.F. Sparling, P.G. Wiesner, W. Cates Jr., S.M. Leman, W.E. Stam (Eds.) *Sexually Transmitted Diseases* (Second Edition) (85–91). New York: McGraw Hill.

32. Thurman, Q.C., Franklin, K.M. (1990). AIDS and College Health: Knowledge, threat, and prevention at a Northeastern university. *College Health,* 38: 179–184.

33. Solomon, M.Z., De Jong, W. (1986). Recent sexually transmitted disease prevention efforts and their implications for AIDS health education. *Health Education Quarterly,* 13(4): 301– 316.

34. New York State AIDS Institute. (July, 1990). Draft: HIV Counselor Training Programs and Course Descriptions. 1–31.

35. (1991). Update: Transmission of HIV infection during invasive dental procedures. *MMWR 40* (23): 377–381.

36. *The Medical Post,* April 10,1990.

37. Harrison, D.F., Wambach, K.G., Byers, J.B., Imershein, A.W., Levine, P., Maddox, K., Quadagno, D.M., Fordyce, M.L., Jones, M.A. (1991). AIDS knowledge and risk behaviors among culturally diverse women. *AIDS Education and Prevention.* 3 (2): 79–89.

38. Aaron, H. Schwartz, W.B. (1990). Rationing health care: The choice before us. *Science,* 247: 418–422.

39. Clements, C.D. (1989). "Therefore choose life": Reconciling medical and environmental bioethics. *Perspectives in Biology and Medicine,* 28(3): 407–425.

40. Jeffery, R.W. (1989). Risk behaviors and health: Contrasting individual and population perspectives. *American Psychologist,* 44: 1194–1202.

41. Stanton, M.D. (1977). The addict as savior: Heroin, death, and the family. *Family Process,* 16(2): 191–197.

42. Menninger, K.A. (1938). *Man Against Himself.* New York: Harcourt, Brace

43. Harsanyi, J.C. (1976). Can the Maximin Principle serve as a basis for morality? *Essays on Ethics, Social Behavior, and Scientific Explanation.* Boston: Kluwer.

44. Walzer, S., Richmond, J.B., Gerald, P.S. (1976). The implications of sharing genetic information. In M.A. Sperber, L.F. Jarvik (Eds.), *Perspectives in Biology and Medicine* (pp. 147–162). New York: Basic Books.

# CHAPTER 2

# Identifying the Systems Impacted by AIDS

## *J. Landau-Stanton, C. D. Clements, A. Z. Griepp, R. Cole*

In order to assess and manage HIV disease, it is important for the health care professional to be aware of the multiple systems levels at which patients and clients function. To begin to show the clinical usefulness of systems theory, let us start with the story of "Mary Porter."*

### MARY PORTER
#### The Beginning

Mary was a woman in her 20s who lived in an outlying rural district with her husband and two small children. Her dreams were about improving her land, owning a bigger farm one day, and being able to stay home to breed her horses and be a full-time mother to her children.

Mary's life changed dramatically when her husband died of cancer. In an attempt to deal with her loneliness, and not yet ready to start another permanent relationship, she had several casual encounters with men she met at the bars. As she became more secure in her widowhood, her confidence increased and she met a man with whom she and her children developed a committed and stable relationship. Life looked great—and then her symptoms started.

She began to experience fevers, night sweats, diarrhea and weight loss. At first, she attributed these symptoms to viral illness and stress, resulting from the two years of turmoil following her husband's death. Naturally thin, her continued weight loss became a source of dismay,

---

*For the protection of patients' and clients' confidentiality, names and identifying material have been changed throughout the book.

which she managed to ignore for as long as humanly possible. When asked about the dramatic changes in her appearance she quickly explained how the extended mourning for her husband, and the responsibility of raising two small children alone kept her thin and constantly exhausted. These explanations convinced even Mary herself for many months.

It was only when her boyfriend complained that there was no longer anything of her for him to hold and that her clothes were falling off her that she accepted that she should seek medical attention. Her rural family practitioner was perplexed by her excessive weight loss. A careful and thorough physician, he meticulously ruled out metabolic disorders, anorexia and bulimia, carcinoma and leukemia, and the malabsorption syndromes. Mary complained that there was not a part of her body left sacrosanct, nor a vein unpunctured—but still there were no answers.

Laboratory tests resulted in changes in diet and exercise patterns, but she continued to lose weight. Suddenly she developed pneumonia. She was hospitalized in the local rural facility where a diagnosis of pneumocystis pneumonia was made. There was no apparent reason for this fit, healthy, 28-year-old to have this form of infection. Both Mary's and the physician's anxiety and frustration grew as her symptoms worsened. In desperation, he sent her for consultation to a tertiary medical center for further diagnosis and management. It was then she learned she had AIDS.

### HELENE DE VILLIER'S CASE
### The Beginning

Helene de Villiers was a gorgeous 23-year-old who had immigrated to the United States from Haiti at the age of seven. Although having acculturated well, she retained some of her traditional Haitian values and superstitions. Her future looked bright, she had a job awaiting her graduation, a boyfriend of whom her parents approved, and much youthful exuberance. Then she was diagnosed with AIDS.

Suddenly darkness descended; a ghost from her past had come back to haunt her. Her traditional superstitions led her to believe that this would not have happened to her had she not done something to deserve it. It took some time for her to admit to her physician that a brief and painful episode from her past might be responsible. When Helene was 21 years old, an older, experienced Haitian partner had been selected for her traditional sexual initiation. Her choices had been limited by her surroundings far from her native land, and she had been forced to make her own selection in the absence of senior family members to do it for her. She was devastated at the realization of what a mistake she'd made. She felt guilty and incompetent and became extremely depressed.

Helene had realized soon after her symptoms began that she needed HIV testing. When the results she dreaded were confirmed, she was embarrassed and ashamed to have to advise her current boyfriend, as well as previous partners and lovers, that they needed to be tested. She had painful genital warts that could not be successfully treated due to the deficiency of her immune system. She felt dirty, undesirable, and frightened that she would lose her current boyfriend because of her illness.

Mary and Helene experienced alterations in their lives when they became infected with HIV. Each changed physically. Each experienced major shifts in mood, sleep and appetite patterns. Each became concerned and preoccupied with health status. Despite the differences in their lives, there were many similarities.

Based on these two cases, we can begin to see how a systemic view provides us with a practical tool for understanding these differences and similarities, and how it helps us understand HIV disease. For example, as we look at Mary's story, it is obvious that it is difficult to encapsulate her struggles or limit the effects to the biological, psychological, or social sphere. Her physical, or biological, infection with HIV resulted from the death of her husband and the social environment in which she coped with that loss. The isolation of her rural area and its false sense of security and denial of risk of AIDS are dependent upon the social level of Mary's life system. That same sense of safety and denial operated on the support network of medical care and its level of education and awareness. Important biological information was not gathered because of the effects of other levels in the system. Her worsening health, her medical problems and her attempts to manage these problems consumed Mary's time, energy, and finances. It is not possible to limit the scope of impact to only the sphere of molecular biology, although that biological level is crucially important.

The diagnosis itself, and the medical care required, produced much stress and anxiety for Mary at many levels, as well as upon her extended family system. Each new test meant pain and going further into debt. Mary's sleep became worse as she worried about paying the bills and lamented the erosion of her plans and dreams, along with the growing threat to all aspects of her existence. Where would one map this on a biopsychosocial model?[1] Is her sleep disturbed because of medical reasons, because of personal anxiety and worry over finances, or because her children are becoming more withdrawn and needy? We can construct a diagram prior to the onset of symptoms for both Mary and Helene, and then diagram the changes that resulted from the diagnosis (Figure 2-1).

As we look at this diagram, it becomes clear that it is extremely difficult to separate out the biological from the psychological and the social spheres.

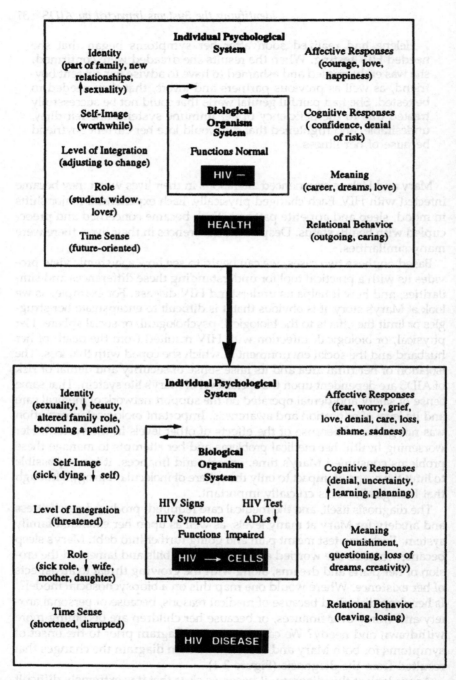

**Figure 2-1.** Development of HIV impact at personal, biological, and psychological levels (Mary and Helene)

HIV underscores the importance of an integrative view. For example, when Helene began to develop painful genital warts and to lose her feelings of sexuality, the biological impact of these symptoms created a major impact on her psyche; anxiety, guilt, and fear took over. The combination of physical debility and psychological symptoms quickly impacted on her social world, both personally and professionally. Also, because Helene was a woman and because the definition of AIDS was originally based on men's opportunistic diseases, the importance of her genital warts could easily be missed. Biological, psychological, and social components were separable for only a brief moment in time.

Figure 2-1 above allows us to look at the impact at an individual level. But individuals don't operate in a vacuum. Helene knew immediately after receiving her test results that she couldn't bear the news of her HIV positivity alone. Her mother had always been a close and trusted confidante. But how could she share this with her? All the rules by which she had been raised seemed to come into conflict with her present situation. Although giving the public appearance of a well acculturated Haitian American, her private life was as loyal to her Haitian identity as she could make it. And now, nothing made sense any more. What could she say to her mother? Had she made a serious mistake in judgment?

Helene was her mother's only daughter. They had always been exceptionally close to the extent that when her father ventured off to America, Helene stayed behind with her mother. The household in Haiti at that point consisted of Mother, older brother, Helene, and her mother's extended family with whom they lived. There was considerable pain at the parting from the extended family when the migration occurred, and clear directives had been given by her grandmother for the family not to forsake their traditional values.

Shortly after arrival in the United States, Helene's mother had a baby boy. Helene assisted her mother in raising him and poured out the love that she could no longer lavish on her grandparents. What would her beloved baby brother say now? Would she have to stop kissing him? Had she already inadvertently exposed him to the virus? Would she be responsible for the death of the people she loved, living in the same home, eating off the same dishes, sharing a bathroom? What had she done?

Eventually she plucked up courage to share her news with her mother. However, once her mother had reassured her of her constant love, her mother begged her not to discuss the matter further, since she didn't believe that there was a real possibility of Helene's dying. Helene's mother insisted on telling her father and older brother herself, and asked Helene not to discuss her illness with them. Helene was also asked not to share her problem with Jean, her baby brother, who was 12 years old at the time of her diagnosis.

Helene was very lonely in her silence in the face of her family's denial of the possibility of her death. Her love for her family gave Helene the strength to maintain her silence.

The desire to protect family members through silence is not uncommon in loving families. Families facing any of a number of significant problems (suicidality, major illness, drug abuse, death) may care deeply for each other, but may talk about everything else except the problem. The issue of secrecy and protection in families will be discussed in Chapter 8. Some family members may even "sacrifice" themselves via suicidality or misbehavior to draw attention away from the families' pain.[2] It is important to understand the dynamics operating in Helene's family. While it may appear that they were "cut off" and isolated from Helene, in reality there was a desire to protect the family from pain and this required everyone's silence. This silence eventually required Helene to seek support outside the nuclear family.

## MARY PORTER
### The Rest of the Story

No two families are configured the same way or have the same orientation towards problems. Unlike the case of Helene, where her mother had difficulty acknowledging Helene's illness, Mary herself was the one not ready to acknowledge her HIV status. What happened to Mary and her family when she began to lose weight dramatically? How did they deal with her hospitalization and subsequent diagnosis?

Mary's live-in boyfriend, James, was troubled from early on. He knew something was radically wrong and didn't know how to convince her to seek medical care. She kept him at arm's length by attributing the symptoms to her husband's death. How could he argue with that, even though he knew it wasn't an adequate explanation? And how could he answer her children's questions when they asked him, "What's wrong with Mama?" He wasn't the only person to notice the dramatic changes in Mary. Her two sons began to play at home more quietly; they stayed close to her, not risking their usual games outside. James finally insisted that she go to the doctor. There she received the information that she was HIV positive. Her mother and stepfather responded the minute James shared Mary's diagnosis with them. They took the children for a few days to allow Mary and James time to be alone together and plan for an entirely different future from the one that they'd envisaged. Mary and James couldn't imagine coping without the support of her parents.

Her illness progressed rapidly. She and James realized that it was time for him to be tested for HIV too. It was no great surprise when he tested positive. The two of them despaired about how they would deal with what was to come. As Mary deteriorated, the family closed ranks and tried to be there for each other whenever possible. Mary's 16-year-old brother was excluded from the family drama. Mary was ashamed of her "sinful" behavior and felt that she had set a really bad example from which her brother should be protected.

Mary's 25-year-old brother, who lived a short distance from the family home, bore his sister's illness with rural stoicism, "She's sick, but I've got to go to work now," he would say. Mary's biological father remained totally ignorant of her predicament.

Mary's parents and James understood very clearly what the prognosis was. They grieved each time she was hospitalized. The children were again excluded from the process. Mary refused to share her imminent death with them. Her younger brother, Bill, eventually insisted on being informed about what was unfolding. She shared her story with him three months before she died, and her worst fears were realized. He fell apart, sobbing uncontrollably at the thought of losing his big sister. He didn't judge her, however, and did his best to be there for her.

Her mother and James were with her every moment possible. They both struggled with Mary's decision to leave her children with their grandparents, and not with James. He would repeatedly beg her to marry him, and make the children legally his. Mary refused to saddle him with a family at the point that she knew beyond doubt that she was leaving him. Also, in the face of his HIV positivity, she refused to place her children with a father who was sentenced to die.

Both her mother and her stepfather, despite their misgivings about their age, supported Mary in her decision. However, they worried about how they would keep up with another generation of young ones. Their own children were all but launched. They had been thinking about buying a trailer and retiring to Florida and reaping the rewards of many years of hard work.

Mary's mother and James stayed with her during her final days on the ventilator. Her mother did her best to comfort James and to be there for him, knowing that, in some ways, his loss was going to be greater than hers. Mary realized that the end was near. As a smoker, her lungs were not pliable and couldn't take excavation. An attempt was made to clear her lungs and remove her tube so that she could talk to her children. The attempt failed and her only means of communication was through writing and pointing out letters on a spelling board. Her mother and her children climbed onto the bed, and she spelled out for them that she would die. Her mother was left with the task of explaining to the children what had happened to their Mama. James was bereft. His worst fears were realized after her death. He had no claim on the children and had to surrender them to Mary's parents.

As we explore Mary's situation, it becomes apparent that there are some limitations to the simple biopsychosocial diagram presented earlier. A more comprehensive approach is needed to denote the reality of the social systems with which she was involved. The limitation of our current diagram is that Mary's entire social system is defined within one small component of the picture. Let us expand on the social component of "biopsychosocial" in order to obtain a more complete and realistic perspective of the social system. Lewin's field theory,[3] on which the diagram below (Figure 2-2) is partially based, allows us to do this in a comprehensive way.

Using this expanded diagram as the basis, let us now try to obtain a clearer picture of Mary's life. HIV disease clearly impacts on many more people than only the infected person. In Mary's nuclear family, the far reaching impact of HIV can be readily seen.

> During Mary's long illness and after her death, James was sad, distracted, preoccupied, and unable to function at his usual high level on his job. Supervisors were confused about why this fine employee was "not on his toes" lately.
>
> Mary's two sons may have been quiet at home out of respect for their mother's illness, but they were not so quiet in the class setting. Joe, the oldest of the two, began to become somewhat aggressive with other boys in his class. Joe's teacher noted changes in his behavior, and when she talked with Joe, he merely stated that, "My Mom's been sick." He did not elaborate on the frequent hospitalizations, his fears, the fact that more often than not they had been spending nights at their grandmother's, or that he did not really understand what was going on. Because of this, Joe's teacher did not understand why Mary did not respond to a note sent home with Joe for his mother.
>
> Mary's mother loved her daughter a great deal, but felt increasingly torn as her condition worsened. Mary's mother had remarried only a few years before, and had begun to enjoy an active social and sexual life that was being limited by the constant presence of her beloved grandchildren.
>
> Mary's brothers and their social systems were impacted by the HIV disease as well. Her 25-year-old brother became more and more remote from the family. He could not bear to see his sister suffer so, and he began taking every overtime shift offered and spending an increasing number of evenings in the local bar. Her 16-year-old brother tried to be as stoic as James and his older brother, but this was not in his nature. He was tearful at times, sensitive, and easily irritable at high school. His team mates began to tease him about how edgy and tearful he was, and began to withdraw from him. His coach noted this change as well and began to play him less (to the team's detriment), suspecting that he was using drugs.

In this one vignette it is easy to see how far the fingers of HIV reached. It is sometimes tempting for health care workers to focus on the individual

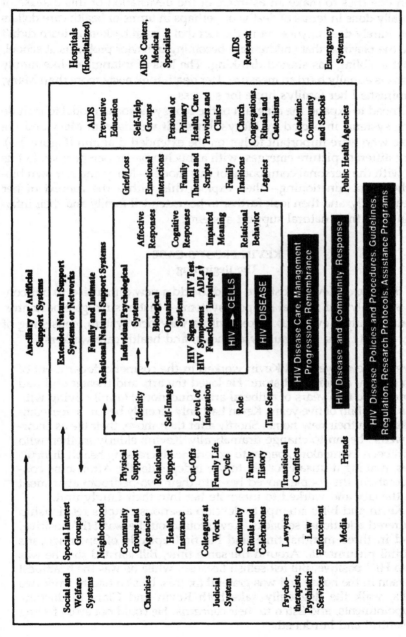

**Figure 2-2.** The addition of the social level: Family and intimate relational natural support systems; extended natural support systems; ancillary or artificial support systems in HIV disease

at hand, but the impact of HIV reaches far beyond the infected individual. When one tries to make an estimate of the devastation of this disease, it is usually done in terms of deaths or perhaps in terms of health care dollars spent. Rarely does anyone count the fact that a rural basketball team didn't make the playoffs, that children are becoming behavior problems at school, or that a sibling has started drinking. The loss of intangibles like family dreams is equally hard to measure. Her death took away more than Mary; it diminished her family's hope for success.

We need to expand the diagram of the biopsychosocial model to include all the systems impacted by Mary's illness. If we diagram Mary and the people who were important to her on the extended diagram (Figure 2-3), a very different picture emerges, with a much broader perspective. Let us start with the personal component of this model—Mary and her own bio-psychological functioning—then explore this within the context of her nuclear family, and then look further to her extended family and their interaction with their natural support systems.

### KEVIN FROST'S CASE
### The Beginning

In the case of Kevin Frost, we need to add a new dimension to our concept of family and natural support systems—that of surrogate or nontraditional family. Kevin was linked with a very rich system, consisting of lover, parent, pets, community agencies, and health care workers.

Twenty-seven-year-old Kevin worked in the cosmetic department of an elegant department store. He loved the arts and theater and had completed two years of a liberal arts education. Happily living with his lover (Bill) of five years, Kevin had only recently begun to feel comfortable in their new home. Shortly after their move, their life as "newlyweds" began to change dramatically. Kevin's elderly mother, who had been living alone, began to experience increasing health difficulties, making it unsafe for her to live independently. After some consideration, the couple moved her into their two-bedroom apartment in the city and worked to integrate her into their family unit.

Kevin and Bill's attempt to develop a serious couples relationship suffered additional setbacks. Kevin found out he was HIV positive, and in three months' time had his first episode of pneumocystis carinii pneumonia. Around the same time, Bill learned that he was also HIV positive. Bill felt selfish because, while he was the healthiest person in the house and was grateful for this, he also had to work two jobs, walk the dog daily, take both Kevin and Clara to doctors' appointments, and listen to their concerns. He could not avoid feeling resentful and burdened.

Tempers began to flare and this once happy unit had constant tension and at least one daily fight, frequently about the lack of money. Clara was terrified to discuss her son's illness–she had lost sons before. Her son, Tom, committed suicide when he was 23, and her younger son, Kelly had been court-ordered out of the home when he was 12. Clara had also lost her husband to a long siege with cancer approximately five years before Kevin's illness.

Kevin felt guilty that he was probably the one who had brought HIV to the couple. He also experienced recurring problems with sinusitis that would eventually lead to bacterial pneumonia, causing him to be hospitalized nearly every three months. Kevin's anxiety began to turn to rage. He was mad at his father for dying, his brothers for being worthless, his mother for being an invalid, Bill for being sick too, and the dog for needing to be walked. He raged at his respiration (which was too compromised to allow him to go up and down the three flights of stairs), at the neighborhood kids for being so noisy, at his primary care doctor for not being able to reduce his anxiety, and most of all at himself for having placed himself at risk for HIV.

Bill's anger was manifested in a different way. He became quieter because he felt that Kevin and Clara were too ill to stand hearing how he really felt about things. He began to hover around them and became overprotective of both of them. Bill noticed that his tips at work were decreasing and realized that he was being less pleasant and friendly to customers.

Bill's temper flared uncontrollably when one co-worker questioned whether he and Kevin had been tested for HIV. Bill began to become increasingly demanding of the family doctor. He would call daily with some concern about either Kevin or Clara. Bill felt it was his responsibility to ensure their well-being, but he was also tremendously afraid and had nowhere to go to talk about his concerns. He considered his HIV status a moot and unimportant point. "I have good T4s and am healthy, so what do I have to complain about?"

The immediate family cluster was not the only one affected. At coffee breaks, Bill's co-workers frequently speculated about what could be wrong with Bill. The small group of friends that Bill and Kevin had begun to cultivate wondered why they were rarely available for social gatherings. Kevin's co-workers wondered what could have happened to have made him go out on disability so quickly. "I think it's AIDS," some whispered.

Dr. Brown, the family's physician, and his office staff were also impacted. At first, the Frosts were among some of their favorite patients—polite, compliant, clean, attractive and good bill-payers. Things were changing. Kevin was increasingly argumentative and stirred up trouble on many of his admissions to the local hospital. "Why am I the only one to receive dinner on paper plates?" he would ask, "They leak and the gravy drips on me. Don't people in this hos-

**Family and Intimate
Relational Natural Support Systems**

Physical Support (parents, lover who is HIV+)

Relational Support (parents, lover, children)

Cut-offs (secret from brother, lover excluded)

Family Life Cycle (child dying before parents)

Loss of Spouse

Family History

Transitional Conflicts (parents retiring, now must care for grandchildren—lover loses family) Brother in high school acting out

Grief/Loss (parents, children, siblings, lover, self)

Emotional Interactions (closeness & leave-taking)

Family Themes and Scripts (stoicism—hope for next generation)

Family Traditions (rural American)

Legacies (farewell to children, giving children to her parents)

**Individual Psychological System**

Affective Responses (sadness, concern)

Cognitive Responses (denial, planning)

Meaning (dream of farm lost, provision for children)

Relational Behavior (secrets, withdrawing, dependent/providing)

Identity (mother, girlfriend)

Self-Image (loss of attractiveness)

Level of Integration (threatened)

Role (sick role vs mother, lover)

Time Sense (end of dreams, future, shortened time with children)

**Biological Organism System**

HIV Signs
HIV Symptoms
Functions Impaired

HIV Test
ADLs↓

HIV → CELLS

HIV DISEASE

HIV Disease Care, Management Progression, Remembrance

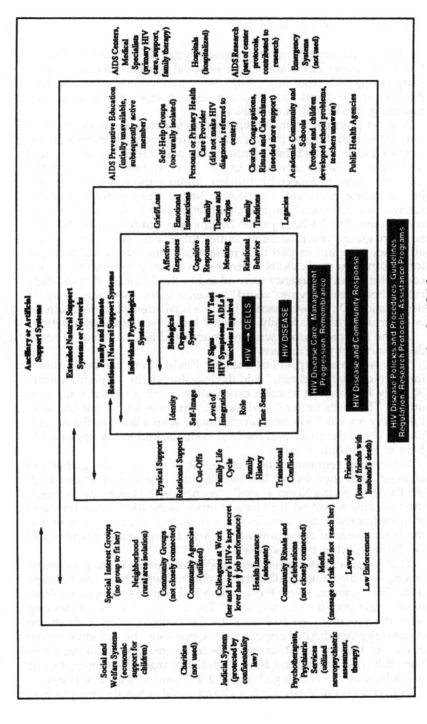

**Figure 2-3.** Mary's HIV disease developed within the entire natural and artificial support systems

pital know that my HIV can't be passed by my dinnerware?" Needless to say, whenever Kevin was in the hospital, Dr. Brown could expect daily phone calls from him complaining about some injustice, from Bill concerned about Kevin's progress, and from the nursing staff regarding Kevin and Bill's attitude.

A good physician, Dr. Brown tried to set reasonable limits. This only infuriated Bill and the nursing staff more; they wanted answers to their questions and they wanted them now. Then, Dr. Brown tried to delegate: "The social worker in the office can best help with that." This also failed to relieve his burden, because the social worker also began calling him daily. Dr. Brown, being creative, thought about referral to a community agency; for a brief time this referral brought some relief. The 24-hour-phone hotline was comforting to Bill. The support group provided some outlet for Kevin. The social service advocacy program helped the Frosts gain some additional coverage for prescription medications. Then, Kevin began to get worse, and the counselors from the agency were added to the list of Dr. Brown's daily callers because of Kevin's "weird" behavior in their support group. In desperation, Dr. Brown reached out in a final attempt to maintain his equilibrium with this family; he asked for a psychiatric consultation.

At the first psychiatric session, an irritated Kevin stated, "I really don't know why we're here."

"You were really upset last Tuesday, Kevin, don't you remember?" instructed Bill. "I was not," said the irascible Kevin. At about minute 30, they had started to calm down after clearing the air with each other. "That feels better," said Kevin, "but now let me tell you who I'm really mad at." The session continued with a laundry list of complaints about the social and medical systems, and many appeared to have at least some validity.

Kevin then requested medication: "It is the only thing that has allowed us to cope for the last two weeks." The session ended with the therapist giving Kevin a small prescription of Valium and suggesting that they might wish to look at other medications once they and the psychiatrist had become better acquainted. An arrangement was made for a second appointment. The psychiatrist made a note to call Dr. Brown within the next week.

That phone call never happened. Within five days, the psychiatric emergency department called the psychiatrist with the announcement that, "Your patient, Kevin Frost is here and requires admission. What floor would you like him to go to?" The day after his initial meeting with the therapist, he had gone to the support group held at the community-based AIDS organization. Once there, he wouldn't get out of the car. He was sure that everyone in the group was talking about him. Bill tried to reassure him, as did staff from the agency, but he was adamant. "I want to go home, I don't want to see those people."

Bill, concerned about such a change, did what he thought was best—he gave Kevin some extra Valium to calm him down. What a surprise when exactly the opposite happened. By the next morning, Bill was awakened by Kevin screaming out of the window at the neighborhood children. Bill gave him another Valium. A few hours later, Bill was interrupted at work by Clara who said, "You have to come home, Kevin's in trouble. I tried to stop him but I couldn't." Speeding home, what should Bill see but Kevin, in pursuit of the neighborhood children, brandishing a butter knife. Bill was able to get Kevin to go to the psychiatric emergency department, where he was believed to be delirious from all the Valium. He required emergency admission to rule out an organic affective illness and/or AIDS dementia.

In cases such as Kevin's, it is abundantly clear that our concept of family needs to include nontraditional family structures. If we fail to include these, we will limit the resources available to health care providers and to patients. Kevin's spouse, Bill, clearly belongs within the nuclear family circle, and Bill's extended family would be integrated with Kevin's in the circle committed to extended family and friends. (See Figure 2-4).

<h2 style="text-align:center">HELENE<br>The Rest of the Story</h2>

Despite the difference between Kevin's non-traditional and Helene's Haitian family structure and experiences, there were some remarkable similarities. Helene's struggle with HIV quickly encompassed many people beyond her nuclear family. Their need for silence and denial drove her into the arms of less intimate extended family members and friends. Since the nuclear family chose not to deal with the issues at that time, her grandparents, aunts, and uncles were not even informed, and another major source of support was thereby excluded.

The only person in the family with whom Helene could discuss her disease was Marie, her brother's new wife. Marie, an earthy and practical woman, who had recently joined the family, did not need the protection accorded those who had loved Helene dearly through time. Marie listened kindly and didn't burden Helene with philosophical problems. She would console her with platitudes, such as, "Don't worry. . . . They'll find a cure in time for you. . . . You'll get better. . . . You look good!"

Shortly after her diagnosis, Helene realized that she needed to share her HIV positivity with both her past and present boyfriends. She had met her previous boyfriend, Don, at college, subsequent to her sexual initiation. She struggled with how to tell him. She would have preferred to handle it face-to-face, but couldn't afford an air ticket and realized she'd have to write or call. Which would be kinder?

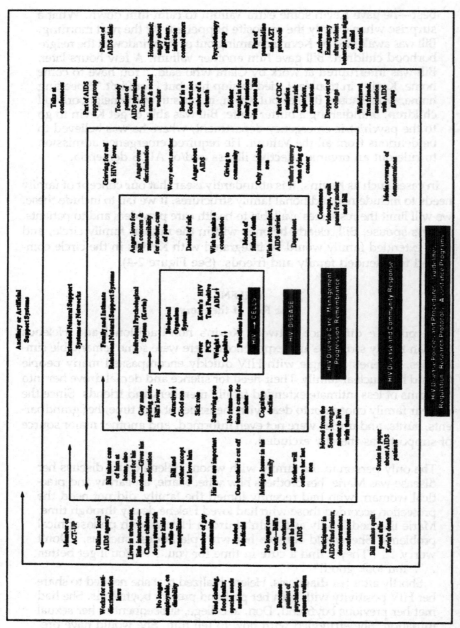

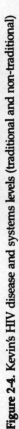

**Figure 2-4.** Kevin's HIV disease and systems levels (traditional and non-traditional)

She called Don to tell him the news and educate him about his need to be tested. A caring person, Helene had already secured the local hotline number for him and had mailed him brochures from the AIDS clinic, since she wouldn't be there to explain everything to him herself. He wasn't easily convinced that he was really at risk, since he was young, fit, and heterosexual.

It took her some months, and lots of literature and cajoling, to persuade him to be tested. Don tested negative, much to Helene's and his own relief. He was able, after his test, to be there for her by letter and phone, and she was very appreciative of having somebody that she could confide in.

Her current boyfriend, Gerard, on the other hand, reacted very differently. He believed her when she told him of her HIV results and quickly went to be tested. When his test came back as negative, both he and Helene were overjoyed. (However, he did not feel it necessary to have a subsequent test six months later.) Helene was thrilled to have a healthy, supportive partner close to her. He professed undying love and protection of Helene in the moment of relief when test results were obtained. Gerard, like many negative partners of HIV positive individuals, was not able to maintain this degree of commitment to Helene over time. Gerard gradually became less and less available to her, never citing HIV as the reason.

Despite knowing that this was her last hope of a relationship, she did not argue when he told her that he had been offered a job in a distant city. She realized that he was not capable of making this last journey with her. She never heard from him again. She wondered whether she had misjudged him entirely or whether he cared too much—whether he couldn't bear the pain of watching her die.

Her next hope for companionship and understanding was her best friend, Eloise, the person with whom she had always shared everything, even her original sexual escapade. Since Eloise, too, was Haitian, she had been very supportive of Helene's attempt to do the traditional thing. Eloise was horrified at Helene's news, which came only three days before the birth of Eloise's first child. Eloise and Helene had practiced together for Helene to be the birthing coach, since Eloise's husband, Louis, felt that a delivery room was no place for a self-respecting Haitian man. Helene waited it out, coached Eloise as planned, trusting that once the baby was born and Eloise settled, her friend would be there for her as usual.

This trust was shattered within 48 hours of the birth. When Louis came into the nursery and found Helene rocking his first son and about to kiss his forehead, Louis screamed. "What are you doing? Do you want to kill my baby? Get out, don't ever come near him again!" Helene fled, distraught, feeling utterly alone. Despite Eloise's calls and attempts to reassure her and reconnect, Helene was too hurt to respond and to risk trusting Eloise as a friend ever again. Eloise, however, was not so easily turned away. She loved Helene dearly, and was very distressed about what had happened. She couldn't bear to think of the pain her friend was feeling, nor to imagine her dealing with her illness all alone. Eloise stayed connected through Marie, and eventually, as Helene lay dying, showed up at the hospital and made her peace with her best friend.

Helene's mood grew increasingly sad. She had shared her HIV positivity with many people so far, but, for various reasons, none of them had been able to provide open communication and support on an ongoing basis. This is not unusual in HIV disease; frequently, the person with HIV must be the strong and knowledgeable one and provide education and support to his or her loved ones in dealing with the disease.

A resourceful person, Helene began to look for other avenues of support where she might talk freely about her fears and concerns. She identified her church pastor as someone whom she respected and whom she believed to be a kind and caring man. Gradually, she made herself better known to him, and let him know that she had "health problems." He was supportive, kind, and always willing to pray for her recovery. Something inside made her hold back on telling exactly what those "health problems" were. She was terrified that "a man of the cloth" would not understand her sexual choices and would lose all regard and respect for her if he knew what she had done, and that she was suffering from AIDS.

Simultaneously, she called the AIDS hotline number that she saw on TV. The listener was understanding and knowledgeable and put to rest many of her fears about the possibility of having exposed her little brother to HIV. The hotline also helped her obtain the number of the local community-based HIV organization.

Her family doctor quickly recognized that he was out of his depth in managing her difficult-to-treat warts, as well as her HIV disease. He arranged for her to visit the AIDS specialty clinic in town. She was nervous and apprehensive as she opened the door. What if someone saw her going into the clinic, or worse yet, what if she saw someone she knew in there? Her fears were allayed when she saw only gay men in the waiting room on her first visit. She was also comforted that her first contact was with a mature nurse who placed her in a private examining room relatively quickly. This nurse was to remain a significant part of Helene's support throughout the rest of her life.

Helene and the nurse, Karen, became very important to each other. After several visits, Karen became aware of the fact that she was thinking about Helene between appointments. Karen was also aware that she was scheduling Helene for appointments that were not medically indicated, but rather for emotional support. At this point, Karen recognized that she was becoming a little too close to Helene, but was unsure how to extricate herself delicately.

Karen identified that Helene was losing weight, having early morning awakening, crying daily, and feeling hopeless and helpless. Karen appropriately sought psychiatric consultation for Helene. Helene, however, was not sure she wanted to see a psychiatrist, partly because the notion was not consonant with her Haitian roots. Besides, she thought to herself, she already had all the support she needed from Karen. A three-way meeting between Karen, Helene, and the psychiatrist helped to smooth the transition.

After a major depressive episode, Helene began treatment that included psychotherapy and medication. She improved dramatically and within a few weeks was able to join a psychotherapy group for women who were HIV positive, and to decrease her individual therapy time. Eventually, she was successfully tapered off her tricyclic antidepressant, so that her only therapeutic modality was the women's group.

Helene blossomed in this group of women who had come into contact with the virus in a number of different ways. As each woman shared her story, Helene felt less and less alone. They all cried as they described abandonment by lovers, the fact that they could no longer feel comfortable in having children, and their embarrassment at meeting new potential partners and having to discuss sex and disease transmission with men they scarcely knew. Helene realized she wasn't the only one feeling dirty, and the women shared practical information about safer sex, how to tell partners, and the latest scientific findings. Helene began to move beyond her own problems and developed a strong sense of altruism, which is not surprising given her academic background in sociology. She began volunteering her time to help others. She decided to integrate women into the community-based organization's gay men's group, and became the "heart" of that group.

As her mood and hopefulness improved, not surprisingly, so did her health. Feeling herself to be too old to be living off the family, she obtained a part-time job while keeping up with her volunteer activities. Her smile and calm acceptance became an inspiration for every patient and caregiver with whom she had contact. She freely processed her feelings about her own impending death and disfigurement with the women in the group, and modeled superb coping skills. When she died, most of the hospital as well as the women's group and the group from the community-based organization went into mourning. She had changed from a sad, frightened girl to an activist, a teacher, a friend and an important member of a new (and unfortunately rapidly growing) community of People with AIDS (PWAs).

As her confidence grew, she was more and more able to talk frankly with the members of her natural support system. She told her mother that she needed to talk about what was happening to her, and her mother was able to listen. She told the family that she believed that her young brother needed to know what was happening to her and that she could no longer tell him lies in answer to his questions. When she told him about her diagnosis, he understandably was sad and confused, but Helene turned this into an opportunity to protect him from becoming HIV positive by educating him about risk behavior. She had utilized her professional supports well, and at exactly the right moment, and now she could more fully return to the more important people in her life.

## LEARNING FROM THE CASES: THE FINAL DIAGRAM

Mary, Helene, and Kevin provide clear illustrations of how important it is to view persons with HIV infection in context. Even though it is critical not to ignore the individual needs of patients and not to forget their own bio-psychological functioning, it is also important to remember that the other parts of their lives are just as critical. When one individual is afflicted with AIDS, many others are impacted by it. The emotional stress and pain, the reorganization of lives, the financial stress, and the eventual loss of loved ones always impact on a large system.

This system includes not only the patient's biological or nontraditional family, but also his or her work colleagues, neighbors, friends, and church community. It also impacts dramatically on the health care community, with specific emotional and physical implications for the health care providers who minister to each patient. Without considering all of these components of the patient's systems of import, one cannot understand or predict the individual patient's reactions, emotions, needs, or behavior. What appears at first glance to be irrational, unpredictable and impossible to deal with suddenly becomes explicable and manageable as one begins to comprehend the complete context in which one's patient lives. Such comprehension allows the health care professional to design treatment and therapy in a rational, logical way, leading to a natural sequence of steps toward preventing spread of the disease.

Figure 2-5 allows us to see the extent of the effects of HIV disease, and the complexity of management and decision-making regarding them. From the ribonucleic acid replication of the virus to the existential coping with human mortality and meaning in end-stage HIV disease, the integrated levels of the natural system of life, or the ecosystem,[4] shape our interventions and goals for AIDS prevention and treatment. Mental health and other health professionals cannot be specialists on all the levels that are important to understanding and therapeutically intervening in HIV disease, but detailed specialist expertise is not always required. Instead, a basic understanding of how to think systemically, and an ability to access and use the available expertise in therapeutic situations is what is needed.[5,6,7,8] The

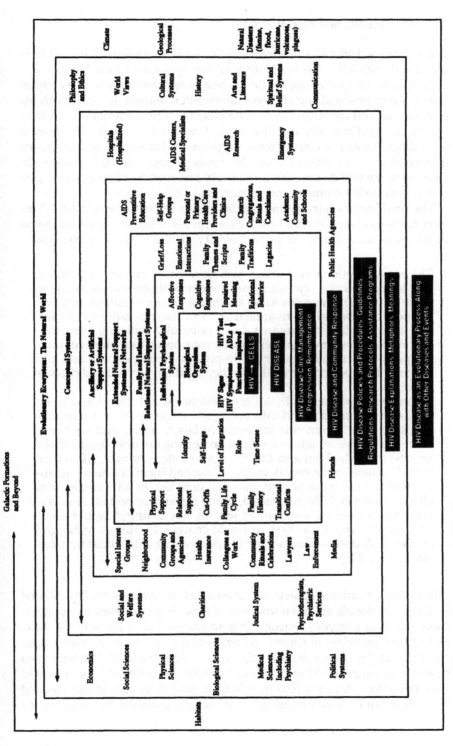

**Figure 2-5.** The complete system of HIV disease

cases of Mary, Helene, and Kevin require a global understanding of how they lived with HIV disease, within all the systems of their lives.

In therapy, diagramming the life system as we have done in this chapter can be a very practical and effective intervention in itself. It allows both the professional and the client to see concretely the interconnections and their effects on the client's life and disease. In Chapter 8, we will fully develop such diagramming of connections, supports, and strengths in therapeutic interventions, and elaborate on the famiy aspects of HIV disease. In Chapter 9, we will discuss the community and macrosystem from the perspective of both treatment and prevention.

The final level of our diagram encompasses the entire ecosystem. This integrative level can give the health care provider a broad, contextual focus in which to understand the impact of HIV. In the words of Sussman:[9]

> The heavy emotional cost of care will force policy makers, legislators, and human service organizations to identify those individuals who relate well to persons with AIDS and to use family members, however defined, as allies in the treatment process. New paradigms of care, and an evolution in human values, hopefully will unite families, friends, human service professionals, volunteers, and other committed persons in a common service to provide the hope, care, and love required by a person with AIDS as they fight for survival and prepare for death.
>
> Families of persons with AIDS experience social stigma and isolation, fear of contagion and infection, guilt, anger, grief, and economic hardship . . . . From this suffering of heart, mind, and soul may emerge a mythic structure focusing on healing not only the ills of the specific individual but also the ills of our modern culture. AIDS then would become, by its very devastation, the harbinger of a new humanity in which the immune systems of all individuals, all societies, and all of nature would be nourished, cared for, and protected. A necessary transformation from "me as self" to "we as unity" would occur and, in turn, the whole system would change. Families—recharged by the AIDS crisis—may well be the catalysts for this crucial transformation. (p. 238)

Sussman's thinking reflects the framework of systems theory. Mental health professionals are often unaware of how frequently they use systems theory in their everyday practice. It is so embedded in the way we think and in how we relate to clients and patients that we apply it almost automatically, as the cases discussed above have demonstrated. We have seen how the assessment and management of Mary, Helene, and Kevin would have been very different had they been regarded as individuals isolated from their families, communities, and cultural contexts. Systems theory may seem very abstract, very theoretical, almost esoteric, but, in fact, it is about people and cases. It allows us to understand the intricate two-way interaction and influence between people and the systems they live in.

Engel, in his description of the clinical application of the biopsychosocial model, extended the biological systems model of Weiss[10] and von Bertalanffy[11] to "everyday practice and patient care."[1] He created a diagram (see Figure 2-6) that has become a classic for visualizing how the interconnections of the biological, psychological and social components of human beings are integral to understanding, and working with, any medical condition.

It was from this base, along with Lewin's field theory,[2] that we developed the systems diagrams used to illustrate the levels of system impacted by HIV disease. Engel accepted Weiss's basic premise that nature is hierarchically organized [1,12] and that each hierarchical level has specific properties and characteristics that at the same time are part of a continuum constituting the system.[1]

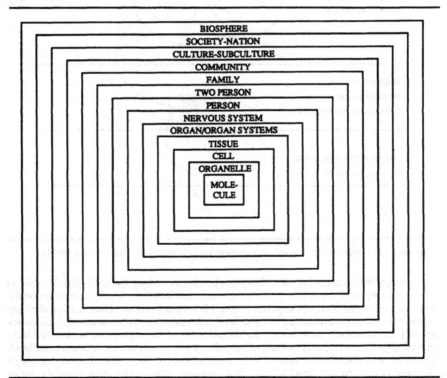

**Figure 2-6.** George Engel's continuum of natural systems

Reprinted with permission from Engel, G.L. (1980). The clinical application of biopsychosocial model. *American Journal of Psychiatry, 137*(5):537.

   In addition to Engel's depiction of systems levels, there are other schematicized drawings to illustrate the systems concept and provide us with a practical understanding of its relevance to medical practice. Von Bertalanffy [11] presented Boulding's and others' models of the levels of systems complexity. Clements and Potter[13,14] propose an alternative way of visualizing system levels aimed at capturing the unified structure of system levels or focuses (Figure 2.7). These models attempt to integrate the various levels, noting that effects impinging on one level also affect the other levels in various degrees.

   Underlying all these schemas is a primary idea, a central concept. That

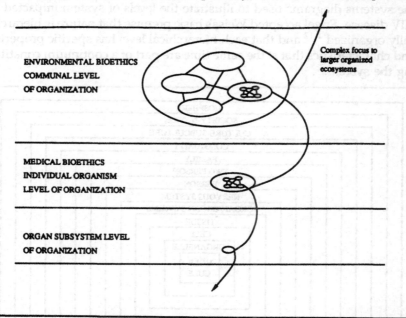

ENVIRONMENTAL BIOETHICS
COMMUNAL LEVEL
OF ORGANIZATION

Complex focus to larger organized ecosystems

MEDICAL BIOETHICS
INDIVIDUAL ORGANISM
LEVEL OF ORGANIZATION

ORGAN SUBSYSTEM LEVEL
OF ORGANIZATION

**Figure 2–7.** Colleen Clements' integrated relationship of subsystem levels

The integrated relationship of subsystem levels (including the individual, medical bioethics level and the communal, environmental bioethics level) seen as recombinations and more complex organizations. New functions or relationships develop at these levels of organization, but the basic integration remains intact and the levels are not dichotomous, as indicated by the position of the organ unit within the individual organism unit, and of the individual organism unit within a communal level. There is no reductionism versus holism dichotomy within this diagram. If major damage occurs to any level within this diagram, there is built-in effect (great or small) within all levels. Miserable survival is a bidirectional flow within an integrated, hierarchical organization.

Reprinted with permission from Clements, C.D. (1985). "Therefore choose life": Reconciling medical and enviromental bioethics. *Perspectives in Biology and Medicine, 28*(3):408.

concept, Engel argues, is of critical clinical importance. It provides the basis for his biopsychosocial model, as well as for other systems views in medicine. Doherty and Campbell note that "Engel's model (and the other models) explicitly reject the one-cause/one-disease/one-treatment approach in favor of a comprehensive view of factors influencing health, illness, and health care."[15] Koop, in his description of his own clinical view, summarized in Chapter 1, highlights the usefulness of systems theory, which he believes gives the foundation for the moralist and scientist to build an integrated approach to AIDS.[16]

For those not familiar with the theoretical basis of systems thinking, the following brief summary has been included.

## A Summary of Applied Systems Theory

Based on our application of systems theory to understanding the HIV infectious disease process and to developing a psychosocial and educational intervention, there are some general statements that can be made to describe this approach.

1. Systems theory is an integrative method at its core, an inclusive way of viewing experience. Although there have been dichotomies, "either-or" forced choices, created between "reductive science" and "holistic systems," a full appreciation of systems theory reveals these as false dilemmas. Systems theory opens the way for a unified understanding of human experience.[17] It provides a "both-and" approach. The basic concept of systems theory is integration and inclusion. And this simple concept is an extremely important rethinking of many of our conventional beliefs.

2. Systems theory describes levels of organization of the same building blocks of reality, or scales of perception of the same basic experience.[18,19] It proposes that our human experiences are made up of both less organized and more organized blocks, or viewed as smaller and larger scale. This organization or scale has a discoverable repetition and style, what some community ecologists are calling a pattern,[20] and what some physicists and physician-researchers are calling chaos theory.[21] Simpler organization has greater stability, less flexibility, and also a tendency to collect together into patterns that create more complex organization. Complex organization has less stability, greater flexibility and response to change, and a tendency to break apart into its simpler components. This ongoing organization and decomposition implies a process view of the world, a dynamism. The control of HIV infection or of any other disease, for example, will not be achieved indefinitely, and we should not have been surprised at the emergence of a new epidemic such as HIV disease.

3. Simpler and more complex levels of organization or scale are fundamentally connected. As systems theory sometimes puts it, there is unity

within diversity.[22] In fact, unity is a functioning state, maintained by mechanisms that communicate between levels and work to achieve controlled state. These mechanisms can allow some disruption at one level without destroying the entire system, but only within limits.[23] The system is not completely self-correcting, and a controlled state can swing into a disintegrating state and eventually collapse the entire system.

This strong integration of the system also implies that an event at one level can be communicated throughout all levels, with either measurable or nonmeasurable effects. This is sometimes oversimplified to say that the flapping of a butterfly's wings in Asia can affect weather patterns globally. But because there are feedback mechanisms for partially controlling effects at one level (the flapping butterfly), it is rare for one small event to send more complex levels out of control. More generally, failure of the controlling mechanisms occurs with an accumulation of atypical events. AIDS prevention and treatment, then, need to address all levels, from microbiological research, to the patient with HIV, to the medical care system, to the family system, to the cultures, to the broad society, to values and spirituality, to world views.

4. There is no value judgment made among the levels of organization or scale. Simpler, less organized levels are not "lower" in any value sense. Nor are more complex levels "higher," assuming a preference. The level of the retrovirus, HIV, is not better or worse, higher or lower, than the family system of the individual who is seropositive; but its effect on the individual's body system and family social system can lead to collapse of both systems. If we wish to maintain the individual and family organization, we need to understand the complete interactive process that occurs at all levels and choose our intervention to accomplish the most with the fewest chaotic effects.[23]

5. Because organization and scale are integrative, our interventions need to maintain a careful balance of all levels of the system. The needs of levels will often be in conflict and a controlled state is not a static steady-state.[24] In fact, complex levels have a built-in mechanism of limit and collapse. As a result, the needs of community health, public health, and the individual who has a communicable disease such as HIV infection can be anticipated to conflict. Interventions will not completely resolve the problem but must try to attain some optimum trade-off between needs.

This balance will be specific to the environment or situation, will need to be continually reevaluated, and will need to be done carefully with an eye to the fragility of complex levels such as social systems. Decisions made about the balance between the needs of HIV infected individuals and the community's health and viability should be made differently in Central Africa and the United States. The risk to social systems in Central Africa is so great and the resources to cope with those risks so limited, that the community level could collapse into chaos and further cause a tremendous loss of individual lives. In such a situation, the risk to a particular individual's needs cannot be given as high a priority as it still can in the United States. The policy implications of systems theory are also clear.

## REFERENCES

1. Engel, G.L. (1980). The clinical application of the biopsychosocial model. *American Journal of Psychiatry, 137* (5): 535–543.
2. Stanton, M.D. (1977). The addict as savior: Heroin, death, and the family. *Family Process, 18(2):* 191–196
3. Lewin, K. (1935). *A Dynamic Theory of Personality: Selected Papers by Kurt Lewin,* Translated by Donald K. Adams and Karl E. Zener, 1st edition. New York and London: McGraw-Hill Book Company, Inc.
4. Auerswald, E.H. (1968). Interdisciplinary versus ecological approach. *Family Process,* 7 (2): 202–215.
5. Auerswald, E.H. (1983). The Gouverneur Health Services Program: An experiment in ecosystemic community care delivery. *Family Systems Medicine,* 1 (3): 5–24.
6. Doherty, W.J., Baird, M.A., Becker, L.A. (1987). Family medicine and the biopsychosocial model: The road toward integration. In W.J. Doherty, C. Christianson, M.B. Sussman (Eds.) *Family Medicine: The Maturing of a Discipline.* New York: Haworth.
7. Bloch, D.A. (1988). The partnership of Dr. Biomedicine and Dr. Psychosocial. *Family Systems Medicine,* 6 (1): 2–4.
8. Bor, R., Miller, R., Perry, L. (1988). Systemic counseling for patients with AIDS/HIV infection. *Family Systems Medicine,* 6 (1): 21–39.
9. Sussman, M.B. (1989). Epilogue—AIDS: Opportunity for humanity. In E.D. Macklin (Ed.). *AIDS and Families.* New York: Herrington Park Press.
10. Weiss, P. (1977). The system of nature and the nature of systems: empirical holism and practical reductionism harmonized. In K.E. Schaefer, H. Hensel, R Brady (Eds.). *Toward a Man-Centered Medical Science.* Mt. Cisco: Futura Publishing.
11. Von Bertalanffy, L. (1968). *General System Theory: Foundations, Development, Application.* New York: George Braziller.
12. Pattee, H.H. (1973). *Hierarchy Theory: The Challenge of Complex Systems.* New York: George Braziller.
13. Clements, C.D. (1985). "Therefore choose life.": Reconciling medical and environmental bioethics. *Perspectives in Biology and Medicine, 28(3):* 407–425.
14. Potter, V.R. (1985). A response to Clements environmental ethics: A call for controlled human fertility in a healthy ecosystem. *Perspectives in Biology and Medicine, 28(3):* 426–433.
15. Doherty, W.J., Campbell, T.L. (1988). *Families and Health.* California: Sage Publications.

16. Koop, C.E. (1991). *Koop: The Memoirs of America's Family Doctor.* New York: Random House.
17. Clements, C.D. (1983). The lesion and the function: Setting up the reductionist problem. *Perspectives in Biology and Medicine, 26*(3): 433–440.
18. Pickett, S.T.A., Kolasa, J., Armesto, J.J., Collins, S.A. (1989). The ecological concept of disturbance and its expression at various hierarchical levels. *Oihos, 54:* 129–136.
19. Levin, S.A. (1988). Pattern, scale, and variability: An ecological perspective. In A. Hastings (Ed.). *Lecture Notes in Biomathematics* (pp. 1–12). New York: Springer Verlag.
20. Pickett, S.T.A., McDonnell, M.S. (1989). Changing perspectives in community dynamics: A theory of successional forces. *Tree, 4*(8): 241–245.
21. Krasner, S. (1990). *The Ubiquity of Chaos.* Waldorf, Maryland: American Association for the Advancement of Science.
22. Gray, W., Rizzo, M.D. (1973). *Unity Through Diversity.* New York: Gordon Breach.
23. Clements, C.D. (in press). Systems Ethics and the history of medical ethics. *Psychiatric Quarterly.*
24. Clements, C.D. (1976). Stasis: The unnatural value. *Ethics, 86*(2), 136–144.

# CHAPTER 3

# Individuals, Families, and Populations at Risk

The systems we have discussed that are impacted by HIV disease are the same systems that determine vulnerability to risk of infection by HIV. They are also the systems that form the focus of the prevention of the spread of HIV disease, clinical care, and healing. In this chapter we will be discussing individuals, families, and populations at risk. In the next chapter we will present issues of risk to the health-care provider, and in later chapters we will deal with the issues of clinical care and healing.

The perspective of prevention allows us to think about risk at primary, secondary and tertiary levels. Prevention is defined as: (1) Primary prevention, that is, the prevention of infection or disease, generally requiring community-wide public health measures, for example, immunization. When completely successful, the result of primary prevention is the eradication of the disease, as was achieved by the monumental worldwide effort and subsequent success with smallpox. (2) Secondary prevention is the prevention of complications of the infection or disease, and (3) tertiary prevention is the prevention of reinfection.

How may this framework be applied to HIV disease? Primary prevention of HIV infection remains the central and most pivotal goal in the management of this disease, as with all other infectious diseases. It is more critical with HIV infection, since there is as yet no known cure or effective vaccine. The AIDS epidemic currently resembles the early experiences with syphilis, tuberculosis, leprosy, and pneumococcus pneumonia, to mention just a few examples from our medical history. It also resembles the current situation of infectivity with Creutzfeldt-Jakob disease and the death sentence that accompanies pancreatic cancer. Because of the unavailability of a vaccine, primary prevention has focused on preventive education rather than on quarantine. HIV disease has also not been classified as a notifiable disease in the way that syphilis and gonorrhea have, which further complicates the institution of public health preventive measures.

As a result, primary prevention depends on the individual's own risk assessment and willingness to change behavior. In order to do this, the individual needs to be made aware of the risk factors. Secondary prevention of the complications of HIV infection is a major task, since the sequelae of the infection itself are life-threatening and the risk of opportunistic infections not only is extremely high in this disease, but, in fact, defines it. Secondary prevention employs the tools of personal lifestyle management and the tools of medical, neuropsychiatric, and psychotherapeutic care. In terms of tertiary prevention, the term takes on a special meaning in the management of HIV infection. Since no cure has, as yet, been developed, the traditional interpretation of tertiary infection (that is, reinfection after cure) does not apply. However, there is some medical evidence that repeated infection can intensify and aggravate a preexisting infection, rendering the virus more virulent and increasing the complications and severity of the disease, as well as hastening the onset of AIDS Related Complex (ARC) and AIDS in those who have had an initial infection. Prevention of reinfection takes the same form as primary prevention, but is complicated by the infected person's certainty that prevention is no longer applicable, and by the health care providers'conviction, or suspicion, that prevention will not significantly alter the course of the disease.

## RISK

### Risk Perception and Awareness

Of the 269 matched pre- and post-evaluations done by our NIMH AIDS Training Project, 57 percent of trainees from all specialties felt at risk because of their professional work and 10 percent felt at risk outside the workplace. The Project sample included a large number of medical students and direct health care givers (69 percent). Physicians made up five percent of the sample. Of the entire sample, 32 percent had either worked with AIDS patients or with patients who were HIV +. This self-reported risk awareness is consistent with other surveys of medical students and residents, which find close to two-thirds of the group very worried about the risk of HIV infection in their professional responsibilities. In the Project results, death anxiety was also raised. Thoughts about personal mortality were already high in medical students and physicians, but were increased by the preventive intervention—a necessary anxiety for the avoidance of risk. (The level of anxiety did not correlate with a willingness to treat the HIV population.)

An individual's perception of personal risk may include not only the realistic probabilities of transmission routes such as needlesticks and blood contact with skin, mucous membranes, and eyes, but also uncommon and/or debatable risk, such as from aerosolized blood, brain biopsy tissue, urine and vomitus, bites from psychotic patients, and even tears from HIV+ babies. Awareness that HIV is found in certain fluids does not necessarily mean that HIV may be transmitted by them; however, many individuals feel safer taking maximum precautions regardless of the level of risk.

Health care professionals may perceive infection control techniques as impractical for a variety of reasons. Statistics from the Centers for Disease Control that stress the low probability of infection are often emphasized in preventive interventions. However, we should not be surprised if this is insufficient to resolve the questions and feelings about risk. An understanding of the probability of HIV infection (less than one percent, less than five percent, less than contracting hepatitis, etc.) only gives part of the equation of risk. It is true that there are more common dangers in the world, and even more likely risks in medicine. But the severity of the consequences is much lower than the severity of HIV disease. The one partially comparable example is Creutzfeldt-Jakob disease (CJ), which is infectious and lethal, and which is a proven risk for clinicians and laboratory technicians.[1] Many nurses working with CJ patients, inside and out of the operating theater, routinely double-glove and still feel that they are at significant risk, even though the probability of infection in terms of numbers is really quite low.

Severity of the consequences of infection must be added to the risk equation. If the consequences are lethal, risk perception will be high no matter how low the probability. Many people fear the risk of flying, not because so many airplanes crash, but because the result of a rarely occurring crash is generally lethal. As severity increases, reluctance to take even a small risk increases. "That single case could be me."

The ability to have some control over taking the risk is also part of the equation. Sadoff[2] has reviewed this and other factors in risk-taking. Jeffery[3] has also given a more systemic view of the risk concept. The risk of lung cancer because of smoking cigarettes, for example, can be divided into absolute, relative, and population risk. The absolute risk for a 40-year old man in the United States of dying of lung cancer in one year is 11 in 100,000. The relative risk for a 40-year old man who smokes compared to a nonsmoker is 10 to 1. Population risk (a function of relative risk and prevalence of a risk factor) is 101,000 lung cancer deaths per year. The absolute personal risk tends to be low. For a 35-year old smoker, the 10 year absolute risk of lung cancer is only .03 percent. Smoking is a behavior under some personal control; the individual does not feel the risk is forced on him from an external source. As a result, the individual is more comfortable with such a risk, even when the severity of the consequences of lung cancer are considered.

Personal control over risk is a very important factor in the equation. HIV infection is seen as an imposed risk, more similar to the risk of nuclear power plant meltdown than to smoking, for a number of reasons that may seem paradoxical. After all, sexual behavior and even intravenous or injection drug use may seem to be personal choices. However, since total abstinence is the only certain way to avoid contracting HIV through sexual intercourse, and yet we depend for survival of the species on procreation, this can hardly be viewed as individual choice.

The sense of the external imposition of risk is clearly seen in the risk to health care professionals. In many countries, professionals are not allowed routinely to know the HIV status of patients and thus feel they have little control over the risks they are assuming. Many health care professionals are not allowed by law or professional oath to refuse to take the risk of caring for an HIV + patient or client. Professionals may also feel that they are not given adequate practical infection control mechanisms and have no effective way of protecting themselves. Further, health care professionals who contract HIV lose considerable control in their professional roles. Many are now concerned that iatrogenic transmission of HIV, as demonstrated in the transmission of HIV by a dentist to his patients, will result in mandatory HIV testing for them although they will still not have control of their personal risk-taking.[4] Because of such consequences and a sense of the lack of control, risk-perception becomes an even more important consideration in risk-reduction.

But even control over personal behaviors such as unsafe sex and injection drug use may be problematic. Our sexual behaviors are not so easily or practically brought under our control, as any teenager can demonstrate. Abstinence is not a viable option. Women may not feel they have sufficient control because of cultural norms that make negotiating for condom use very difficult. Addiction to drugs can remove self-control over risk-taking. Economic pressures (as in prostitution) can also dilute control.

A systems view of the factors constituting risk makes it easier to understand how people perceive and evaluate risk-taking, and to appreciate that probability figures alone provide an oversimplified view of the process. By analyzing the risk equation of *Probability of Risk + Severity of Risk + Personal Control of Risk Exposure*, a more realistic picture may be gained without prejudice or judgment.

## Risk Assessment and Willingness to Treat

One of the prevalent fears of AIDS experts has been that, as the awarenesss of health care professionals about the risk of infection increases, there would be a deleterious effect on patient care. It was thought that high risk-perception led inevitably to unwillingness to treat or work with individuals who are either at risk for HIV, are HIV +, or have AIDS. In support of this, a survey of medical students and residents showed that a third of the group consider refusing to treat individuals who fall into those categories.[5] However, emergency treatment or treatment of someone who is already a patient was excluded from this refusal decision. Many physicians, as reflected in their professional codes, want the freedom to accept or reject an individual as a patient. In light of these facts, there has been concern that preventive education that fully and openly discusses the risks of HIV infection by occupational exposure might decrease an already tenuous willingness to treat.

We were relieved to find that the training evaluation data of our NIMH AIDS Training Project did not support this concern. In fact, our data showed that the educational process highly increased both willingness to treat and perception of competence. The increase in these categories was highest for women who, as a group, had been initially less willing to treat these individuals than had the men. However, despite the gender difference, there was a global increase in willingness to treat. This increase in willingness occurred even though fear of infection and death anxiety also increased. Therefore, a thorough presentation of risk perception and risk-taking did increase the sense of risk and death anxiety, but it also increased the willingness to assume that risk by treating the populations who present it.

As a result, it is safe to conclude that the interaction between risk assessment and willingness to treat populations that present a risk of HIV infection is more complex than is assumed. One hypothesis that can be suggested is that thorough discussion of realistic risk assessment (which includes all the components of risk evaluation) increases the trainees' sense of trust and their sense of personal control of the risks. The trainees' sense that the trainers understand and validate their concerns about risk and provide them with practical problem-solving skills further increases their feeling of competence and their capacity to face risk.

## Levels of Risk

We will now examine the risk to and by individuals, families, communities, natural support systems, and professional support systems from a systemic perspective.

Therefore, while discussing the biological vulnerability of a hemophiliac, we still need to be aware that hemophiliacs also need to be discussed under the heading of social level, since they form a class of individuals and families. In the same way, biological risk, such as the failure to use a condom, invariably implies the presence of behavioral risk factors, and may be based on cultural, philosophical, economic, or political factors as well. When we discuss the social level and identify the groups at particular risk, remember that within these groups are individuals, with biological and psychological functions, embedded in family and social relationships. From this perspective, levels are not separate and distinct entities. While reading this section it might be useful for the reader to anticipate the connections across all the levels and the impact that an event at one level inevitably has on all the others.

## THE PERSONAL-INDIVIDUAL-BIOLOGICAL LEVEL

### Infection Control in the Delivery of Health Care and at Home

Infection control has always been an integral component of infectious disease management. AIDS, however, has reinforced the need for very strict infection control procedures; the Centers for Disease Control (CDC) now recommend *universal precautions* as the ideal infection control procedure. Universal precautions require the assumption that all patients are HIV positive. Precautions can vary from gowning and gloving to eye-protective goggles to total protective body suits with self-contained ventilation systems, depending on the context of patient care. Universal precautions can, unfortunately, be unwieldy and they depend on careful individual behavior in handling *sharp objects* such as knives, safety-pins, needles, and high-power drills; *body fluids* and excreta such as expectorant, vomitus, dirty diapers, and spurting blood; and during *invasive procedures* such as surgery, bone tissue and aerosolized blood.

Infection control within a private home is easier to employ than within larger institutions such as hospitals, community health and mental health agencies, hospices, community AIDS agencies, transportation services, and day care facilities. It is also easier to maintain if service is not being delivered in an *emergency setting* such as at a roadside accident where an emergency medical technician (EMT) may need to act with great speed to save a life, and may not have special gloving immediately accessible. The same constraints may apply to emergency police and prison situations.

In the home, members of the family usually know the HIV status of the individual. Therefore, in addition to being prepared for universal precautions, they have a specific situation for which they know precautions are needed. In addition, they do not have to use them all the time, for all members of the family. A major impediment to the use of universal precautions is that people who are told that precautions need to be exercised all of the time become casual, since they have no idea when they are particularly at risk. People tend to lower their guard when a situation becomes routine.

Also, realistically, in institutional settings, it is not always possible to use good universal precautions.[6] Gloves may not be immediately at hand, or a physician or nurse might arrive in the ward or emergency department and need to become instantly involved in lifesaving measures. It is really difficult under those circumstances to question, "Is this patient HIV positive? Do I risk his/her life by not taking all measures—just in case?" Sharps containers for needles may not be located close enough to where the needle is being used, while a technician who takes blood for a living might feel that the risk of the occasional needle stick from the rare visit of an HIV-positive person does not warrant the use of a procedure that renders her hands clumsy and insensitive. Even with the meticulous practice of universal precautions, risk may still occur in the instance of glove failure. Some hospital and police personnel have begun double-gloving in order to eliminate the danger of a faulty glove.

There are solutions to many of these risk problems. It is possible to manufacture gloves, both for emergency medical personnel, surgeons, nurses and EMTs and for the home, that are strong enough to resist most regular usage, if not puncture wounds. EMTs can be encouraged to ascertain when they check their packs that their heavy-duty gloves are right on top and have to be put on prior to any other task. Barriers can be used in the application of cardiopulmonary resuscitation (CPR) in the field, and should be a standard component of the emergency pack carried by anyone trained in the use of CPR. Protective goggles should also be standard in any emergency setting where there is the likelihood of spurting blood.

Needles can be designed that do not require removal from the syringe and hazardous disposal. Staff of institutions can be taught the importance of reliable universal precautions and the dangers of regarding their jobs as routine. People in homes or institutions can learn the applicability of general hygiene to their daily activities. Few people would touch an infant's feces or vomitus with their bare hands; why then do it if one is also risking HIV infection?

The other situations described above are more difficult to deal with in a manner certain to ensure infection control. Personnel performing invasive procedures can wear masks and goggles to avoid aerosolized blood and bone; however, face masks allow the passage of the virus; a self-contained body suit is really the only safe answer. Researchers working with blood that contains a high concentration of HIV require not only laboratory hoods, but self-contained suits and a range of special containment levels.

Infection with HIV should not be the only concern of people dealing with this population. Opportunistic infections may be transmitted as well, so that infection control needs to be concerned with prevention of the spread of these infections. Active tuberculosis, as an example, is a rapidly spreading opportunistic infection.[7] It is airborne and hence requires considerable attention to infection control. Further information about the risks of opportunistic infection will be given in Chapters 5 and 6.

## Specific Dental and Hospital Procedures

HIV disease has demonstrated that a newly discovered disease may hide many surprises. Dental procedures had been considered to put people at relatively low risk. With dentists using masks and gloves, and following routine sterilizing procedures, it was assumed that infection control would be adequate. The Florida cases (described in Chapters 1 and 5) dispelled this false sense of security and taught us that very tight infection control procedures were needed in all health care settings. There is now concern for aerosolized blood, which can be produced during dental or medical procedures, for the adequacy of gloves as a barrier to transmission of the virus, and for sterilization of instruments and their handles, which have been shown to contain minute particles of blood and bone tissue.[8]

Orthopedic surgery is one of those hospital procedures with particular risk of infection. Orthopedic surgeons have been discussing this for some time. Although recent voluntary HIV testing of this group showed that only two out of 3,420 surgeons were HIV positive,[9] the consensus now is that orthopedic surgery requires special precautions even though these do not completely remove the risk of infection. These same precautions could be applied to all operating rooms to reduce the risk to medical staff during surgery. Aerosolized blood is in suspension in the operating room theater and will continue to raise questions about the risk to staff and subsequent patients.[10] Suggestions have been made about exchanging the air after each procedure; however, there is no statistical evidence at this time for the employment of such measures. The delivery of aerosolized pentamidine has also been thought to expose the health care provider to risk of tuberculosis infection.[7] Recent pharmacological developments have led to alternative methods for the administration of this drug, not only for reasons of safety, but also because the aerosolized form was not thought to reach all areas of the lungs.

In addition to orthopedic surgeons, individuals specializing in obstetrics and gynecology who work in the wards, outpatient settings, or delivery rooms and operating rooms need to take particular precautions to prevent infection by HIV. Since their field of work includes dealing with large amounts of blood, amniotic fluid, or mucous membrane, effective barriers such as heavy gloves, aprons, and goggles should be used to reduce risk. Neurosurgeons are especially at risk during routine brain surgery or biopsy of neural tissue, since they use high-speed tools and deal with tissue that can be highly contaminated. Similarly, but to a slightly lesser degree than the specialties mentioned above, all surgical staff are at risk and need to ensure that they are employing effective universal precautions. In addition to operating room staff, postanesthesia nurses should also take precautions in dealing with postoperative body fluids in the recovery room.

**Blood and Organ Donation and Artificial Insemination**

In Chapters 1 and 10 we discuss the history of *blood transfusion* as a source of HIV infection, and the fact that 12,000 transfusion recipients became infected with HIV before blood banks began the Enzyme Linked Immune Absorbent Assay (ELISA) and Western Blot screening. Currently, screening identifies the majority of HIV-infected blood but, because of the average six-month window between infection with HIV and the development of antibodies that the ELISA/Western Blot tests for, some HIV infected blood does get through the screening process. Further information on the current testing procedures will be presented in Chapter 6. A direct test for HIV in blood, the Polymerase Chain Reaction Test (PCR), is being refined for more general use, but, since the reading of the results is extremely delicate, quality control needs to be further standardized before it can be applied on a mass scale.[11] Cost factors also come into play in the decision to use PCR for blood bank screening.

Blood transfusion has always presented some risk. For example, prior to effective screening, hepatitis could be transmitted and, currently, routine screening procedures are not available for HTLV-I and CJD. However, the small risk needs to be balanced against the need for blood transfusion; in cases where blood can be lifesaving and there is no effective alternative, the small risk should not preclude the decision to transfuse. The transmission of infection through the blood factors needed as a lifesaving measure by patients with hemophilia resulted in a high percentage of hemophiliacs becoming HIV+ prior to the availability of screening measures. This will be discussed below.

*Organ donations* of tissue such as kidney, bone marrow, cornea, heart, liver, and skin can also transmit infectious diseases such as HIV. Tissue can be tested for HIV prior to transplantation; however, the urgency of some organ transplantation precludes this. In some instances, for example where the donation of an organ has been prearranged (such as in the case of a live related donor of a kidney), the donor may be pretested by the standard ELISA/Western blot. In the case of cornea and skin donation, the cadavers can be tested, and there is time to wait for the results, since corneas and skin are generally stored in a bank. However, in the case of heart, liver, and nonrelated donor kidney transplantation, the results of the ELISA/Western Blot test are unlikely to be available in time. It is hoped that within the near future a test capable of producing immediate and accurate results will be devised.

Two known cases of multiple organ donation from cadavers that have produced HIV infection in recipients have been reported. One, reported in 1991, indicates that screening still does not entirely obviate the risk, since the cadaver tested negative on the ELISA/Western Blot test, perhaps due to the window period. Still, the risk must be balanced with the urgent need for a transplantation to save the life of the recipient.

There has been a marked change in the management of sperm for *artificial insemination* during the past few years. Sperm stored in liquid nitrogen is capable of transmitting HIV,[12] so most sperm banks are now routinely testing for HIV. Prior to such screening, however, there were cases of HIV infection through artificial insemination and one could argue that sperm banks took too long to begin routine HIV testing.

## Sexual Risk Prevention

Abstinence is the only guaranteed way to prevent the acquisition of HIV through sexual activity. While abstinence is hypothetically possible, it is not likely that the entire population will practice it in the near future. The history of syphilis indicates that even a serious and potentially fatal disease will not curtail sexual behavior. Winston Churchill's father died of syphilis, showing the world that it was not a disease only of the socioeconomically deprived and the morally depraved. In the same way, sexual activity puts people at risk of HIV regardless of class, color, creed, marital status, or lifestyle. Since the virus knows none of these boundaries, it indiscriminately crosses mucous membranes, infiltrates blood, and infects those exposed.

The biological line of defense rather than the behavioral (which is presented later in this chapter), consists of barriers to prevent the infiltration of the virus. Such barriers include condoms, dental dams, and HIV-toxic spermicidal jellies.[13] The use of condoms in combination with such jellies has been found to be relatively effective if used properly. The jelly most commonly in use contains Nonoxynol-9 and is available across the international market. However, it has been implicated in vaginal and urinary tract infections. Condoms, much to the surprise of many, vary considerably in their efficacy as barriers. Also, frequency of exposure and HIV prevalence, even with careful condom use, increases the risk. It has been estimated that the risk of a single act of unprotected intercourse with an HIV + partner is one in 500 of contracting AIDS. With a condom, the risk becomes one in 5,000. However, after 500 acts of intercourse, the risks are two in three without a condom, and one in 11 with a condom.[14] In high prevalence areas, the risk will be increased; in low prevalence areas it will be similarly reduced.

Counselors need to ensure that they are extremely specific in their education of their clients, not only to the proper use of condoms, but also about the types likely to be most effective in the prevention of spread of the virus. Only latex condoms will prevent the passage of the virus across the condom material. Condoms made of other materials are ineffectual. Even latex condoms are more effective used with HIV-toxic jelly. Latex condoms do, unfortunately, have a failure rate, based on manufacturing quality control, so we need to be aware that we are talking about safer sex, rather than safe sex. Some counselors may not be comfortable educating their clients about safer sex measures. It is advisable for these counselors to ensure that their clients will be receiving the necessary education from their primary care physicians or nurses. If this appears unlikely, or if the counselor is unable to effect a referral, then referral to the local sexually transmitted disease clinic is advisable.

In educating clients, couples, and their families about the use of condoms, it is critical to ascertain that they know that condoms do not store well in extreme heat or cold, and that the usual carrying place (that is, the man's pocket) is likely to be too warm to maintain condom efficacy. It is also important for clients and families to be aware that unused condoms wear out and they should be advised to read the package instructions very carefully so that they can replace them in good time. Condoms may also not be reused, a simple fact that many clients do not know. They are also rendered ineffectual if they are blown into in order to test them for holes, or if stretched excessively prior to application. They also fail if applied to a flaccid penis or not pulled up to the junction with the groin.

It may be helpful to demonstrate the correct procedure for putting on a condom by using a banana or dildo. There are many new and playful condoms now on the market. However, tasty as they may be (some are fruit-flavored), shine brightly as they might (some glow in the dark), they are not safe enough if they are not stamped with the approval of the Federal Drug Administration (FDA). It is advisable to use only water-soluble lubricants (such as KY Jelly), and not petroleum products and lubricants that are not water-soluble, since these may render even a latex condom permeable to the virus.

Even though the mechanical application of condom use may be effective, the individual and social context of condom use may render it an ineffective means to prevent transmission of HIV. Condom use assumes an intelligent, in control, mature individual, who thinks carefully and plans his or her sexual encounters. That is not the usual description of adolescents, who generally believe that they are invulnerable and tend also to act impulsively. In addition, frequently there is a high level of embarrassment. For these reasons it is critical to educate adolescents who are currently at extremely high risk. There are several books written specifically for this population and their parents. A particularly popular and easily read book is *Risky Times: How to Be AIDS-Smart and Stay Healthy* (a) *A Guide for Teenagers* and (b) *A Guide for Parents*.[15]

Certain religious, political, and cultural constraints may also make condom use an unsatisfactory method for the prevention of HIV infection. The debate over condom availability through the school system highlights this. Despite the potential efficacy of condom use (if we could ensure that adolescents would use them reliably), there have been considerable obstacles raised to the installation of condom dispensers in schools and colleges or condom distribution by school personnel. The arguments against this condom availability have ranged from religious and moral objections to political concerns about the authority of state versus family.

Those who have raised moral objections are concerned that the availability of condoms would encourage the adolescent population to become promiscuous; religious objectors either have strong taboos against the use of condoms in any setting, or believe that sex outside marriage is wrong or sinful. Political objectors feel that public institutions should not be involved in such intimate family matters and that the sexual activities of children should remain within the private domain of the family system, subject to parental, not educational, control.

The realities of condom use are also impacted by economic and cultural constraints. The reality in Africa was expressed by President Museveni of Uganda at the International Conference on AIDS in Florence, Italy in 1991:[16]

> "In countries like ours, where a mother often has to walk twenty miles to get an aspirin for her sick child, or five miles to get any water at all, the practical question of getting a constant supply of condoms, or using them properly, may never be resolved."

Women as a special group also present difficulties with condom use. They may not be in control of the decision to use condoms, because of cultural and gender issues, which will be discussed both later in this chapter and in Chapter 9.

When we consider oral sex in the form of cunnilingus, there is no really effective physical barrier. It has been suggested that dental dams may perhaps lessen the risk of infection by this route. However, the use of dental dams as an effective means of prevention has not been demonstrated. Counselors, although they should certainly mention this suggestion, should be clear about the lack of evidence of their efficacy and should not give their clients a false sense of security. In the case of fellatio, condoms are clearly the preventive of choice.

## THE INDIVIDUAL-PSYCHOLOGICAL
## PLUS FAMILY-RELATIONAL LEVELS

### Vulnerability

Individuals and their families may be particularly vulnerable to placing themselves at risk of acquiring sexually transmitted diseases, including

HIV, because of psychological dynamics and family relational factors. Individuals may place themselves at risk with little awareness of doing so. Or they may be put into positions of risk, while relatively unaware of it, by their personal or family situation. It is important to identify the factors leading to vulnerability in order to be able to enhance prevention efforts. Examples of factors increasing vulnerability at the personal-individual-psychological and family level are *personal loneliness and isolation, psychiatric disturbance, personal and family losses, and severe family stress.* All of these may lead to diminished awareness of risk or to a lack of capacity to go to the lengths needed to avoid it.

*Personal loneliness and isolation* are extremely common in our society, where families live far apart, and friendship, neighborhood, and collegial systems may not hold up well over weekends or after dark. With divorce having become a common phenomenon, and the presence of bar and lounge social-ization a more common meeting ground for singles than the church picnic, many people search for relationships in dangerous arenas.

Mary, whom we discussed in the last chapter, was a bright, sociable indi-vidual, living a very stable life in her nuclear family, who resorted to social-izing in bars only after the death of her husband. However, this behavior resulted in her contracting AIDS and dying. Mary's experience may be seen as the heterosexual equivalent of what has been common in the homosexual community, the use of gay bars and bathhouses as a means of building social relationships. In a similar way, adolescents who are not, and perhaps should not be, ready for permanent relationships and marriage are vulner-able to repeated, brief relationships in their quest for experimentation and learning about love.

*Psychiatric disturbance* that places individuals in vulnerable positions may range from mild depression and anxiety to personality disorder to severe psychosis and dementia, with concomitant lack of awareness of danger, sex-ual or other. People who are severely depressed are particularly vulnerable to risk-taking behavior. They may not care whether a condom is used or whether their partner is HIV positive. This behavior may take the form of deliberately placing themselves at risk, since their will to live is no longer strong enough to ensure survival. People with passive-dependent person-alities may be unable to stand up for themselves by asking the HIV status of their partner or by requiring the use of a condom, for fear of losing the relationship. Psychotic or demented individuals may be totally unaware of risk and quite unable to avoid it if aware. The clinical management of these types of problems will be presented in Chapters 7 and 8.

The stress created through suffering serious *personal and family loss* may also account for an increase in vulnerability through diminished self-protection. Mary is a good example of the effect of catastrophic loss. The death of her husband resulted in her unintentionally becoming infected with HIV because of her increased vulnerability. In a similar way to psychiatric disturbance, people suffering from grief may place themselves in this position. This is discussed further under the heading of risk-taking behavior and in greater detail in Chapters 8 and 9.

*Severe family stress* may be caused by the family having to deal with multiple concurrent lifecycle transitions, often including loss or potential loss of an important member of the family.[17-21] In our own work, we have found that more than three major transitions occurring concurrently or within close proximity result in major family stress and may precipitate symptomatology.[22] It can also include economic loss caused by loss of job, early retirement, chronic illness, divorce and single-parenting, cultural change, major geographic moves, or the aftermath of a natural disaster such as earthquake, flood, or hurricane.

Multiple family losses may also be seen as belonging in this category. The disorganization, instability, and insecurity engendered under these circumstances render the individuals in the family particularly vulnerable to not taking adequate care of themselves, since that seems a minor priority in the face of major disaster. This area will also be elaborated in Chapter 8, where the techniques and principles of treatment will be presented.

### Risk-Taking Behaviors

Increased vulnerability may result in risk-taking *behaviors that are potentially self-destructive*, inappropriately *wagering with life and death*. Certain individuals and their intimate others place themselves at great risk with little concern for those left behind or for those who may become infected along the way. Other decisions are made on the basis of a willingness to gamble for a constructive end or goal. Little is gained without any risk. However, decisions made on the basis of pathological gambling may include a carelessness about whether the result may be death.

People take risks that are potentially self-destructive for many reasons. An individual may unconsciously sacrifice himself on behalf of the family. Self-sacrifice and risk-taking go hand in hand and it is not uncommon for the "black sheep" of a family to be, in reality, the identified "savior" of the family.[23] Such a pattern of self-destructive behavior may become entrenched in families over time (see Chapter 8). Another factor in self-destructive risk-taking is that of loneliness and poor self-image, resulting in a search for human contact at any price.

*Sexual risk behavior* with HIV might entail something as simple as "forgetting" to put on a condom or as dangerous as prostitution. It might entail not ascertaining that the condom used is FDA approved, cruising the streets, choosing an injection drug-abusing partner, indulging in anal sex, or changing partners frequently. Sexual risk behaviors are the ultimate method of risking self-destruction through infection with HIV.

The health care professional needs to be able to talk freely with her or his patients or clients about sexual practices and behaviors. If professionals are easily embarrassed, unacquainted with the local sexual jargon, or ignorant of common practices, they may be allowing their patients or clients to place themselves at unnecessary risk. Frequently, patients or clients place themselves at risk through ignorance and can be educated not to do so. In the case of deliberately self-destructive behaviors, or overt dismissal of the dangers of infection, the role of the counselor may be key—in fact, potentially lifesaving. It is sometimes difficult to talk about sexuality in a relaxed and empathic way. However, it is far more effective to be spontaneous and honest, rather than to deliver a canned speech or a lecture based on published literature.

Brochures, bulletins, and other literature can be helpful when combined with a good therapeutic alliance, particularly where the health care provider does not fully understand the client's culture or language. Acquiring access to these will be discussed in Chapter 5. Health care providers might consider finding a lexicon, or dictionary, of terms used in the communities that they serve and, if necessary, working with a language or cultural interpreter. In instances where this is not possible, referral to the local community agency or to the patient's primary care service might be the answer.

However, none of these adjuncts can adequately replace a comfortable acceptance of human sexuality on the part of the health care provider. In fact, this is often more important than a detailed understanding of the virology and epidemiology of HIV. Courses on sexuality are freely available through county, state, provincial, and federal governments in most countries, as well as through university courses.

Once one is comfortable talking to one's patients or clients, how does one evaluate what types of behavior constitute greater and lesser risk of HIV infection? We have listed a number of behaviors below and invite the reader to rank them from lowest to highest risk. Keep in mind that absolute precision beyond the three categories of low risk, moderate risk and high risk is unrealistic. Table 3A following the list will enable you to check your accuracy.

In order to further complicate your decision as to the risk of certain behaviors, the epidemiology of HIV varies from one country to another. In 1991, the year that Table 3-A below answering your problem about ranking of risks was compiled, the gay population in the United States had the highest number of members with AIDS. The inner city minority populations followed closely behind, with the most rapidly increasing statistics, and the figures for adolescents as a group were also rising significantly. However, in Central Africa, HIV was highest in the heterosexual population, as was the case in a Thailand, India, and other parts of Asia. Therefore, bear in mind that the accuracy of your ranking is specific to time and place and that you might want to repeat this exercise, checking your own answers against current statistics instead of Table 3-A, at a later date. Methods for staying abreast of these rapidly changing demographics will be given in Chapter 5.

## LIST OF SEXUAL BEHAVIOR RISKS—UNRANKED

Fellatio protected by a latex condom

Unprotected anal sex with one homosexual partner in Zambia

Unprotected vaginal intercourse with prostitutes in Kinshasa or New York City

Anal intercourse protected by latex condom and spermicidal jelly with nonoxynol-9, in a long-term, completely monogamous relationship in Zaire and India between partners who have tested negative for HIV every six months for the past three years

Protected intercourse with multiple heterosexual partners in France

Deep or French kissing with any partner

Unprotected vaginal intercourse with one intravenous drug-abusing partner

Vaginal intercourse protected by latex condom and spermicidal jelly with nonoxynol-9, in a long-term, completely monogamous relationship in Great Britain, Australia, or New Zealand between partners who have tested negative for HIV every 6 months for the past 3 years

Unprotected intercourse with multiple intravenous drug-abusing bisexual partners

Cunnilingus with a lesbian partner

Unprotected vaginal sex with one heterosexual partner, in the United States or Western Europe

Unprotected anal intercourse in a gay bath-house in the US

Protected intercourse with multiple homosexual partners in Uganda

Unprotected fellatio with a heterosexual partner in Denmark

Abstinence

Unprotected vaginal or anal sex with a bisexual partner

Unprotected vaginal intercourse with multiple partners in Africa

Unprotected fellatio with a single partner

Unprotected anal intercourse with multiple partners in Canada

It is clear from Table 3-A that an individual can be a member of more than one risk group, putting himself or herself at *double jeopardy* for HIV

**TABLE 3-A**
**Ranking Sexual Behavior Risks for HIV Infection**

Abstinence

Vaginal intercourse protected by latex condom and spermicidal jelly with nonoxynol-9, in a long-term, completely monogamous relationship in Great Britain, Australia, or New Zealand between partners who have tested negative for HIV every 6 months for the past 3 years

Anal intercourse protected by latex condom and spermicidal jelly with nonoxynol-9, in a long-term, completely monogamous relationship in Zaire and India between partners who have tested negative for HIV every 6 months for the past 3 years

Deep or French kissing with any partner

Fellatio protected by a latex condom

Cunnilingus with a lesbian partner

Unprotected fellatio with a heterosexual partner in Denmark

Unprotected vaginal sex with one heterosexual partner, in the United States or Western Europe

Unprotected anal sex with one homosexual partner in Zambia

Protected intercourse with multiple heterosexual partners in France

Protected intercourse with multiple homosexual partners in Uganda

Unprotected vaginal intercourse with one injection drug-abusing partner

Unprotected fellatio with a single partner

Unprotected vaginal or anal sex with a bisexual partner

Unprotected vaginal intercourse with multiple partners in Africa

Unprotected anal intercourse with multiple partners in Canada

Unprotected intercourse with multiple injection drug-abusing bisexual partners

Unprotected anal intercourse in a gay bath-house in the United States

Unprotected vaginal intercourse with prostitutes in Kinshasa or New York City

---

infection. In a case that will be discussed in greater detail in Chapter 8, a young woman, Emily, recovering from drug and alcohol addiction, had unprotected sex with a recovering intravenous drug user, who was also bisexual. Both Emily and her partner were already at double jeopardy for HIV based on their individual behaviors, being promiscuous and drug-abusing. Added to this was her partner's bisexuality. Subsequent events proved that the combined risk was extremely high to both Emily and her partner. Her partner eventually died of AIDS and Emily herself became infected with HIV and went on to develop AIDS Related Complex (ARC). It is important to understand the cumulative effects of multiple risk behaviors, as well as the potential impact of relationships on vulnerability and risk of acquiring HIV infection.

## Relational Risk

Health care providers should keep in mind one of the truisms of AIDS prevention: The individual is hypothetically (and certainly in terms of vulnerability to infection) having sex with every other sexual partner that his or her current sexual partner has slept with over the past few years. If one of those people happens to be at high risk for HIV disease, that means that your patient or client may, unwittingly, be involved in a *relationship with a high-risk individual.* In Emily's case, her relationship with a bisexual intravenous drug abuser astronomically increased her risk of infection. When relationships are extremely important or when there is a disparity of power in the relationship, an otherwise careful individual may engage in high risk-taking behavior. Similarly, a younger person (and this is the age group currently most at risk for HIV infection) might be too shy or embarrassed and not want to risk losing a new relationship by asking for the use of condom and jelly. Or, as in the case of Emily, the person may feel that she herself is not part of a risk group and, therefore, not think of asking her partner whether he is particularly at risk. In the same way as universal precautions are advised for home and hospital, *universal sexual precautions* should be used at all times for all relationships other than one in which both partners have been absolutely monogamous for at least 15 years and have had at least two sequentially negative HIV tests with at least a six-month interval between them.

When we think of relationships, we tend to characterize them as adolescent or adult relationships. But *pregnancy* is the beginning of a potential relationship with a child-to-be.

In Emily's case, not only had she been part of a risky adult relationship with a bisexual recovering intravenous drug user, but she had married and became pregnant after the break-up of that relationship. During her pregnancy, Emily began experiencing odd symptoms. For one thing, she noticed that her waterbed was soaked every night and she asked her husband to repair the "leak." When she visited her obstetrician, she complained of swollen glands and lethargy. He attributed these symptoms to the pregnancy and told her not to worry. She also developed an unexplained rash, which he explained to her was not uncommon in pregnancy.

Emily was dissatisfied with her obstetrician's answers and asked her primary care physician whether she should consider an HIV test since she was beginning to realize that she might be in a group at risk of infection. He agreed with the obstetrician that the symptoms were a normal part of pregnancy, reassured her, and sent her home untested. Except for these symptoms, that bothered her intermittently throughout, the pregnancy was uneventful, and she delivered an apparently healthy baby boy.

During the early months of her son Mike's life, he developed persistent diarrhea, as well as troublesome thrush (candidiasis). Emily herself did not feel well. When she began to experience sweats in the day time and her husband assured her that the waterbed was repaired, she realized that she was ill. In addition, Mike continued to get rashes, his thrush would just not go away, and he began to run an unexplained temperature, particularly at night.

Emily went back to her primary care physician and demanded an HIV test. He did not feel he was able to do such a test and advised her to find an appropriate test site, even though he was not really in agreement with the need for testing. Emily's test was positive and she realized that her nine-month-old baby was also at high risk. Mike's test also came back positive. He had received a PCR test, which saved the family the agony of waiting two to three years before his own HIV infection could be confirmed.

Emily's case illustrates the *special problems for women* (who are a recently added HIV high-risk group) and the particular problems for women of childbearing age. The criteria for ARC or AIDS were based on the male population and, until the recent recommendations of the CDC, did not include the typical opportunistic infections of women: pelvic inflammatory disease, cervical neoplasia, and aggressive, recurrent vaginal candidiasis. With the CDC's proposed AIDS-defining standard of CD4 cell counts below 200 cells/cubic mm., many of the women with female opportunistic infections would be included.

Since ARC and AIDS were initially defined based on opportunistic infections in male patients, physicians have been slow to see women as being at risk for HIV infection. For women of childbearing age, this is particularly critical. After her experiences, Emily strongly recommended that physicians routinely do HIV testing for women considering pregnancy and for women who are pregnant.[24] She felt that by being unaware of the 13–33 percent risk of her baby being infected with HIV, and also of the fact that her own HIV positivity could make *breast milk a source of infection*, she had put her baby, at double risk. Even if he had been fortunate enough not to have become infected in the uterus, her breast-feeding could have exposed him to the virus. It is hoped that Emily's obstetrician and family doctor, as well as other professionals in their position, have become aware of the necessity of being alert for early symptoms of HIV disease in women and children, and that they also now advise routine testing in line with Emily's recommendations.

Emily wished that she had known her HIV status during the pregnancy. She also felt that she should have had the necessary knowledge to enable her to make the decision to terminate the pregnancy. Emily's problem is shared by many other women, particularly those from minority cultural groups and resident in the lower socioeconomic areas (inner city in the United States, and outer city in South America). Many of these women are adolescents. The statistics indicate that approximately one-third of children born to HIV-infected mothers will also be HIV-infected and that two-thirds will not become infected. At birth, all these children will have the mother's antibodies to HIV and will test positive on ELISA/Western Blot. Only the PCR test, or direct virus culture, can distinguish which babies are themselves infected.

Becoming pregnant while HIV + is a gamble that raises multiple medical, economic, and ethical dilemmas. For some inner city women, a two-thirds possibility of a good outcome may appear to be good odds, whereas other women might decide not to take the risk. The decision to pursue the pregnancy is similar to the decisions that genetic counselors have helped parents make about congenital birth deformities, autosomal genetic diseases, and chromosomal abnormalities. Inherited diseases such as Huntington's, Marfan's syndrome, and cystic fibrosis, with a range of risk probability that might be as high as 75 percent, raise all the same issues for genetic counselors and parents. In some of these congenital problems, as in the case of Marfan's syndrome, babies might inherit the abnormality, but have a relatively good prognosis and be able to lead normal lives. They might, alternatively, have a very poor prognosis with major problems resulting in early death. In the case of HIV disease, however, if the baby has the infection, there is no possibility of its being mild. The baby will become seriously ill and will not live beyond childhood. Even if the baby is uninfected, he or she has a good chance of losing one or both parents. This further complicates the counseling process.

## THE SOCIAL LEVEL

The social level, for purposes of this discussion, refers to groups of individuals and their families within their natural and artificial/ancillary/professional support systems. The following groups have been identified through demographic and epidemiological research to be at special risk: Substance Abusers; Sexually Transmitted Disease Population; Inner City Low Socioeconomic Status Populations; Ethnic Minorities; Women, Infants, Children, and Adolescents; Prostitutes; Prison Populations; Hemophiliacs; and Gays and Lesbians. Individuals, many along with their families, have gained membership in these groups:

   a.  by inheritance of particular traditions or culture;

b. because of specific high-risk behaviors;
c. by genetic inheritance;
d. as a result of family dynamics and stress;
e. by situational means, such as living in high-risk areas or low socioeconomic status;
f. because of their relationships;
g. because of their lifestyle; and
h. because of any combination of the above.

Since the CDC has recognized the specific vulnerability of certain groups, we will discuss them individually, although they clearly overlap. The heterosexual population currently has a higher rate of increase in HIV infection than the gay population, so we have elected to deal first with them. Emily's case represents two of these high risk-groups (substance abusers, women and children); in addition, she was at risk because of many of the factors discussed earlier in the chapter.

**Substance Abusers**

In April of 1992, CDC figures for heterosexual male and female injection drug users indicated that the cumulative total of AIDS cases in this group was 48,312, or 23 percent of total AIDS cases in the United States at that time. The category of male homosexual/bisexual contact with injection drug use accounted for 13,823 AIDS cases, or an additional 6 percent. Injection drug use accounts for 41 percent of AIDS cases in New York State, while accounting for only 23 percent of AIDS cases in the rest of the country.[25]

According to Osborn,[26] in 1989 in highly urbanized areas in New York and New Jersey, 50 percent of intravenous drug users were estimated to be infected with HIV and the infection rate of their sexual partners was estimated to be higher than that of partners of bisexual men. However, in a collaborative study of people in drug abuse treatment programs in six regions of the United States in 1988, the following HIV seroprevalence was found: (i) New York City area 61 percent of samples obtained in late 1986, up from 50 percent in early 1985; (ii) Baltimore 29 percent; (iii) Denver 5 percent; (iv) San Antonio 2 percent; (v) Southern California 1.5 percent; (vi) Tampa 0 percent. There was no difference between these groups in reported lifetime needle sharing, which ranged from 70 percent in New York City to 99 percent in San Antonio.[27] In clinics treating drug abusers the incidence of HIV positivity ranges greatly, depending upon the prevalence of the virus in that specific community, and not dependent on the statistics of needle sharing. It ranges from 0 percent in Tampa to 45 percent in the central substance abuse clinic in Belgrade, Yugoslavia to as high as around 70 percent in some clinics in New York City. The rise of seroprevalence of substance abusers in Argentina is a clear example of why there should be cause for alarm. In 1980, it was 0.3 percent; in 1985, 30 percent; by 1988 it was 45 percent.*

These figures indicate that HIV is spreading rapidly among the injection drug-using population and that its ripple effect puts the immediate families and close and remote sexual contacts of substance abusers at significant risk. The spread of HIV among this group and their sexual partners is accelerated by the common sharing of needles in communities with a high HIV prevalence, promiscuity while under the influence of substances, and a relatively high incidence of bisexual episodes while actively using.

According to David Smith, the *sharing of needles* is "associated with socialization, communal feeling, and protection in the drug culture."[28] He discusses a Dallas study in which the researchers warned that merely increasing the availability of needles without educational intervention might have limited effect, since needle sharing is part of a drug culture ritual and not simply due to needle shortage. He outlined the risk of needle sharing in three patterns. In the first pattern, intravenous drug users (IVDU) shared needles with one partner 140 times. In the second, users shared 70 times with each of two partners, and in the third, they shared twice with each of 70 partners. The last pattern produced a significantly higher cumulative risk than the other two.

Despite Smith's doubts about the efficacy of free clean-needle programs, some states in the US have legalized free needle programs to attempt to reduce the rate of spread of the virus. Gillian Walker also states that clean-needle programs have proven effective in reducing HIV infection in heroin users in Amsterdam and Liverpool.[29] Smith also cites another study indicating that intravenous drug users have a heightened awareness of the risk of sharing dirty needles and were using a number of techniques to clean needles and works (or outfits). However, although addicts stated that their needle sharing was more controlled, they added, "Except when they got too stoned or junk sick."[28]

The situation is more complex than sharing needles, however. In most situations, intravenous drug users do not share needles at all, but draw needles from a pool of used needles kept by the shooting gallery (a place where addicts pay to gather or pay to use the facilities to "shoot up" or inject substances), and this is equivalent to sharing with possibly unknown partners who previously used those needles.[30] In addition, shooting galleries provide "dirty water" (water provided for cleaning purposes) and "clean water"

---

*Data communicated by Aldo Josef, M.D., Assistant Secretary for Prevention, Department of Health, Argentina to author (Judith Landau-Stanton) while scholar in Argentina (Fulbright and USIA. October, 1991).

(water drawn to mix with drugs). With cocaine, which is not cooked during mixing, whatever pathogen is in the "clean water" will be injected into the shooter, so that even if the drug user has a new set of works, the water mixed with the drug could be infective. The jars of "dirty" and "clean water" are communal and many draw from their contaminated water. The needles, also, are communal. When the population of a Miami shooting gallery, 230, was tested for HIV, 47 percent were positive (p. 75).

Health care professionals should not only educate their patients and clients and families about the dangers of sharing needles, but should also teach them about using individual jars of water and how to sterilize their needles and works (or outfits). A common and easy method is to immerse them in dilute bleach. It is important to remember that parts of the works such as the cotton ball can transmit HIV and need to be discarded, and never shared. Unfortunately, many addicts will use the small amount of drug captured in the ball, if no other drug is easily available. It is critical to maintain the intensity of education in a shooting gallery. The proprietors are generally the best target audience, since they are completely in control of the practices in their galleries. Constant reinforcement is needed, or the compliance rate will drop. The owner of a shooting gallery in the Page study admitted to a commitment to reducing risk amongst his clients, several times expressing his desire to keep them alive because his livelihood depends on their returning to his galleries.

Research has also shown that other substance abusers (in particular those using noninjected cocaine, but also those using alcohol and other substances) appear to be at high risk. For example, drinking alcohol is thought to lead to disinhibition.[31] Other researchers have studied both drug and alcohol use and showed that drinking while engaging in sexual behavior was significantly associated with higher-risk sexual behaviors in San Francisco gay men.[32,33] Other studies are not as consistent. A study of the role of drinking among heterosexual adolescents found a significant association between alcohol, lack of condom use, and casual partners only with regard to first-time intercourse, with the relationship to risk behavior diminishing with subsequent episodes.[34] Martin and Hasin's study also failed to detect any relationship between alcoholism and anal intercourse.[34]

The use of multiple drugs, however, is associated with higher-risk sexual activities. Doll studied urban gay men and found that the use of multiple drugs was significantly associated with higher-risk sexual behavior, but that alcohol consumption alone was not.[31] Martin and Hasin suggest that the discrepancy in these findings may be due to the definition and measurement of sexual risk-taking and the possibility that unusual, or episodic, heavy drinking may result in increased risk-taking.[34]

The substance abuse alone may put people at risk, but, beyond this, the risk of becoming far more ill once HIV is acquired is higher in this group, particularly if cirrhosis is present, since this may result in an alteration of the immune system. In addition, many drug users and alcoholics use multiple substances, varying them according to their finances and current associates. Disinhibition can result in risk-taking that the individual would not ordinarily consider. Also, a large percentage of this population may be self-destructive, not really caring what the outcome of the infection might be.

Once the addict is infected with HIV, health care providers may be tempted to ask, along with the addict, why bother with drug treatment when the HIV will kill him or her anyway. Many professionals believe that methadone treatment is the treatment of choice for this group. Others believe that active management, including fellowship programs and family therapy, in freeing the addict of the addiction improves the quality of life and allows for growth, even within the shortened time that the disease allows. Active treatment programs, in encouraging the addict to recover, also provide the family with hope for their future and for the ultimate eradication of addiction in their descendants. This will be further discussed in Chapter 8.

Emily, for example, was able to stop both cocaine and alcohol use, then describing her life with HIV infection as far more productive and satisfying than it had been. She said,"HIV has given me back my life, because it helped me avoid my addiction." Emily used her opportunity of working with her family to resolve her own self-destructive behavior and their difficulties. A New York City Puerto Rican couple, Carmen and Pedro, who had both been intravenous drug users, also developed AIDS. But it was very important for them to become "clean" and they too described their life with HIV after drug treatment as the best time in their marriage. They were among the first to break the silence within their own Hispanic community. Instead of ostracism, they were met with invitations to provide education in churches, prisons, and schools. One can only guess at the number of lives they may have saved and the number of lives Pedro may have redeemed as he walked the alleys of the shooting galleries encouraging addicts to seek treatment or at least learn to sterilize needles. Their experience with HIV is discussed further in Chapter 6.

## Sexually Transmitted Disease Population

People with risk behaviors for sexually transmitted diseases, or a prior history of sexually transmitted disease (STD) are at higher risk for HIV disease. These STDs include gonorrhea, syphilis, herpes, genital and anal warts, and Clamydia infection. The link between STD's and HIV infection has been well established. A population, called the STD core population by some, has been identified demographically in certain American cities as being at higher risk of sexually transmitted diseases than is the general population.[35] This population tends not only to have a higher base rate of STD, but is also more prone to reinfection and is therefore vulnerable to having multiple STDs. Not only is HIV a sexually transmitted disease itself, but infection with other STDs increases the risk of HIV transmission. Syphilis and gonorrhea, in fact, can be used as a marker for the spread of HIV infection.

Dr. James Chin, chief of the office of research surveillance of the World Health Organization's AIDS program, told the 7th International Conference on AIDS in Florence that the expectation is that:[36]

> HIV will spread more widely through populations where sexually transmitted disease rates are high, and increasingly heterosexual transmission will become the predominant mode of transmission throughout the world. (p. 24)

The scenario for the third world is described as frightening, and the prediction is that the same decimation seen in parts of Africa will soon hit Asia and South America. Based on current projections, Sub-Saharan Africa will have about 10 million cases of HIV infection by 1995; Latin America two million; and Asia more than 2.5 million; while the industrialized countries will have two million. Therefore, the total number of cases of HIV infection projected by 1995 is 15 million conservatively, and 120 million within 8 years, less conservatively.*

The STD core population as described by Brunham[35] is found predominantly in certain areas of the inner city, is of lower socioeconomic status (SES), and for these reasons tends to be overrepresented by ethnic minority groups. The core population comprises 70 percent of individuals with higher-than-average rates of multiple partners. It also has a higher degree of transiency and a disproportionate percentage of prostitutes. This population also has a higher distribution of recidivist polysubstance abusers. In addition, STD reinfection rates are higher in this core population. This group is therefore seen to be at multiple jeopardy.

Public STD clinics are therefore not only responsible for managing STDs, but also encourage, and in some places insist, on providing HIV testing for all their patients. Certain STDs are notifiable in many countries, which means that the health authorities are informed of its existence and take responsibility for tracing, notifying, and testing all sexual contacts. Unfortunately, in the United States and many other countries, HIV does not fall into this category. The basis for this is both political and pragmatic. Significant political actions blocking routine notification were undertaken

*Harvard School of Public Health.

on behalf of specific populations at risk, in order to avoid stigmatization of those groups. Added to this has been the extreme practical difficulty imposed by the length of the testing window between actual infection and seropositivity, resulting in an inestimable number of potential sexual contacts. In a city in Argentina, where intimate contacts have been traced, an average as high as 46 contacts has been found.[37]

## Low Socioeconomic Status Populations (U.S. Inner City)

Low socioeconomic populations are at risk for both substance abuse and sexually transmitted diseases. In the United States, the inner city lower socioeconomic group is also disproportionately represented by ethnic minority groups. The economic factor is significant. Given the current number of the homeless in our crowded urban areas and the large number of people living below the poverty line and without health insurance, a dangerous public health situation is building in our society.

A predictive model for the result of this dangerous situation may be one given at the Florence 7th International Conference on AIDS. Professor Vulimiri Ramalingaswami (All India Institute of Medical Sciences) demonstrated how HIV infection rates in one small area of the third world can skyrocket. In the Indian state of Maipur, in October of 1989, only one tested blood sample was HIV positive.[36] By May of 1990, 54 percent of 1,500 blood samples were HIV positive. In allowing conditions in U.S. inner cities to resemble third world environments, we are increasing the danger of a rapid spread of HIV. In addition, in the inner city, families may have several members with AIDS, thereby increasing the overall risk of this group.

In other parts of the world, the overcrowded low SES group at high risk may be found on the periphery of cities, as in South America. Low SES can be the result of discrimination, catastrophic family events, job loss and chronic illness, recent immigration or migration, and lack of opportunity. This group, whether inner or outer city, forms part of the most rapidly growing exposure to HIV category. Health care professionals wishing to contribute to the efforts of AIDS prevention might be well advised to concentrate their energies within this population. Unfortunately, all the factors that render individuals and families part of this group also make them extremely hard to reach. Both financial and physical efforts needed for this task often daunt professionals. However, the potential impact of successful preventive education and early diagnosis makes the effort worthwhile. All of the populations we have considered so far, due to historical accident and economic forces, converge into a composite group at risk.

**Ethnic Minorities**

Ethnic minorities predominate in the lower socioeconomic areas of cities worldwide. Therefore, the specific groups at risk in this category vary from one country to another. In the United States, Hispanics and African-Americans constitute the majority on the East Coast, while on parts of the West Coast Asians form the largest proportion. In Germany, the inner city minorities tend to be Turkish and in Holland they consist primarily of Surabayans. As we mentioned earlier, the chief factors leading to this concentration of minorities in inner cities are forced migration from countries of origin, urbanization (resulting in a move to the cities from rural areas that can no longer support them), discrimination, and job availability.

Inner (or outer) cities are frequently the only available haven for this group, since they offer cheap accommodation and the company of earlier migrants from their own population group. Cheap accommodation is frequently the major determinant of this choice, since migrants and immigrants rarely possess the qualifications or credentials for higher-paid jobs. Discrimination based on skin color is another key factor, a factor that makes it more difficult for these groups to leave the inner (or outer) city than in the case of other migrants or immigrants. Cultural markers such as dress, language, values, traditions, and religious beliefs also render this group more vulnerable to discrimination. Language barriers alone may make it almost impossible for them to acquire good jobs or blend with the local population.

The lower socioeconomic areas of cities are crowded, hygiene is less easy to maintain, and facilities such as washing and cooking are often communal. Infection control is far more difficult. In addition, race and culture can complicate AIDS preventive education. Not only may there be cultural differences that make communication difficult, but a previous history of discrimination may make minority groups suspicious of any outside intervention. The history of sickle cell anemia testing is an historical example of a public health measure that did not sufficiently include the minority community in its planning or educate them adequately.[38] This resulted in a rejection of the testing as "discriminatory"and even "genocidal." In terms of discrimination, there was some truth to this perception, since known carriers of the sickle cell gene were excluded from certain occupations.

Health care providers need to be extremely sensitive to what may appear to them to be paranoid fears, while at the same time remaining sufficiently confident in the public health goals and individual needs of AIDS prevention. Interpreters of language and culture should be used wherever possible and the minority communities should feel a sense of ownership in the program. Connecting with community leaders prior to establishing final goals can be extremely helpful in achieving these aims.[39] Mays et al., in their book *Primary Prevention of AIDS: Psychological Approaches*, include several chapters on ethnic minority groups and their particular problems with AIDS, making it a useful resource to the health care provider.[40]

### Women, Infants, Children, and Adolescents

In the United States, the women primarily infected with HIV are African-American (53 percent of women with AIDS) and Hispanic (21 percent), reflecting that population's overrepresentation in the inner city. However, this does not mean that other social and ethnic groups are immune, as we have seen in the examples of Mary and Emily. We have talked about some of the issues of women at risk previously and would underscore the importance of HIV testing for all sexually active women. According to the CDC, the total number of women with full-blown AIDS in the United States in April, 1992 was 22,607 out of a cumulative of 218,301 total cases. The number with HIV infection is a great deal higher. Approximately 84 percent of this group were either injection drug users or the heterosexual contacts of injection drug users and bisexual males. Heterosexual women represent 50 percent of injection drug users with AIDS.

In a study done by Harrison et al, surveying AIDS knowledge and risk behavior in culturally diverse women, including African-American, Hispanic, Caucasian, and Haitian, women in general did not see themselves at risk for HIV infection.[41] Risk perception and attitudes towards prevention also varied culturally. Haitian women believed that AIDS could be acquired from casual contact or from insect bites. Hispanic women believed themselves to be at greatest risk through unprotected sex with primary partners (whether heterosexual or bisexual) and unprotected sex with partners paying for sex. In general, however, unprotected sex with the primary partner occurred across all racial and ethnic groups. Using a condom for AIDS prevention was not acceptable to over 40 percent of Hispanic and Haitian women, and 20 percent of African-American women, even if the partner was HIV positive. Caucasian women reported greater prevalence of intravenous drug use risk behavior. The study concluded that Hispanic women ranked highest for risk factors, followed by Caucasian, African-American, and Haitian.

Pediatric cases of AIDS, as Chapter 1 discussed, are not a new development. But there was resistance to considering this as one of the exposure categories until quite recently. Most children infected with HIV were infected in utero, and as a result are also predominantly (90 percent) from the minority populations discussed above.[42] In a study done on blood specimens of all newborn infants in New York State (for the routine detection of genetic diseases), the overall seroprevalence rate of HIV was 0.66 percent, but with 1.24 percent in New York City, and 1.72 percent in the Bronx.[43] Protecting children from HIV infection, therefore, involves preventing the spread of infection to women. This needs to be achieved prior to pregnancy, since pregnant women are reluctant to be HIV tested even after successful prenatal AIDS education and increased knowledge about risk.[44]

Children are, therefore, at physical risk both through breast milk and through vertical transmission (mother to fetus), but have not been demonstrated to represent a significant risk of HIV transmission to others through horizontal transmission. Despite the furor caused in various school districts by the presence of a child with AIDS, such spread has not been shown to constitute a significant threat. In Emily's case, as in other families, apart from school concerns, there is always an additional concern of HIV spread from baby to adults caring for the baby, and spread to other siblings, relatives ànd playmates.

Emily had a best friend, Sandra, whom she had known for seven years. Both Emily and her friend delivered their babies within a few weeks of each other. When Emily's friend was told that Emily's son, Mike, was HIV positive, it did not affect her relationship with either Emily or Mike in any way. She hastened to read the literature and reassured herself that she was perfectly, and easily, able to keep her baby safe from HIV.

However, the husband of Emily's friend was not as sanguine. He called the local AIDS community service agency and was horrified to be told by the person manning the telephone hotline that she "wouldn't dream of allowing her baby to play with anybody with AIDS." When Mike cried, his friend's father took his baby away, stating that the tears could kill him and he never wanted him to be near Mike again. Fortunately, after considerable education of Sandra's husband, Sandra was able to persuade him that she would not allow their baby to be exposed to Mike's excreta or body fluids and that she would keep him safe when in contact with Mike and Emily.

Emily had been desperately hurt that anyone could think of her as someone who might put a friend or child at risk of dying.

Health care providers who are in the position of manning hotlines or providing AIDS education need to be extremely careful about brief telephone contacts. They also need to take special care not to react personally to the questions raised, but rather to offer a range of reliable information that can be substantiated, and then to help the caller arrive at his or her decision. It is also helpful to follow up such calls with written material and the offer of an individual appointment or participation in a group.

Adolescents are a special group since many of the unique biological, psychological, and social factors of adolescence warrant specially designed HIV prevention programs. The attitude of adolescents toward their own mortality is a major factor. Their need and desire to experiment with the world around them and their need to assert some level of independence from the various forms of social control add to their vulnerability to sexual risk behavior and, therefore, to HIV infection.[45] We have mentioned the particular problems of substance abuse amongst adolescents and their vulnerability as part of the inner city group above.

Another category of adolescents at special risk is that of runaways. A study of seroprevalence in clients of a facility for runaway and homeless adolescents in New York City found that, as of 1989, 5.3 percent of adolescents tested positive.[46] Hispanics had the highest rate (6.8 percent) followed by Whites (6.0 percent) and then African Americans (4.6 percent). Seropositivity in these cases was linked with intravenous drug use, male homosexual/bisexual activity, prostitution, and sexually transmitted disease other than HIV.

Another study questioned the effectiveness of educational efforts to avoid pregnancy and sexually transmitted diseases such as HIV disease in young African-American female adolescents.[47] During a clinical intervention conducted with adolescents, the use of condoms was discussed as a preventive intervention. The girls expressed disgust, fear, and the sense that condoms belonged in the male domain. These factors would interfere with the girls' use of condoms and place them at high risk for sexually transmitted diseases, including HIV disease.

## Prostitutes

Prostitutes are generally found in the sexually transmitted disease core population, which was described by Potteratt et al.,[48] and later by Brunham,[35] as a group that maintains the endemicity of sexually transmitted diseases. It is likely that this group will also maintain an endemic reservoir for HIV. In South Florida, of the women studied by Harrison, 21 percent obtained a living from prostitution, while 44 percent had engaged in prostitution, with nearly two-thirds of these trading sex for money or drugs.[41]

Prostitution may be either male or female. Ironically, female prostitutes are more at risk from HIV positive clients because it appears that the virus passes more easily from male to female, but the short history of HIV in Africa indicates that women prostitutes can certainly spread the virus to male clients—in Kenya, 85 percent of prostitutes were found to be HIV+. Additionally, this group generally represents a higher than average percentage of substance abusers, and prostitution is frequently a method for making sufficient money to support a habit. Many of these prostitutes are young, frequently adolescent (often runaway adolescents), and commonly in the childbearing age. Hence, not only are they themselves at risk, but so are their clients and their babies.

The legal system may often require HIV testing after an arrest for prostitution and, in countries where prostitution is legalized such as France, HIV testing for all prostitutes is a mandatory component of their regular health checks. In the only place in the United States where prostitution is legalized, that is Nevada (excluding Reno and Las Vegas), routine checks for HIV and other diseases are performed. In our own local area, Rochester, New York, a recent police sweep of a city area noted for its numbers of prostitutes resulted in the arrest of a significant sample. The presiding judge, Judge Walz, informed the media that, based on the reports on those women, he estimated that approximately 50 percent were HIV positive.

**Prison Populations**

This population has been deemed to be at high risk of HIV infection, but this has to be qualified. In a study of individuals entering the Iowa prison system, all inmates entering between January 1st to April 30th, 1986 were tested for HIV. None of these serum samples was reactive to the Western Blot even though there was high prior intravenous drug use (22–50 percent). This was a predominantly young white male population with a very low rate of homosexuality.[49] However, the prison population in New York State has 1,548 reported cases of AIDS, a severe problem with treatment-resistant TB/HIV, and a law that prevents obtaining HIV prevalence data in the prison system, since mandatory HIV testing is prohibited. Part of the explanation for this discrepancy may be that New York City African-American male drug abusers, who form a substantial part of that prison system, have an average HIV seropositivity rate of 67 percent.[27] Women are also a high risk group in prison populations in New York State. In 1988, a seroprevalence study on New York female prison entrants found that 18.8 percent were HIV seropositive. Seroprevalence was highest in the 30 to 39-year-old age group, 25 percent, and also varied by ethnicity (Hispanics, 29.4 percent) and residence (New York City, 23.8 percent). Nearly half were intravenous drug users and a third were also positive for syphilis.[50]

Prison populations are overrepresented by groups at high risk for HIV infection. For example, we have mentioned the substance-abusing population. However, there is also a disproportionate number of inner city dwellers, minority groups, and prostitutes. Whether certain prisons are more at risk than others because of the prison environment itself has not been shown, but there is no doubt that prisons within high-risk areas do have an extremely high prevalence rate. Prisons may provide the opportunity for AIDS preventive education since they are a means for reaching these high-risk groups. In addition, people being admitted to prison in a high-risk area are exposed to high risk, since the presence of sexual behavior in prison is a given. Therefore, preventive education and encouragement of inmates to take precautions is critical in our fight against the virus."The legal and ethical responsibility of prison officials to protect the health and safety of inmates includes protecting against possible transmission of HIV by infected prisoners and protecting HIV-infected prisoners from persecution and possible violence by guards and other inmates."[51] (p. 65.)

## Hemophiliacs

Hemophiliacs constitute a special group of iatrogenic transmission of HIV. Hemophiliacs have a genetically inherited deficiency in their blood clotting mechanism due to the absence of certain factors present in blood. Factor VIII is the factor most commonly required for hemophiliacs to correct their blood clotting deficiency (classic hemophilia). Factor IX (Christmas Disease) is far less common. These factors are produced by the combining of numerous blood donations. The Centers for Disease Control and particularly, Don Francis, M.D., had suspected that HIV might be transmitted through blood and the CDC monitored requests for pentamidine for hemophiliac patients to investigate this possibility. When the first request was made, the CDC realized that HIV was blood transmitted and that hemophiliacs were at extremely high risk because of the multiple exposures to blood products.

In fact, in this population, high rates of infection happened quickly. An average of 70 percent of hemophiliacs who received clotting factor prior to screening and treatment of blood are HIV positive. The breakdown for hemophiliac men in the United States ranges from 33 percent to 92 percent HIV positive and 14 percent to 52 percent have been reported among those diagnosed with hemophilia A and hemophilia B. It is also estimated that 5 percent to 20 percent of hemophiliac spouses are infected.[52] Blood screening with the ELISA/Western Blot, and heat treatment of the blood to kill the virus has solved this problem for hemophiliacs. In addition, the clotting factors have now been genetically engineered and hematologists are hoping that they will be commercially available within the next five years. However, significant transmission of HIV occurred before this new technology was available. Newly diagnosed patients with hemophilia are not at significant risk, but all those who received human blood products prior to the development of safe factors in 1985 are still at risk.

After the introduction of heat treatment, hepatitis (non-A non-B) is the largest killer of hemophiliacs. Hepatitis C has now been identified. Many people with hepatitis live a long time with a chronic illness. Arthropathy is another major difficulty that this population faces; it has a clearly economic basis. Those who grow up in a developed country, such as the United States or South Africa, can anticipate a normal baseline life expectancy and minimal arthropathy. This is largely attributable to accessibility of treatment. Those living in developing countries cannot be treated for each minor episode of bleeding and suffer far higher rates of arthropathy. The bias for morbidity is, therefore, largely economic.

The contribution made by hemophiliacs to our understanding and prevention of AIDS can be grasped by naming Ryan White, or by recalling the three young boys in Florida who all developed HIV disease. Ryan White, who had been a controlled hemophiliac, developed AIDS as a young schoolboy as the result of receiving HIV-contaminated Factor VIII, and died in his late teens after having become a role model for AIDS education and prevention. Ryan's mother is currently very active in the field of AIDS prevention. This is a very special group in that hemophiliacs have needed to develop an enormous trust in the medical system in order to continue surviving. The fact that it was a failure of the medical system that resulted in their being at risk for a major lethal illness has threatened their relationship with the system upon which their lives depend. John Rolland's contribution, exploring the meaning of illness, and specifically dealing with hemophilia, is a seminal work in the field.[53,54]

### Gays and Lesbians

It may seem strange that this group, which was initially the major risk group and is still extremely vulnerable to HIV Disease, should be considered so late in this listing. As we mentioned above, we elected to group heterosexuals at risk together. Since they form the fastest growing group with HIV infection, that meant listing them ahead of the gay population, even though, in the United States, the morbidity figures for this group still outweigh the others, as do the seroprevalence figures. In April 1992, the CDC figures for AIDS cases among male homosexuals/bisexuals was 124,961, or 58 percent of the total of AIDS cases. Therefore, although the gay population may not currently be suffering the most rapid infection rate, they still constitute the group with the largest incidence of the disease and the greatest actual risk in the United States. As gay activist Cleve Jones said, after being briefed by Dr. Conant on January 14th, 1982, "We're all dead."[55]

Many of the cases discussed in this book are stories of homosexual individuals coping with HIV disease. Some of those risks include unprotected anal sex; bathhouse sex with anonymous partners; the sexual freedom that was linked to gay rights and gay pride, but which resulted both in multiple sexual partners and in an exploration with new, different, and fortuitously dangerous sexual practices; and discrimination that confined much gay socializing to bars, streets, and lounges. They tend to live in urban areas, partly because of discrimination, and partly because of lifestyle, which in turn puts them at greater risk.

Initial preventive educational efforts were targeted largely at the gay population and their health care providers. For a brief time, the rate of infection in this group appeared to stabilize. However, it is once again on the increase. Young gay men have not had the benefit of being part of the older generation's culture and experience with HIV disease; they have to relearn what older members of the gay community now know. Also, many of the younger members also fall into the double or triple jeopardy groups, being adolescent or young adult, being from ethnic minority groups, and living in the inner city. Individuals from this group are also involuntarily involved in sexual sharing with member(s) of a high-risk (high-prevalence) population.

This is a group whose members, similar to those of the ethnic minority groups, have been heavily discriminated against. They frequently are afraid that their families will reject them, and often do not feel that they have that support system available to them. Secrets abound in their daily lives, many of them are not out of the closet about being gay, and the risk of HIV compounds an already difficult social situation. In Chapter 8, we will discuss some of these issues as they apply to therapy with this group. The courage of some members of this community in coming out of the closet and embarking on a mission of AIDS prevention has been remarkable. It has been, in no small measure, responsible for the change in rates of infection of this population, and for alerting the rest of the world to the seriousness of this disease.

Health care professionals need to be, or to become aware, of their own feeling about sexuality and homosexuality, in order to be able to work with this group with respect and professionalism. There is a great deal of literature on AIDS in the gay community, and several excellent papers on therapy with this group.[56,57,58] In addition, gay writers have described the experiences of this disease in screenplays, movies and novels, and these can give the health care professional a full sense of the human beings at risk for suffering from HIV disease.[59,60,61,62,63,64]

## Worried Well

The worried well, as they have come to be called, consist of individuals who, despite being at no higher risk than the general population, have developed an acute fear of HIV infection. Some members of this group are ignorant of the vulnerability and risk factors for HIV transmission, although some are intellectually aware of current knowledge on HIV, but they are individuals who are uncomfortable with anything but zero risk.

For example, a man in his middle forties, who had occasion to visit a drug abuse facility, sat on the toilet seat. Knowing from the media the rate of infection among substance abusers attending such a facility, he panicked about being infected. A health care provider who was unconcerned about the possibility that his fears might be reality based might have sent him away to suffer emotionally. He was fortunate to meet a counselor who advised him to be HIV tested, both immediately and six months later. The counselor informed him about the epidemiology and routes of transmission of the virus, and explained her rationale for the testing regimen. He was reassured, and able to go on with his life. His fears had not been ignored but, instead, had been adequately addressed.

Gentle and considerate handling, adequate education, and consistent knowledgeable reassurance are frequently all that are needed. Some of the worried well, however, unlike the man discussed above, develop full-blown AIDS phobias, and psychotherapy may be required since the AIDS phobia is likely to represent something entirely different within the individual and family system that needs attention. AIDS, like any other illness, might become a metaphor for the expression of underlying problems. Le Roux et al. describe the principles of this phenomenon in regard to a case of hypertension.[65] AIDS phobia is most clearly defined as a wholly unfounded fear of becoming infected with HIV despite repeatedly negative HIV test results.[66] In the only article describing subsets of this population, two to five percent of the worried well who approach AIDS counselors approximate the symptoms of AIDS phobia.[67]

## THE CONCEPTUAL LEVEL

Risks at the conceptual level can include risks caused by spiritual or religious belief systems, risks resulting from public policy decisions, risks generated by economic reality, risks caused by ethical positions, and risks caused by cultural traditions and practices. For example, if the religious beliefs of an individual preclude the use of condoms and if adherence to strict abstinence is not realistic (as it seldom is), then those beliefs can put the individual at increased risk of HIV infection. Another example would be that of cultural tradition (for example Hispanic) that does not view the active partner in homosexual behavior (the one who penetrates the other) as homosexual, or as in any way less heterosexual. This individual will not see himself as either homosexual or bisexual, and will therefore not perceive himself as belonging to a risk group or as engaging in high-risk behavior.

This culturally bound misperception can be fatal for the individual and members of his family.

In a similar way, Helene, whom we discussed in Chapter 2, was placed at risk of HIV infection by her attempt to maintain her cultural traditions as best she could in a foreign country and cultural setting. She did not feel that she was in any way exposing herself to danger, but that instead she was doing her best to honor the traditions of her ancestors. As in Helene's case, migration has amplified the danger of culturally appropriate behavior that is practiced in a foreign setting putting members of that culture at risk in unprecedented ways.

Apart from the religious taboos, many cultures stress the importance of childbearing or fertility. In these, the virility of men may be judged by the number of children their wives bear, or there may be a critical need to produce sufficient children to provide the parents with caretakers and subsistence in their old age. When one of the mates is HIV positive, that alone may not be sufficient cause to break with tradition, regardless of the risk of HIV infection to both parents and to their unborn children. This dilemma will be discussed at greater length in Chapter 8.

Public policy decisions can enhance the spread of HIV as well as impede it. If insufficient funding is provided for disposable needles in hospital and clinic settings, HIV can spread through a population very rapidly. Policy decisions concerning injection drug users' needles and works can also place drug users at higher risk. Such decisions can also place the general population at greater risk because the abuser's risk can be a source of infection breaking out from the contained group. Policies regarding HIV testing are still being debated and it is not yet clear which policy decisions will actually be better public health measures than others. Chapter 11 will explore some of these policy decision questions.

In this chapter we have talked about economic realities that are creating ghetto conditions, not only in most metropolitan areas in the third world, but in cities within the United States and the United Kingdom. These ghetto conditions are perfect settings for the rapid spread of multiple infectious diseases: HIV, tuberculosis, cholera, typhus, for example. Tuberculosis is in itself becoming a major health hazard in urban areas in the United States, both in HIV-positive persons and in the general population of the inner city. The medical aspects of this will be presented in Chapter 6.

The economics involved in the policy debate about testing cannot be overestimated. There is currently a shortage of laboratory facilities and personnel, and the cost of worldwide testing would be enormous. This is only one of many policy decisions that are driven by, or influenced by, economic choices. It is frequently difficult, if not impossible, to separate economic considerations from policy decisions, or from ethical evaluations. For example, the announcement by Magic Johnson (the U.S. basketball star) that he was HIV+ triggered an immediate increase in requests for HIV testing across the United States. As a result, many testing facilities quickly exhausted their annual operating budget.

Decisions to "Do the Right Thing" are difficult and may have unexpected consequences, as Spike Lee's movie so well portrayed.[68] Those decisions will also have an effect on either the spread of HIV or its curtailment. One of the most difficult decisions is the choice between the good of an individual (who has not been tested for HIV and does not wish to be) and the good of the social system (which may need to have that information in order to prevent a lethal disease from becoming a pandemic on the scale of the Black Plague). We have to understand that if we choose exclusively one or other of these poles, without considering a balance or compromise, we may hasten the spread of the disease. If we choose mandated testing, it may drive individuals to try to avoid being tested rather than volunteering to be tested, and this lack of information can spread the disease more quickly. If, however, we opt exclusively for the needs and interest of the individual, and do not press for testing and informing about the results of the test, the disease can also continue to spread rapidly. These dilemmas will be further elaborated in Chapter 10.

## REFERENCES

1. Brown, P., Cathala, F., Raubertas, R.F., Gajdusek, D.C., Castaigne, P. (1987). The epidemiology of Creutzfeldt-Jakob disease: Conclusion of a 15–year investigation in France. *Neurology, 37,* 895–904.
2. Sadoff, M. (1982). On markets for risk. In D. Teichler-Zallen, C.D. Clements (Eds.), *Science and Mortality: New Directions in Bioethics* (pp. 205–222). Lexington, Mass.: Lexington Books.
3. Jeffery, R.W. (1989). Risk behaviors and health: Contrasting individual and population perspectives. *American Psychologist, 44,* 1194–1202.
4. American surgeons scoff at CDC proposals on HIV. *Medical Post, 27* (39): 7, 1991.
5. Medical resident study presented at the American Federation for Clinical Research 1990 meeting. *The Medical Post,* October 17, 1989.
6. Barman, M.R. (1990). AIDS precautions in practice. *Medical Laboratory Observer,* pp. 24–33.
7. (1990). TB is now back with a vengeance. *The Medical Post,* p. 15.
8. Lewis, D.L. (1991). Letter to the editor. *American Society of Microbiology ASM News, 57* (8): 393.
9. (1991). *The Medical Post, 27*(26), 25.
10. Swift, D. (1990). AIDS O.R. shock. *The Medical Post, 26*(30): 1 and 36.
11. Gibbons, A. (1991). Hoffman-LaRoche's PCR push. *Science, 253:* 627.
12. Shaw, G. (1990). Artificially inseminated woman gets AIDS, sues. *The Medical Post:* 5.

13. Centers for Disease Control (1988). Condoms for prevention of sexually transmitted diseases. *Morbidity and Mortality Weekly Report, 37*(9), 133–137.

14. Appelbaum, K., Appelbaum, P.S. (1990). The HIV antibody-positive patient. In J.C. Beck (Ed.) *Confidentiality Versus the Duty to Protect: Forseeable Harm in the Practice of Psychiatry.* Washington, D.C.: American Psychiatric Press, pp.121–140.

15. Blake, J. (1990). *Risky Times: How to Be AIDS-Smart and Stay Healthy (a) A Guide for Teenagers and (b) A Guide for Parents.* New York: Workman.

16. (1991). *The Medical Post, 27*(27): 24.

17. Hill, R. (1971). *Families Under Stress.* Westport, CT: Greenwood Press. (Original work published in 1949).

18. Holmes, T.H., Rahy, R.H. (1967). The social readjustment rating scale. *Journal of Psychosomatic Research, 11*: 213–218.

19. McCubbin, H. (1979). Integrating coping behavior in family stress theory. *Journal of Marriage and the Family, 41*: 237–244.

20. McCubbin, H.I., Boss, P.G. (Eds.) (1980). Family stress, coping and adaptation. *Family Relations. 29*(4).

21. McCubbin, H.I., Figley, C.R. (1983). *Stress and the Family: Vol. 1: Coping with Normative Transitions.* New York: Brunner/Mazel.

22. Landau-Stanton, J. (1982). Therapy with families in cultural transition. In M. McGoldrick, J.K. Pearce, J. Giordano (Eds.) *Ethnicity and Family Therapy.* New York: Guilford Press, Inc.

23. Stanton, M.D. (1977). The addict as savior: Heroin, death and the family. *Family Process, 16* (2): 191–197.

24. Clements, C.D. (1991). A dying mother's plea: Test all pregnant women as part of good prenatal and postnatal care. *The Medical Post, 27* (24): 28–29.

25. Smith, P.F., Mikl, J., Hyde, S., et al. (1991). The AIDS epidemic in New York State. *American Journal of Public Health, 81*: 54–60.

26. Osborn, J. (1989). Public health and the politics of AIDS prevention. *Daedalus, 118*(3): 123–145.

27. Lange, W.R., Snyder, F.R., Lozowsky, D., Kaistha, V., Kaczaniuk, M.A., Jaffe, J.H., and the ARC Epidemiology Collaborating Group. (1988). Geographic distribution of human immunodeficiency virus markers in parenteral drug abusers. *American Journal of Public Health, 78*(4): 443–446.

28. Smith, D. (1987). The role of substance abuse professionals in the AIDS epidemic. In L. Siegel (Ed.), *AIDS and Substance Abuse* (pp. 181–188). New York: Haworth.

29. Walker, G. (1991). *In the Midst of Winter.* New York: Norton.

30. Page, J.B., Smith, P.C., Kane, N. (1991). Shooting galleries, their proprietors, and implications for prevention of AIDS. In D.G. Fisher (Ed.) *AIDS and Alcohol/ Drug Abuse.* New York: Haworth.

31. Room, R., Collins, F. (Eds.). (1983). *Drinking and Disinhibition: Nature and Meaning of the Link.* NIAA monograph No. 12, Washington, D.C.: U.S. Government Printing Office.

32. Stall, R., McKusick, L., Wiley, J., Coates, T.J., Ostrow, D.G. (1986). Alcohol and drug use during sexual activity and compliance with safe sex guidelines for

AIDS: The AIDS behavioral research project. *Health Education Quarterly, 13:* 359–371.

33. Stall, R. (1988). The prevention of HIV infection associated with drug and alcohol use during sexual activity. *Advances in Alcohol and Substance Abuse, 7:* 73–88.

34. Martin, J.L., Hastin, D.S. (1991). Drinking, alcoholism and sexual behavior in a cohort of gay men. In D.G. Fisher (Ed.), *AIDS and Alcohol/Drug Abuse.* New York: Haworth Press.

35. Brunham, R.C. (1991). The concept of core and its relevance to the epidemiology and control of sexually transmitted diseases. *Sexually Transmitted Diseases, 18:* 4–6.

36. (1991). *The Medical Post,* 27(27): 24.

37. Silvia Suevez de Gine, Asistente Social (personal communication, City of Salta, Province of Salta, Argentina, October 13, 1991).

38. Reilly, P. (1978). Sickle cell anemia legislation. *Journal of Legal Medicine, 1* (4 and 5): 39–48, 36–40.

39. Landau-Stanton, J. (1985). Competence, impermanence, and transitional mapping: A model for systems consultation. In L.C. Wynne, T. Weber, S. McDaniel (Eds.). *Systems Consultation: A New Perspective for Family Therapy* (pp. 253–269). New York: Guilford Press, Inc.

40. Mays, V.M., Alber, G.W., Schneider, S.F. (Eds.) (1989). *Primary Prevention of AIDS: Psychological Approaches.* London: Sage Publications.

41. Harrison, D.F., Womback, K.G., Byers, J.B., Imersheim, A.W., Levine, P., Maddox, K., Quadagno, D.M., Fordyce, M.L., Jones, M.A. (1991). AIDS knowledge and risk behaviors among culturally diverse women. *AIDS Education and Prevention, 3* (2): 79–89.

42. Walker, G. (1991). Pediatric AIDS: Toward an ecosystem treatment model. *Family Systems Medicine, 9*(3): 221–227.

43. Novick, L.F., Glebatis, D.M., Stricol, R.L., et al. (1991). Newborn seroprevalence study: Methods and results. *American Journal of Public Health, 87:* 15–21.

44. Berrier, J., Sperling, R., Preisinger, J., Evans, V., Mason, J., Walther, V. (1991). HIV/AIDS education in a prenatal clinic: An assessment. *AIDS Education and Prevention, 3* (2): 100–117.

45. Hein, K. (1991). Fighting AIDS in adolescence. *Issues in Science and Technology, 8*(3): 67–72.

46. Stricof, R.L., Kennedy, J.T., Nattell, T.C., et al. (1991). HIV seroprevalence in a facility for runaway and homeless adolescents. *American Journal of Public Health, 81:* 50–53.

47. Demb, J. (1990). Black, inner-city, female adolescents and condoms: What the girls say. *Family Systems Medicine, 8* (4): 401–406.

48. Potteratt, J.J., Rothenberg, R.B., Woodhouse, D.E., Muth, J.B., Pratts, C.I., Fogle, J.S. (1985). Gonorrhea as a social disease. *Sexually Transmitted Diseases, 12:* 25– 32.

49. Glass, G.E., Hausler, W.J., Loeffelholz, P.L., Yesalis, C.E. (1988). Seroprevalence of HIV antibody among individuals entering the Iowa prison system. *American Journal of Public Health, 78*(4): 447–449.

50. Smith, P.T., Mikl, J., Truman, B.I., et al. (1991). HIV infection among women entering the New York State Correctional System. *American Journal of Public Health, 81*: 36–40.
51. Hepworth, J., Shernoff, M. (1989). Strategies for AIDS education and prevention. In E.D. Macklin (Ed.). *AIDS and Families* (pp. 39–80). New York: Harrington Park Press.
52. Needle, R.H., Leach, S., Graham-Tomasi, R.P. (1989). The human immunodeficiency virus (HIV) epidemic: Epidemiological implications for family professionals. In E.D. Macklin (Ed.), *AIDS and Families*. New York: Harrington Park Press.
53. Rolland, J.S. (1987). Family illness paradigms: Evolution and significance. *Family Systems Medicine, 5*(4): 482–503.
54. Tiblier, K., Walher, G., Rolland, J. (1989). Therapeutic issues when working with families of persons with AIDS. *Marriage and Family Reviews, 13*(142): 81–128.
55. Shilts, R. (1987). *And the Band Played On: Politics, People, and the AIDS Epidemic.* New York: St. Martin's Press.
56. Gonsioreh, J.C. (Ed.) (1985). *A Guide to Psychotherapy with Gay and Lesbian Clients.* New York: Harrington Park Press.
57. Baer, J.W. (1989). Study of 60 patients with AIDS or AIDS-related complex requiring psychiatric hospitalization. *American Journal of Psychiatry, 146*: 1285–1288.
58. Patten, J. (1988). AIDS and the gay couple. *Family Therapy Networker, 12*(1): 37–39.
59. Cunningham, M. (1990). *At Home at the End of the World.* New York: Farrar Strauss Giroux.
60. Kramer, L. (1985). *The Normal Heart.* New York: New American Library.
61. Monette, P. (1990). *On Borrowed Time: An AIDS Memoir.* New York: Avon.
62. White, E., Mars-Jones, A. (1988). *The Darker Proof: Stories from a Crisis.* New York: NAL.
63. Reed, P. (1991). *The Q Journal: A Treatment Diary.* Berkeley, California: Celestial Arts.
64. Rene, N. (Director). (1990). *Longtime Companion* (Film).
65. Le Roux, P., Bakker, T., Lasersohn, B., Van Zyl, J. (1987). Symptoms as therapeutic metaphor: A case of hypertension. *Family Systems Medicine, 5*: 7–30.
66. Jager, H. (Ed.) (1988). *AIDS Phobia: Disease Patterns and Possibilities of Treatment.* New York: John Wiley and Sons.
67. St. Lawrence, J.S. (1990). Book Review. *Clinical Psychology Review, 10*: 607–609.
68. Lee, S. (1989). *Do the Right Thing.* (Film).

# CHAPTER 4

# Health Care Providers at Risk

There are many kinds of risks that health care providers can and do encounter. HIV disease highlights these risk factors for health care providers and illustrates the many levels at which risk can be encountered. These risks can be divided into personal risks (to health care provider and his or her family) and risks encountered in the health care delivery system itself. Personal risks can be either real physical risks or emotional risks. In addition to the risk of infection and concern about infection control, families of health care providers can feel vulnerable. There is also the uncommon, but always possible, risk of injury due to violence in health care settings, particularly mental health. Health care providers who do a significant amount of psychotherapy are already cognizant of issues of emotional risk, such as counter transference. Other health care providers are often more accustomed to dealing with the issues of personal grief around chronic illness and the loss of their patients.

Risks in the health care delivery system include the over involvement, or triangulation, of professional (or artificial) support systems and the ubiquitous question of how to arrange the disposition of patients with dementia. In addition, there is legal risk of malpractice or breach of confidentiality. Economic constraints are a growing risk to the health care provider who has to find some way to provide quality of care while having inadequate facilities to easily achieve that goal. Problems with the health insurance of this population aggravate the economic difficulties. All of this can lead to the "burnout" of health care providers in any setting and with any disease.

What HIV disease has done is turn its bright spotlight on all of these risks, so that health care providers are more painfully aware of them. What this chapter will provide is an understanding of both personal and health care delivery system risks. Suggestions and techniques will be given to help the health care provider in minimizing the risks to him or herself wherever possible, as well as in learning to develop a sense of those risks that cannot be moderated and need to be accepted in order for one to treat and manage patients at risk for, or with, HIV infection.

97

## PERSONAL RISK

### Physical Risk

Ever since July 27th, 1990, when the Centers for Disease Control reported possible transmission of HIV from a dentist to a patient,[1] the range of physical risk has increased from a fear of contracting HIV infection as part of daily health care delivery to a fear of transmitting it to patients. There has been an increasing concern in medicine with malpractice suits and potential loss of professional licence in medicine. HIV introduces the risk of profession and life itself. The health care provider should have a reasonable concern about all infectious diseases, but should also remember that he or she is specially trained to handle problems of infection control and personal protection.

We have discussed the physical risk to health care providers in Chapters 1 and 3, and will discuss the implications for health policy and medical ethics in Chapter 10. We have talked about universal precautions and their limitations in Chapter 3. The risk of acquiring HIV infection from a violent patient who bites, scratches, or throws excrement is accentuated in the case of AIDS dementia or with psychiatric patients who are HIV positive. Violence in patients is always frightening; with HIV-positive patients, it can be terrifying. Mental health care workers can forget both what they have learned and how competent they are in handling difficult situations, unless they remain acutely aware of the principles of managing the violent patient.

HIV disease, as any other infection, is a normal risk in the health care profession and is not so atypical that health care providers should be helpless or immobilized in the face of its threat. Unfortunately, many of the younger health care providers of this generation made their choice of career without considering the dangers of personal infection and vulnerability. By the time they began their graduate education, the risk to them of severe infectious diseases such as smallpox, tuberculosis, the plague, typhoid, cholera, typhus, and leprosy appeared to have been eliminated. Antibiotics, public health measures and infection control seemed to make the dangers of these diseases a thing of the past.

Tuberculosis, while still present, particularly in third world countries, was no longer a certain killer, and its lethal qualities were a generation removed from the experience of young health care providers. In fact, in first world countries such as the United States, routine immunization and testing are not even performed, other than for immigrants and refugees. The irony of the current problem with AIDS is that tuberculosis is once more becoming a major public health problem in the United States, and antibiotic-resistant strains are proving lethal to AIDS patients and the elderly, with a 72–89 percent mortality rate.[2] The history of tuberculosis can be symbolized by

Cottage Hospital, a TB sanatorium in Gravenhurst, Ontario. When it opened in 1896, it had a mortality rate of 50 percent. It was later sold and the buildings razed once tuberculosis was no longer a public health hazard. Tuberculosis of the future can be symbolized by the reopening of sanatoriums in Central Africa. In a pattern similar to the plague, the cycle returns.

A famous psychiatrist, John Romano, M.D., who was a medical student prior to the emergence of isoniazid for tuberculosis and of antibiotics during World War II, recalled his experiences of those times:[3]

"Sixty years ago I came to medical school. There was a decrease in tuberculosis from around the 1900's because of the improvement in housing, sanitation and water supply. However, it was still a very common disease. I remember in my medical school days, two of my fellow students in a class of forty contracted TB and died. One young man was a friend of mine.

"In this school (University of Rochester School of Medicine), 12 percent of a class would contract tuberculosis. Gordon Meade (who had recovered from tuberculosis himself) found it came from the dissecting room. Students were touching diseased tissue without gloves. (After instituting precautions) he got (the rate) almost to zero the following years. He also introduced BCG and vaccination for tuberculosis in 1943."

Dr. Romano also remembered personal experiences with tuberculosis:

"In my childhood days tuberculosis was rampant. It was a very common disease, and the primary cause of death in children as well as adults. The son of my neighbors, who was a friend, had it. I remember his illness, and going to the sanatorium, leaving school, and dying. I knew some of the people who worked in the sanatoriums. What comes to mind most is my own sadness with the promising young people I knew. I saw, as a student, tuberculosis meningitis of children that killed them, tuberculosis of bone, tuberculosis of brain. It was called consumption—had a pejorative view and people talked about it in hushed tones. A lot of young people died.

"(This all changed) 10 years after I left medical school when streptomycin was discovered and introduced in the treatment of TB with considerable success. Then isoniazid was introduced and brought about a very considerable change in the reduction of TB."

The feeling of contemporary health care providers (that they led charmed lives after the development of antibiotics and prior to the emergence of AIDS) was a false sense of security, however, since medical care by its nature involves physical risks. Creutzfeldt-Jakob Disease, meningococcal meningitis, Rift Valley fever, Ebola fever and HTLV-I leukemia and lymphoma were all transmissible during this time, and some are always fatal. Medical history of diseases other than tuberculosis further underscores the dangers. Doctors treating patients with the plague had to resort to primitive infection control measures. They wore a white outfit that encased their bodies, with a hood over the head, and a mask.[4] Not only were the physical dangers rampant, but the physical discomforts were extreme. The suit had an elongated beak-like projection that contained sweet herbs, both as a measure of infection control and in an attempt to control odor.

Detached from the medical history of the past, many of the contemporary health care providers feel betrayed by the emergence of AIDS, and have not been able to normalize it as a typical part of health care work that requires standard health care practices and expertise. Perhaps the emergence of AIDS is a reminder to health care professionals that precautions should always be taken. Dr. Romano continues:

"I think there is a natural concern about AIDS. This one doctor in Milwaukee took a stand that he would not operate on AIDS patients, he owed it to his family. The American Medical Association (A.M.A.) has taken a positive stand that a doctor's responsibility is to take care of the sick, regardless of risk. It's part of his basic oath to care for people to prevent disease, to prolong life. The surgeon still is at hazard. . . . the risk of being a physician."

As a result of HIV disease and its risks, health care providers currently enrolling in the field will now more closely resemble their earlier counterparts. It is important to understand what their feelings and responses might be. Our AIDS Training Project elicited written emotional responses from the health care providers who had taken our preventive educational program. The program was directed at changing attitudes, in addition to providing concrete knowledge, since the acquisition of knowledge alone has not been shown to change behavior. Some of their typical responses appear in Table 4-A:

These attitudes and feelings need to be validated. The following is a list of the scientific and professional concerns of the health care providers:

1. Realistic and unrealistic fears of HIV infection in professional role or personal life.
2. Concern or unwillingness to take certain risks, based on Probability of Risk + Severity of Risk + Personal Control of Exposure to Risk.
3. Concern or unwillingness to treat or work with HIV+ individuals.
4. Desire to know the HIV status of patients or clients, uneasiness about mandated revelation of the HIV status of health care professionals.
5. Conflicts between personal standards of compassion and tolerance,

personal values, professional values (especially values concerning sexuality) and service to HIV-positive clients and patients.
6. Distrust of current knowledge and information about HIV disease.
7. Sensitivity to threats to professional roles, competence and control.

Despite the threat of this infection, health care professionals are not leaving patient care because of the risk of HIV infection, and students are enrolling in the same numbers as usual. In our study of the willingness to treat, in general, health care workers after attending our training sessions reported a willingness to care for people with AIDS. In addition, many felt that working with AIDS patients and HIV-positive individuals was satisfying and rewarding.

Those health care workers who had already cared for people with AIDS or were HIV positive reported a greater willingness to treat these patients. It is not clear whether this willingness preceded their actual experience or whether treating AIDS patients had changed their attitudes. It is most likely that both effects were operating. Having a close friend or relative who is HIV positive or has AIDS is also related to the participants' willingness to treat. This lends support to the notion that personal contact with individuals who are HIV positive does affect health care workers' attitudes. Neither the participants' perceptions of their job-related risk of exposure nor their personal off-the-job risk were related to their willingness to treat.

The participants were less certain about their safety than they were about their willingness to treat. Prior professional experience working with AIDS patients or HIV-positive individuals was not related to this concern. Those individuals who reported that they had friends or relatives whose behavior puts them at risk for infection reported less fear of contagion than those whose friends were not seen to be at risk. It is quite possible that the workshop participants with less fear of contagion share certain beliefs about con-

**TABLE 4-A**
**Emotional Responses to AIDS Preventive Education**

| EmotionalResponse | Positive | Negative |
|---|---|---|
| Anger, Resentment, Defensiveness | "Expand my understanding when dealing with people who suffer from stigmatized diseases." | "Too much editorializing and value judgments." |
| Safety, Comfort with Self-Relevation, Expression of Emotions | "Sharing with friends, family; being more aware of how an HIV+ person feels." | "I wish this was a safer place to discuss things; I couldn't be open." |
| Fear and Frustration | "I think I will be able to work with HIV-infected persons with renewed confidence." | "There are many medical personnel who would like to refuse to work with AIDS patients." |

tagion with their friends that permitted their friends and relatives to engage in admittedly risky behavior.

There were no differences between African-Americans and Caucasians in fear of contagion, nor between men and women. Medical students and nurses involved in direct patient care, however, were substantially more concerned than physicians, mental health workers, or community agency personnel. Nurses were the most concerned. This is quite understandable as they are the most likely to come into contact with body fluids.

Program participants differed greatly in their fear of death. Women and African-American participants acknowledged somewhat less anxiety than male or Caucasian participants. Those participants who had worked with AIDS patients or HIV-positive individuals were far more likely to acknowledge anxiety than those who had not. There were no relationships between the perception of personal risk, either on or off the job, and death anxiety. There were no relationships between the perceived risk of trainees' friends or relatives and death anxiety. Apparently, perceptions of one's own risk do not affect fear, but working with patients faced with death does.

Interestingly, there were no differences attributable to the discipline or training of the participants. Physicians, nurses, mental health workers, medical students, and community agency workers all reported comparable levels of anxiety. Administrative and support staff reported less anxiety, but the number of individuals in these categories was so small that this difference may not be reliable.

These results reflect the numerous personal decisions that health care workers make about infection control and assumption of risk. As a nurse working in a high-risk maternity unit described, in an interview about attitudes towards dealing with AIDS:[5]

> "The most difficult thing in my practice was changing my habits as far as using gloves and the universal precautions we're now using. I think that the habit of using universal precautions is a major step forward, but it isn't something that's second nature to me in the care that I deliver to my patients."

This particular nurse was ready to use precautions and realized the importance of doing so. However, there is a phenomenon that occurs among professionals, not just in the health care field, who have worked in a dangerous situation for a lengthy time. Familiarity can breed not only contempt, but a sense of routine, and of almost magical invulnerability. Such professionals no longer follow strict guidelines for their safety, placing both themselves and others at risk.

Even though health care providers may be willing to put themselves in a vulnerable position, attitudes can change when there is a risk of exposing loved ones, especially children, to possible infection by their own activities. Bringing home an infectious disease is a much different situation. A labor floor nurse shared her feelings about her own safety, and that of her child:[5]

> "In the past I felt comfortable without gloves. Now I feel comfortable with gloves. It is second nature now and I trust the information from the CDC. . . . (however, with regards to her child) . . . . I received a flyer about HIV-positive children being admitted to my child's day care center. This brought up a new issue for me. While I'm very comfortable in caring for these patients—but when the question comes up, what about your child in a day care setting with these people?"

Family members may have difficulty understanding the mission of the health care provider and feel that he or she is wantonly exposing him or herself in a search for personal glory or fear of refusal to work with this population, regardless of the family's wishes or vulnerability. These are genuine concerns within the family system since HIV is sexually transmissible and, if the health care worker did become infected and did not use proper precautions in the home setting, the family would indeed be vulnerable.

## Emotional Risk

In addition to the provider worrying about infecting the family, the family may worry about the physical risk to their professional member. This can cause emotional consequences to the family that the health care provider may not be willing to accept. Unless the health care provider keeps the family well informed, not only about the risk of infection but about his or her feelings, serious emotional difficulties for both may arise. A psychiatric nurse described her relationship with her family around the issues of her work with AIDS cases:[5]

> "Home can be very supportive, and this is a place where I can discuss the feelings I've had with my family, and receive some support. But, of course, my family's afraid that I could contract the disease. I share with them the precautions we've instituted."

The concerns of health care providers and their families should not be simply ignored or treated lightly. They need to be validated, and a sense of personal control acquired. The best way of achieving this is by ensuring that health care providers and their families are well educated about the realities of HIV transmission and the means to prevent and control it. Where institutions and agencies do not provide adequate education in this area, health care providers should find out what courses are locally available and avail themselves of the help. They should include family members in their educational efforts, since nothing is more terrifying than ignorance and exclusion. Some hospitals have formed support groups for health care workers dealing with many HIV patients; groups that allow families to work with their concerns are also valuable. A forum for discussion is critical, since it is often extremely difficult for health care providers to admit their fears and emotional vulnerability. Health care providers are, after all, meant to be invulnerable.

In fact, this feeling of invulnerability has its origins in a need to feel safe in dealing with situations that may put the health care provider at actual risk. In order to achieve a magical sense of safety (frequently going beyond the real safety of undertaking adequate precautions and remaining well educated about risk), health care professionals may attempt to separate themselves from the "patients" emotionally, as well as physically. This leads to a false concept of being truly separate, and therefore invulnerable.

Health care professionals are, by definition, not patients, and patients are thought of as not being health care professionals, creating a safe separation between the two. This separation can lead to an apparent callousness, such as Dr. John Romano described in his interview. This boundary is meant to protect the worker from feelings of helplessness, grief, and loss. However, it can also protect the worker from feelings of empathy, and a lack of empathy can be detrimental to good health care. This distancing technique can also place the health care provider at risk in his or her own social setting. If he or she feels over-safe with patients, he or she may also take unnecessary risks with friends and lovers. Striking a healthy balance between involvement and distancing can be very difficult.

The separation between professional and patient is at times highly spurious. Doctors and nurses do become patients, as was so well illustrated by William Hurt in the film, *Doctor*, based on the book *A Taste of My Own Medicine*. [6] In fact, the fear of becoming not only a patient, but a patient with AIDS, can be overwhelming. The high-risk maternity unit nurse mentioned above described her struggle between being empathic and distancing from her patients, and how she resorted to judgmental techniques to assist her in the distancing: [5]

"Whether it is a self-inflicted disease or not—certainly all AIDS is not—it is difficult not to be judgmental. You realize their lifestyle brings them to the situation of becoming HIV positive, or even having AIDS because of their patterns of drug abuse, multiple sexual partners, or promiscuity. At the same time, I have had the personal experience of receiving multiple blood transfusions at the time of having open heart surgery. I only came to the decision to be tested last summer."

Health care providers not only have patients with AIDS, but may become patients themselves, and may also have friends and family members who have been diagnosed HIV positive. When this happens, it becomes impossible for them to remain distant from their patients. Empathy becomes a given. In fact, it may be very useful, if you do not know anyone who is HIV positive, to ask around your family and friendship circle whether they know anyone whom you could meet and talk to, not as your own patient, but as a person with AIDS. When talking about her feelings about the issue of boundaries, distance, and closeness, the high-risk maternity nurse said:[5]

"I have friends and people I'm close to in the gay community, so it's (AIDS) a presence here too. I know how I would want them to be treated and how I hope they are being treated. So I hope I can bring that kind of sensitivity to the cases of my patients."

Empathy not only is important to the health care provider, but is an integral component of health care delivery. It is very useful to spend time with administrative and support staff, educating them about the diseases of the patient population that they interact with, and giving them tools to deal with the possible difficulties that they might experience. An intake worker in an AIDS Clinic, who had received this kind of training, described her attitude:[5]

"They seem friendly and nice, and the fact they have AIDS doesn't bother me because I've got to know them as people. I just think that if more people can get to know them on a sort of one-to-one basis, there wouldn't be a lot of the feelings people have about people with AIDS."

Health care providers have a constant struggle: Distancing can dehumanize the patients and interfere with care, empathy can lead to overinvolvement and countertransference problems. Countertransference, the complex feelings of professional to client or patient, is an integral facet of the relationship, as opposed to transference, which is the mode in which the patient or client relates to the professional. Both are moderated by the individual's earlier experiences, real, intrapsychic, and in their families of origin, and result from identification with important figures and experiences from the past.[7] The relating to these "introjects" can determine the way in which client and professional interact with each other.

Countertransference, and overidentification with the clients and patients can lead to overinvolvement. This may be based also upon a sense of mission and an unwillingness to face vulnerability and impose personal limits.

Counselors may be reluctant to admit to themselves or their patients that they are indeed scared, and may overreact (by reaction formation) as heroes and martyrs, working day and night, and failing to take the necessary infection control precautions. They may even be prepared to sacrifice themselves on the altar of AIDS—an unnecessary and futile exercise, since keeping themselves alive and fresh, in order to serve more clients and patients, would be far more fruitful. One of the psychiatric nurses in the videotaped interview talked about wanting more training in AIDS, because in addition to her nursing position, she wanted to work as an AIDS volunteer in the community. She was prepared to work around the clock in this field no matter the cost to herself, her family, or her patients.

Overinvolvement is not restricted to health care providers, but includes their staff as well. One of the secretaries for psychiatric residents who saw numerous HIV-positive patients, said:[5]

"I want to work more closely with AIDS patients. I feel well prepared. I worry about going away on vacation, about how other secretaries will take care of these patients. What if a family member calls?"

This secretary could benefit from some assistance in dealing with this population of patients. She clearly feels overly responsible, and at times helpless, as do many health care professionals. Discussion and support groups can be used in health care settings to develop self-awareness and deal with these kinds of issues. Family-of-origin groups are also helpful in understanding responses to these kinds of situations and learning to deal with them differently and more effectively. Staff need to learn their own limits and to realize that staying within those boundaries enables them to provide better care. Where this is insufficient, personal therapy should be considered. It can be brief and problem-focused, and health care providers and their support staff should be able to access the therapy system with ease and no embarrassment.

Dealing with the chronically ill and/or dying patient is never easy. When the normal life cycle is upended, and the dying are young (as will be discussed in Chapter 8), it goes against the natural order and challenges one's inner sense of competence. Early death is an extremely powerful existential question for everyone. This is reflected in some of the statements health care workers made about death and dying during their interviews. One of the psychiatric nurses who had worked with AIDS patients for two years, said:[5]

"I find one of the most difficult things is the feeling of utter hopelessness that I perceive that they have, and I find when I look into their eyes at times, that they seem to be very empty and almost to the depths of their soul without any hope left. I feel part of my job is to instill some semblance of hope and—maybe not a cure—but an ability to relate to their illness with dignity, and perhaps some grieving, achieve some resolution and the best death possible. But there are times when people aren't doing well, when they're dying, that is really stressful."

The secretary said:[5]

"I'm aware of the optimism of the people in the Infectious Disease Clinic and the therapists. Sometimes I don't always share that, sometimes I feel that we're looking at death and that's hard for me."

The intake worker said:[5]

"I don't know how it is going to be when some of the real favorites come to the end. It makes me feel like I want to cry when I think of what they have to face."

Sadness is not the only way to express feelings about death and loss. Denial and anger are also very common. In fact, health care providers go through the same stages in dealing with death and loss as do their patients, the patients' family members, and their friends. Kubler-Ross advised health care providers to learn about death and dying from their patients—unfortunately, AIDS provides an excellent example. In her classic work with the dying, she described discrete stages that the patient and family went through: Denial and Isolation; Anger; Bargaining; Depression; Acceptance.[8] Parkes develops this model further.[9] In our work with both cancer and AIDS cases, we have found these stages to occur, not necessarily sequentially, but frequently in a cyclical manner, in patients, family members, their friends, and their health care workers.

Health care providers are no more immune to denial than persons hearing that they are HIV positive, or their families. Denial in a health care provider can be very risky to both the health care provider and the patient. It may result in inadequate precautions against infection being taken, or it may result in serious illness not being recognized or treated. A health care provider in denial may expose his or her patient, and his or her own family and friends, to unnecessary risk. Denial may be accompanied by false bravado. If this occurs, it is important to take your colleague aside, help him or her understand the seriousness of the episode, and advise education and/or counseling.

Beyond risk-taking, there is also the danger that the health care provider will not accept the imminent death of a patient, and hence not give him or her an opportunity to say farewell to loved ones or tidy up unfinished business and legal affairs. The health care provider may unwittingly also expose him or herself in this way, to unexpected grief and loss. It hurts when one lets a patient and family down—and it hurts not to be able to say goodbye.

Anger was a major part of the response of a psychiatric nurse to the illness and subsequent death of a close friend:[5]

"I had a friend who died in New York City. He was the first person I knew with AIDS. He never told anybody until right at the end—I remember how angry I was—I'm still angry at him for that—I'm very angry!"

This same nurse described an experience with a patient:

"One of the biggest surprises was with a patient who was so ready to go—he was ready to die—and the rest of us weren't. The big learning process was teaching myself to let go of somebody. He'd reconciled, the family had reconciled."

Again, ignoring anger or suppressing feelings is not a healthy response. Repression may appear to be constructive, and often is in the short term, since anger should not be allowed to interfere with the relationship between professional and client. However, lying or pretending to clients is not constructive. Professionals and patients may be going through the same stages at the same time; however, the primary role obligation of the professional is to the client. Health care professionals should practice sharing their emotional state with their clients, but learn how to do this appropriately. Support groups and counseling can be extremely effective in this learning process, and the clients and their families can be superb teachers.

If health care providers find that they are constantly angry or grieving, they should consider a consultation session with a therapist trained in this area. It may be that they have issues of unresolved grief in their own families of origin, or other issues within their current relationships or natural support systems that are triggering these responses. Therapy or family of origin study can be helpful.

In addition to grief, helplessness, and anger, there are differences in culture and belief systems, secrets, and taboos that can also raise feelings in the health care provider that are difficult to deal with. AIDS has raised the issue of moral and ethical judgment because it has touched upon certain social and cultural taboos in a way not seen since syphilis was prevalent. The population groups originally most affected by HIV have generated their own taboos and secrets. In many families and communities, homosexuality was hidden and lesbianism was not allowed to exist in consciousness. In fact, homosexuality has been illegal in many countries until very recently in our history, and still is in certain places.

AIDS professionals may attribute homophobia to the individuals who are to be given AIDS education and/or treatment, although our evaluation research indicates homophobia is not a significant occurrence even in pre-testing, and other studies have not shown homophobia to be a significant factor. The history of HIV in the United States was intimately connected to the gay community and gay civil rights. Many effective AIDS professionals have a personal commitment to two goals: prevention of the spread of HIV and social equality for homosexuals of both sexes. In the same way that professionals are socialized into a Them/Us dichotomy, members of the gay community have difficulty avoiding a Them/Us construction of the social world. Negative responses and interactions may be presumed to arise from homophobia. This will automatically create an adversarial relationship, with anger and resentment on both sides. Unless professionals are aware of their inclination to interpret an individual's beliefs and views in a homophobic fashion, and conscious of their difficulty in accepting individuals who have negative feelings about some homosexual (and also heterosexual) behaviors, they will not be able to avoid the adversarial relationship. Our training evaluation research looked at the question of homophobia, and did not find it a significant factor for the health care professionals who were our subjects.

The health care provider enters a minefield of potentially emotional responses based on personal beliefs and cultural positions, which may interfere with good medical care. Substance abusers, even if the family admits to recognizing the addiction, traditionally have been hidden by their families. Issues of contraception have created religious and spiritual dilemmas for many centuries, and abortion is still a difficult issue, even if the baby or mother is at risk. Prostitution and sexual promiscuity have always been taboo, and responsibility for the straits of inner city dwellers has long been abrogated. Strongly held beliefs that prevent the practice of currently held standards of quality medical and clinical care can lead the health care provider into many, apparently insoluble, dilemmas. As one of the psychiatric nurses said with an air of self-righteousness:[5]

> "Another very hurtful aspect is the prejudice I experience among the caregivers I work with. Sometimes very cruel things people say or do to people who have AIDS. I find a lot of my job is working with people to help them understand where their judgmental and moralistic views are coming from—helping the caregivers work through their problems."

In Dr. Romano's historical interview, he compared AIDS with "the leper of yesterday."[3] He pointed out that when Paul Ehrlich developed the arsenical 606, it was opposed on moral grounds because it was felt that "those who sinned should be punished," and that the same position was being repeated with HIV-positive people.

In instances where the health care provider feels incapable of administering modern care or is overwhelmed by his or her feelings and beliefs, he or she should consider referral to someone who deals more easily with this population. This same solution has been used for the abortion question. Health care professionals who sincerely feel that their beliefs make medical intervention impossible for them may be excused on the grounds of conscience from participating in such interventions. This level of decision should not be undertaken lightly. It is advisable to explore the emotions attached to the beliefs and question deeply whether they are, indeed, morally firm, or whether they have developed as a way of avoiding difficult situations. Again, group discussions and consultation with a spiritual adviser or therapist might be useful. It is also important to decide what the minimal obligations of the professional role require. For example, in an emergency situation, where the professional is the only one available, a resolution through referral may not be possible.[10]

The more promising resolution is to focus on the health care needs of the individual without feeling the necessity of either accepting that individual's values as one's own or rejecting the individual for having a different perspective from the health care provider's. In some instances, health care providers are uneasy about being tolerant, since they may feel at risk of appearing disloyal to their families' belief systems. In such instances, we have found that families are generally a great deal more permissive than the health care provider expects, particularly in the face of honesty and the good of the patient. It is always worth asking, rather than presuming, before becoming rigid on the family's behalf; family members also grow and change in the face of a changing world and new circumstances.

AIDS presents a particular problem in countertransference and transference. The professional may either be manipulated or be so fearful of manipulation that he or she may become rejecting of the patient. A patient may say, "Nobody will hug me, you're the only one that cares. I don't have any family. My parents don't care about me. You are it. Are you going to leave me alone in my last dying days?" The professional could be influenced by a need to "save," by a need to respect a dying person's last wish. Or he or she could overlook a cultural difference and become inintentionally rejecting.

For example, one of our cases involved a gay man who wanted to kiss the therapist before and after each session. Culturally, gay men are sometimes a little more flamboyant and emotionally demonstrative. For him a handshake was insufficient. For several sessions, client and therapist exchanged handshakes. However, after one of the therapy sessions and without asking, he actually kissed the therapist on the lips. The issue was not about contagion, but rather about therapeutic boundaries. The client wanted to interpret the therapist's attempt to set limits as being the result of fear of HIV infection. A less experienced therapist might have fallen for this and hastened to commence the kissing routine in an attempt to reassure the client, and exonerate herself. This therapist asked, "Do you really think the reason that I care about you not kissing me is because you might give me HIV?" The patient replied, "No." She responded, "Correct." This interchange opened the way for a discussion about what the kiss was really about.

Compassion can also raise questions about transference and countertransference. Another of our AIDS cases involved Latisha, an African-American woman in group therapy. She had become infected through a blood transfusion during the delivery of one her babies. She told her therapist that she was going to work so that her children would have social security to take care of them.

The therapist was impressed that here was a woman who had never worked in her life, who at 30-plus was going out to get a job in order to be a good mother and provider. It was Christmas time and the woman had no money. The therapist could easily have afforded a donation of $500 to help this woman do something nice for her family. She also knew that she could do it anonymously through the AIDS Center, so that the patient would never know where the money came from. However, the therapist realized that she herself would know. The therapist decided against making the personal donation because it would be an infringement of therapist/client boundaries as she perceived them. The therapist's resolution was to call the AIDS Center and suggest that they set up a Christmas donation list for AIDS clients. The client was one of the recipients—and the therapist had not overstepped her boundaries.

Apart from the boundary issue, there was also the question of making the woman dependent upon the therapist. Unless a significant effort is made to mobilize the family and natural support system, health care professionals might find themselves taking personal care of a lot of people, with an exhaustive Christmas list. Once one gets to know and understand families, they are rarely all bad. Techniques for involving the extended family and natural support system will be presented in Chapter 8.

Apart from financial aid to patients, there are several boundary issues, applicable to any patient or client, that are accentuated in the case of HIV positivity or AIDS:

Visiting the patient in the hospital
Hugging and kissing
Visiting the patient at home
Meeting the patient at a fund-raiser

Participating in functions and fund-raisers
Attending patients' funerals
Being politically active
Sharing eating and drinking utensils
Communicating with family members, members of the natural support
    system, and other health care providers
Sex education—for example, how to put on a condom

Boundary issues, such as those listed, can be efficiently dealt with by any and all of the techniques described above. Health care providers should not feel unduly secure that they've "seen it all" because some issue that challenges their assumptions about boundaries and poses the need for new solutions is bound to arise out of the blue.

Health care professionals may also have unexamined feelings of hostility toward other colleagues, either toward those in highly credentialed professions, such as the medical profession, or toward those who do not appear to have adequate credentials. This is, unfortunately, a common bias. Extraneous biases such as this may drive the interaction between colleagues and influence the quality of their patient care. Someone who resents experts might feel, "Physicians think they're God. Experts are elitists. Licensed professionals are not better, but get paid more. Credentialed professionals keep everyone else off their turf for power reasons. Experts are frauds." When this feeling is combined with frustration about the economic and bureaucratic limitations of the health care system, it can be result in negative assumptions. The professionals may be judged as failing to meet an idealized professional standard only slightly lower than Mother Teresa, and the AIDS expert can then engage in a subtle attack on the professional's role ideal and personal ideal.

Similarly, the highly trained professional might feel, "The community worker is too involved and doesn't understand the seriousness of the situation. The AIDS agency staff need to learn about the disease, they're being too casual. They always dump the patient on us when they've messed up. How can they desert their client at this time?" The professionals might judge the community workers for their lack of scientific knowledge, their promise to take care of it all and then not being able to follow through, and for not being as self-sacrificing as Mother Teresa. These attitudes reinforce the natural Them/Us impediment to effective intervention.

The AIDS professional may be globally judgmental, presenting a "correct" way to think and feel about HIV disease issues, thereby directly or indirectly condemning individuals who deviate from that view. Direct judgmentalism shuts off positive interaction and creates an adversarial relationship. Indirect judgmentalism is more insidious in its effects, creating undercurrents of guilt, fear, and resentment in those judged, whether they be trainees or patients. This may precipitate a passive-aggressive response that blocks effective attitude and behavior change in ways that are difficult to undo. Hidden conflict is set up and not resolved.

The professional may also deny the validity of scientific reservations about risk guidelines, routes of transmission, and personal risk assessment. This denial is accomplished by labeling all questioning and scientific skepticism as generated by foolish ignorance. The professional may present consensus opinions about HIV disease as firm, proven facts that should be accepted with conviction. Unfortunately, because HIV is new to medical science and scientific knowledge is only probable, not certain, the AIDS professional is likely to be presenting conclusions that other professionals will find difficult to fit into their clinical experiences and that cannot be proven to be correct. As the professional dismisses their questions as foolish ignorance, the adversarial relationship becomes heated.

One of the common assumptions made by professionals is that all individuals are hypersensitive to the risks of HIV infection. This assumption usually refers to people's fears about "casual contact" with HIV-positive persons or about iatrogenic transmission of HIV (patient-to-physician, physician-to-patient, patient-to-patient). Criticizing people for fearing risk, and then emphasizing the presence of risk so as to teach them that risk reduction is essential to their safety create a strange inconsistency and result in a double bind. Emphasizing HIV risk encourages individuals to see one act of unprotected sex as high-risk (because the individual's life is at stake). Belittling individuals' fears about HIV risk (that there is a low probability that he or she will be the person who contracts the virus) submerges their personal risk within group statistics, negating their feelings and devaluing them. The professional may also ignore the important question of the trainee or patient being able to exercise personal control over accepting or taking risks. Individuals perceive a higher risk (or resent the risk) if they have no control over it. Risk perception and assessment are very complex and professionals should avoid drawing arbitrary and conflicting conclusions since the ambiguity can result in a lack of trust and an adversarial relationship.

Professionals may also make assumptions about the capacity of others for empathy and compassion. They may see themselves as exemplars of these virtues and fail to see the virtues in others who are not AIDS experts. This skewed sense of self versus others gives satisfaction to the expert and limits empathy for others. A feeling of superiority also creates distance and potential conflict.

The areas in which professionals are most at risk of making assumptions are the emotional issues of sexual values, sexuality, and gender identity. They may have hidden agendas, such as changing sexual mores or conventions. They may have differing comfort levels concerning sexual openness or privacy. They may or may not be sensitive to cultural as well as personal variations in intimacy, privacy, and kinship. Discussions about sexuality may even be used as a weapon. On such an emotional subject, there is always the possibility of unexamined bias. Some common assumptions include: "His value system is rigid." "She can't deal with her sexual issues." "He is so immature about sex." "She doesn't realize what is normal." "He won't be able to relate to homosexuals."

Since the state of knowledge about sexuality is controversial, the unexamined feelings and motivations of AIDS experts can make the situation even more precarious. Consider the example of homosexuality. It has been explained in many ways throughout history. Classic psychoanalysis described it as the arrested development of genital maturity, a psychological abnormality requiring treatment to correct sexual orientation.[11] Some family theorists regarded homosexuality as a delay in resolution of the leaving home stage. John Money's explanation is that it is half biologically determined, half environmentally determined.[12] Simon LeVay suggests an early biological variance manifested in CNS development.[13] Certain religious or moral views attribute it to the moral agent's choice.[14] The American Psychiatric Association in 1973 removed homosexuality from its Diagnostic and Statistical Manual (DSM-II), eliminating the pathological label.[15] One of the unwitting contributions made by the advent of AIDS is the increasing openness with which homosexuality and lesbianism are viewed and discussed, the diminution of prejudice, and a greater understanding and sensitivity to sexual orientation.

Or, consider the example of heterosexuality. If we look at studies of heterosexual behavior in primates, we see a wide range of behavior options: gibbons with pair monogamy, chimpanzees with group matriarchy and multiple matings, gorillas with dominant silverback males and harems, orangutans with solitary or mother-child units and multiple matings.[16,17,18,19] Thus in less complex species, sexual behavior norms exhibit a range of possibilities. These ethological animal studies can be used to help us better understand the more complex human sexual behaviors. There are still many unexplained areas. When we combine the complexity of sexual behavioral norms with the accoutrements of culture, the picture becomes even more varied. Add to that the current threat that sexual behavior may be lethal, that is, " Sex equals Death," and the task of the health care provider becomes a real challenge.

## RISKS IN THE HEALTH CARE DELIVERY SYSTEM

The health care delivery setting may also engender risks that are not always appreciated by the health care provider. However, once identified, these risks are easily recognized as the common complaints and difficulties of professional life, leading to confusion, frustration, emotional stress, and burnout. For example, one of the most frustrating problems for providers is arranging disposition of a case. Disposition involves providing a good outcome for the patient or client and his or her family by: (1) providing adequate placement, either through home care, institutional setting or the mobilization of social support systems; (2) assuring ongoing adequate follow-up and clinical care; and (3) securing the financial means, by health insurance or other solution, to provide the above.

Achieving these goals is often difficult, as any health care professional knows from daily experience. Disposition of an Alzheimer's patient is extremely difficult; placement of a patient who has AIDS dementia may approach the impossible. Finding good placement and services for crack and cocaine babies is a challenge; placing babies with crack cocaine and AIDS is a nightmare. Frustration has to be accepted as a normal response to these difficulties, but frustrations that mount up and make health care work an unhappy experience can lead to demoralization and exhaustion. This will be discussed further under the heading of burnout of health care providers who are advised to extend their support systems, make friends with people in positions to help them with disposition, and work toward changes in the system.

We have mentioned the issue of sex education as a challenge to therapeutic boundaries. It also presents a problem with interdisciplinary teamwork. Who has the responsibility for teaching patients and their families to use condoms and jelly, and how to use them effectively? Who is responsible for informing them of the dangers of transient relationships or certain sexual practices? Unless responsibility is clearly assigned, it tends to evaporate in team settings and nobody provides the necessary sex education. The team has to negotiate who is best equipped and trained for the job or, if nobody is, who should be assigned to gain the necessary background. For health care providers working alone, it becomes necessary to build a referral network if the provider does not personally want to undertake this task or feels that it would create a boundary problem (if the provider is a psychotherapist, for example). If this issue is not satisfactorily resolved, the health care provider runs the risk of providing inadequate care, having to deal with the aftermath of team dissension, or of being blamed by patients who have not received adequate education.

HIV disease often has produced economic devastation for the individual, as well as raising serious questions about the economic means to pay for adequate health care at a nationwide level. AIDS patients eventually become the responsibility of the government. In the United States, medicaid reimbursement is not sufficient to recoup the cost of care. Even where it covers medical care, there is never enough to cope with the mental health needs of patient and family. Psychotherapy is a luxury that can become dependent upon the goodwill of the health care delivery system and of the individual provider. Health care professionals are acutely aware of the economic constraints to the quality care of any disease. This increases their frustration and sense of helplessness as they try to find ways around economic constraints, sometimes with success, often with failure. This represents to them a lack of control in their professional lives and may lead to disillusionment and despair.

Perhaps the most visible perceived risk to the health care provider in working with HIV disease is the legal one of breach of confidentiality and ensuing malpractice suit. Professionals are very nervous about meeting the requirements of confidentiality with HIV patients. Different countries and states have varying laws on AIDS confidentiality. Those that do not have laws to guide the practice of confidentiality place the professional at risk of either failing to warn (duty to warn) or failing to safeguard confidentiality. As a result of this perceived risk, some health care professionals become immobilized and unable to share health information when it is both necessary and legal. Confidentiality requirements can also create a sense of secrecy in the system. As one of the psychiatric nurses said:[5]

> "There's still a lot of secrecy bound by confidentiality. Some people have signs on their doors. What does it mean for other patients when you share a bathroom with a patient who is HIV positive? So there's a lot of unanswered questions for the unit."

Her dilemma occurred on an inpatient unit, but this issue is certainly not restricted to inpatient settings. Professionals are often reluctant to give each other information about their clients or patients if they happen to be HIV positive, even when that information is necessary for good health care or for the efficient functioning of the system. It may even be critical for saving the patient's life, or protecting his or her lover or spouse.

Maintaining effective teamwork and collegial collaboration is an essential for providing quality care for all cases, but it is crucial for patients with HIV infection. Because of all the difficulties described above, HIV disease challenges the concept of team cooperation, communication, and collaboration as no other disease does. It represents a risk to the therapeutic system itself, and health care providers will inevitably be impacted by that risk.

It is very tempting, at times, to become overinvolved with one's HIV clients, to buy into the story that one is the only person who can help them, that they have nobody in their natural support system, and that secrecy about the infection must remain absolute. It is also easy, in the face of the current economic system, to believe that financial resources are absent, and that informing a colleague about the HIV status of your patient will place one at risk of legal suit. It might be helpful, when faced with all these dilemmas, to remember the principles of Chapter 2. Patients and clients are not truly isolated; there is generally somebody out there if one explores the natural support system thoroughly.

It is imperative that we learn to talk to our colleagues, trust them in their endeavors with our patients, and avoid secrecy and triangulation that can only be destructive to our relationships with both our clients and our colleagues. Psychiatrists need to work with social workers and infectious disease specialists. Internists and surgeons need to trust family members and community agencies. Teamwork and continuity of care are essential to good health care practice.

Wherever possible, the health care provider should assemble a list of resources available in his or her community. The case management model has been developed in an attempt to assure that the patient is followed from agency to hospital and to private provider so that there is continuity of care and protection against different people administering diametrically opposed measures to deal with the same problem. Maintaining a network of referrals and resources, while staying in touch with them about one's cases, helps to obviate this. Community agencies can be helpful in this regard. They tend to know their clients well and to make natural case managers and go-betweens.

Calling meetings of everyone involved in the care of a particular client can achieve good results.[20,21,22] Providers generally struggle about the same clients and their issues; they may be surprisingly willing to attend such a meeting, or at least be available for a conference call.[20] The issues raised by HIV disease are also too big to deal with alone. We need our colleagues to provide support not only for our patients and clients, but for us as well. How can this be available for us if we are sworn to secrecy? When can we share, what can we share, without infringement of law and ethics?

Perhaps it will be reassuring to remember that the principles of quality care override most others, and that modern quality care implies teamwork and collaboration. It is also possible to discuss patients while not revealing identifying information, if colleagues are available for discussion who are not involved with that particular client. Allowing clients to become dependent on us alone as individuals undercuts the work that our colleagues are invested in, renders the natural support system incompetent, and ultimately places our clients and ourselves at risk.

## HEALTH CARE PROVIDER BURNOUT

The temptation to become overinvolved with one's HIV-positive clients is one of the prime hazards of working in the field of HIV disease. The health care workers we have quoted above also had to deal with the risk of burnout. One of them (the high-risk maternity unit nurse) saw the early warning signs, and took positive steps to care for herself as well as her patients and their families:[5]

> "I just worked nights for three months to take care of my mental health. Nursing is a very stressful job. All of nursing is stressful in the eighties: Nursing shortages, sicker patients. In my own case I did it because I felt I had no more to give. We're very busy at night, but it's strictly physical. Once in a while you get involved with the emotional side, but you're so busy that you don't have time to worry about the families, the social worker, and child protective conferences—and it's a different kind of busyness."

Two of the other health care workers that we described above were not as observant of the danger signs of burnout. The secretary for the psychiatric residents was not listening to the signs of overinvolvment and potential burnout:[5]

> "I don't know them personally, just from phone calls and the reports I type up. That's when I get sad, and that's when I take it home with me. I feel sad for the residents because they're grieving, and I feel sad for myself—because I don't have the actual therapy contact it leaves me more confused."

This secretary expressed her desire to increase her work and contact with AIDS patients, saying, "I feel well prepared." This is very similar to one of the psychiatric nurses who expressed her wish to work with AIDS patients during the day in her job, and then to volunteer to work with AIDS patients in the evening and on weekends. Both are missing the early signals that will lead to burnout. The intake worker, during her interview, while indicating early signs of burnout, also had begun to discover some methods for alleviating it:[5]

> "We know who these people are, and we don't get crazy because we're dealing with them. They're just regular people. We have each other."

The intake worker had discovered two of the lessons in dealing with burnout: regarding the HIV-positive patients as normal patients and applying the same principles to them as to others; and learning to depend on collegial support and discussion. The labor nurse had also applied these principles: "We need to have people to talk to and share things with."

When exploring the issue of burnout it is useful to think about it both at the personal (individual and family) level of individual health care worker, and at the level of agency, hospital or institution.

## Warning Signs

If the early signs of burnout are attended to promptly, burnout can be a protective mechanism and accomplish positive results for the health care worker, his or her family, and the patients. On the personal (individual and family) level, there are some typical warning signs of burnout that health care workers should be monitoring.

If the noncompliance of a patient is beginning to generate strong feelings and an expectation of continued noncompliance, the fault may not be with the patient. It may indicate overinvolvement of the health care provider, laying him or her open not only to frustration, but to a feeling of personal betrayal of trust and disloyalty. Any rescue fantasies can be seen as an early warning sign. It may be that the health care provider wants to rescue the patient from his or her family, or from his or her other health care providers, not trusting anyone else to be there. This may lead to lengthy hours at work and replacement of one's other significant relationships with the therapeutic relationship. If the health care provider finds that his or her entire social life is with HIV-positive people, or that one particular patient has become a personal and intimate favorite, warning lights should go on.

If the health care worker begins to overidentify with patients or clients, this is also a warning sign. Examples of overidentification are: feeling severely depressed when the situation looks grim; finding that sleep or eating patterns are disturbed; or becoming angry or frustrated with the patient's family and feeling that one knows more, and could take better care of the patient than they are doing.

If the health care worker (or supervisor) is constantly exhausted, finds work less exciting, and gets out of bed in the morning only with difficulty, burnout may be occurring. In some instances, persistent headaches, stomachaches, psychosomatic illness, or frequent infection with influenza may occur. In the extreme, this may result in days of work being lost or even a decision to leave the field of AIDS or the profession itself. Similarly, if the health care worker is working longer and longer hours and avoiding social and family events in favor of work (as the psychiatric nurse above was planning to do), this too is a sign of burnout.

Conversely, if the health care worker finds reasons to avoid patient contact and distances himself or herself from patient and family members, he or she should realize that burnout is occurring. Typical feelings of distancing include (a) general emotional numbness: "I'm not going to allow myself to be hurt again," or, "I can't attend any more funerals," or, "There's no point in relating to . . . It doesn't change anything"; (b) pride in being tough, impersonal and objective; (c) overintellectualizing and generalizing about the clients and patients; (d) following protocols to the letter and not allowing for individual variation; or, (e) claiming not to be personally touched by HIV disease.

Feelings of passivity and hopelessness, along with a loss of faith in the efficacy of any intervention, are warning signs that can be particularly dangerous to quality of care as well as to the health care professional. The health care provider may start feeling: "There's no point in doing anything," or, "Why treat him, he is only going to die later anyway," or, "Why waste money on her," or even, "Why prolong the suffering, so he'll recover from the pneumonia, then what?"

Increasing fear of infection and dread of going to work each day are also major signs of burnout. However, many professionals working with AIDS patients report having what has come to be called an "AIDS dream" at the beginning of working in this field.[26] Typically, such dreams are about being diagnosed as HIV positive or having AIDS; having a loved one diagnosed; dreaming of a loved one's funeral from AIDS; having feelings of dread and panic; having a terrible skin disease spreading all over the body; or of dying. What the health care provider needs to keep in mind is that one or two such dreams are normal and do not indicate burnout. If this type of dream should recur frequently, however, it should be regarded as a warning sign.

Should a health care provider who has previously experienced no difficulty in serving members of other cultures or subcultures gradually become aware of an increasing dislike or prejudice against a particular group, this may also be a sign of burnout. The provider may not be at all prejudiced, but may have to deal with the prejudice of colleagues, friends, and family. Labelling can occur as a part of this: "You must be gay to want to work with these people," or, "I didn't know that you took drugs." Becoming prejudiced or noting that other people are making this kind of remark should draw attention to the possibility of burnout.

It may be that the health care provider is not experiencing the feelings associated with burnout, but that his or her family is having difficulties with the AIDS work. The family may be resentful of time spent with the patients, and family fights may be generated by the typical demands that professionals expect to meet. The family may keep asking that the professional find another position, and may even make threats about it. Individual family members might be anxious about becoming infected. For example: "How can you expose our baby to AIDS?" "I'm not going to make love to you ever again." "Grandmother's too frail to let her risk something like that!"

Family members may be split around the issues of safety, time commitments, and emotional commitments. Members of the extended family may be brought in or volunteer to be involved, leading to triangulations and family crises over these issues. Friends may alter their relationships with the health care provider or with his or her family in an attempt to protect their own families, as well as out of ignorance.

At the agency, hospital or institutional level, all the warning signs shared by members of the agency apply, and also create, through the interrelationships within the system, additional types of burnout warning. Employers, administrators, and service directors should monitor their staff and themselves for signs. Staff also should monitor their colleagues and their directors in a similar way. Burnout is not necessarily reserved for those in the trenches, but applies equally across the health care system. It is important to remember that a true systems perspective includes monitoring *all* the staff. We saw earlier how an intake worker and a secretary became overinvolved in their dealings with the HIV-positive patients on their respective services. Housekeepers, gardeners, laboratory technicians, radiographers, and cleaning personnel, to mention but a few, are no less exempt.

For an administrator, a high personnel turnover is one of the most concrete warnings. A plethora of employees coming late for work or taking excessive sick leave or days off is another. Should there be an unusually high rate of incident reports, particularly involving health care providers taking unusual physical risks, burnout should be assumed. The administrators are at particular burnout risk as a result of the pressure of trying to run a system at maximum capacity and with inadequate funding. A general principle of systems is that disasters occur when complex systems are run at (or above) full capacity. The hospital administrator, trying to meet state and federal requirements, trying to pay for much needed facilities, trying to maintain fiscal responsibility and simultaneously practicing cost containment and seeking employee satisfaction, has a perfect blueprint for burnout. His or her professional and support staff are affected as well, further amplifing the tasks.

At the next level of organization, the whole raison d'être of the medical care system is at risk. Instead of seeing themselves as providers of compassionate, quality care, health care professionals are at risk of having to see themselves as economic gatekeepers and triage decision-makers who cannot supply what their patients need. The incongruity between the way we prefer to view ourselves and the way we need to behave may result in the burnout of self-denigration and helplessness.

## Prevention and Management

The primary prevention of burnout and its early and effective management when it does occur are crucial to the well-being of both health care provider and client. The major principles underlying both prevention and management are:

a. Normalizing
b. Awareness and Identification
c. Anticipation of Problems
d. Mobilization of Support Systems
e. Clear Definition of Roles and Boundaries
f. Realistic Goal Setting
g. Taking Care of Self
h. "Claiming the Gift"[23]

*Normalizing.* One of the important advances to be made is placing HIV disease upon the normal spectrum of illness, regarding it as an infectious disease, with epidemiology, diagnosis, and clinical management that may be specific to it, but nonetheless sharing principles with other infectious diseases and life-threatening illnesses. HIV-positive patients are patients. They have physical needs, emotional needs, and social needs similar to any other class of patient. In principle, the minute a patient or class of patients is treated as different, health care is compromised and health care providers are at risk of burnout.

The general expertise of health care providers is the expertise needed to treat HIV-positive patients or any other patients. Skills and competence that providers have displayed in their management of other illnesses are the same skills and competence required for HIV disease. For health care workers, HIV presents issues and conflicts similar to those of other illnesses such as alcoholism, tuberculosis, hepatitis, cancer, serious renal disease, genetic diseases, progressive neuromuscular diseases, progressive neurological disorders, leprosy, or schizophrenia. Health care workers who have very astutely travelled the road of these disorders with success seem at times to lose their way when dealing with HIV. They are often unaware that the same skills that allow for good treatment of cancer or schizophrenia also work for HIV disease.

There have been other diseases with lethal outcome. Skills and competence on the part of the health care provider do not necessarily ensure immortality, or even longevity, but working toward quality of life is an essential responsibility. The more closely care of the HIV-positive person resembles other health care, the better for health care provider and patient, along with their families. Burnout occurs when situations or clients are regarded as special or different, and when health care providers (and hence their clients) lose confidence in their skills and competence.

In order to take care of yourself and your colleagues, and to ensure viewing AIDS cases and HIV infection from a "normal" perspective, you may find it useful to imagine the identical scenario, but caused by another disease or infectious agent. In other words, substitute any other diagnosis for the current symptoms that appear overwhelming and unmanageable. "Take AIDS out of the sentence."[24]

*Awareness and Identification.* As we mentioned above, there are many early warning signs of burnout, and it is useful to maintain a watch for these in order to prevent them leading to full-blown burnout. The early warnings are there to protect us and our patients; attending to these warnings can improve the capacity of the health care provider to deliver quality care. Every effort should be made to attend to any or all of the warnings listed in the warning section of this chapter, at both individual and agency level. They can be physical or emotional; both deserve attention. Self-monitoring or monitoring of one's colleagues may not be sufficient, and group discussion or some personal or family therapy might be indicated.

Miller and Bor[25] list potential sources of stress. They divide sources of stress into three categories:

1. Unanticipated and stressful tasks, such as talking to patients about sex and death, having to help young people face disfigurement, or giving information that is uncertain;
2. Management and organizational difficulties, such as not having enough counseling rooms, poorly defined work boundaries between staff, or lack of support and supervision; and
3. Personal and home issues that intrude into the work situation, such as anxiety of the professional and/or family about becoming HIV infected, overidentification with young patients, or balancing home and work time.

*Anticipation of Problems.* One of the most effective means of preventing burnout is to anticipate difficult situations before they arise. By gaining some command of the situation, the professional is able to plan his or her actions, and avoid some of the crises. It might be useful to make a list for yourself of the areas that are likely to generate the most stress and plan how you might deal with them should they arise, or preferably how to prevent them. Winiarski, for example, has a list of questions that a patient or client is likely to ask the health care provider.[23] His questions include: "Wouldn't you kill yourself if you were me?" "Why would God put me through this?" "Why me?" "What will happen to my family?" "Will I die alone?" "Can you stand to look at me?" "Why should I tell anyone?"[23] (pp.120–124). These are extremely common but difficult questions to answer on a personal or professional level. They require some forethought and it is unlikely that a health care provider can give a satisfactory answer off the cuff.

Anticipating questions like these can head off frustration, anger at the patient, and despair.

The problems that can be anticipated might be difficulties with the patient, his or her family or support system, the health care delivery system, or other professionals involved. Many of the potential problems have been listed in Chapter 2 and earlier in this chapter. The ones that are likely to provide the greatest difficulty are the ones that it might be helpful to list specifically. If you have difficulty preparing your responses, discussion with colleagues might prove fruitful.

*Mobilization of Support Systems.* HIV disease is a field that is extremely difficult to traverse alone, whether you are a health care provider or a patient. We ourselves as providers need access to support beyond ourselves. We need to become comfortable in sharing our feelings with our colleagues and our families, and in facing the really tough issues with support, rather than alone.

As mentioned above, collegial groups can be helpful. We have found that these are best designed on an interdisciplinary basis and servicewide, assuring that all levels of staff are included. At times, in really hierarchical settings, it may be necessary to separate upper administrative levels from other staff to ensure emotional safety and the freedom of expression. A blend of these two can also be highly effective. For professionals working alone, groups may be arranged with people from similar settings—remember, they are also feeling isolated. Groups may be designed as a brief, circumscribed series of meetings or as an ongoing experience. Alternatively, or in addition, ad hoc meetings may be called when stress in the system rises or when you feel that you have a particular need.

Whatever the design, we strongly recommend that some system be devised in the workplace for collegial sharing and support. Generally, it is possible for these to be leaderless groups. However, if problems arise or your particular setting requires it, a group leader may be assigned, either from within the group or from outside. For example, in our AIDS Clinic, a weekly staff group was designed, attended by all staff and run by the Clinic psychiatrist.

Health care professionals often view themselves as tough and resilient, believing that they need to cope on their own, and also feeling that they are required to protect their own families from their work issues, particularly stress. Taken to its natural conclusion, this would mean that the health care professional remains isolated from his or her own family when work stress rises, and that the family may feel excluded and helpless, noticing the level of stress, but not having any means to help alleviate it. Conversely, family members who are concerned about the professional's work setting are unable to share their concerns with the one person who might be in a position to resolve them.

There are several effective ways of dealing with this. Groups in the work setting may be opened to family members on a regular basis, say once a month, or may even include them on an ad hoc basis when issues arise that are bound to concern them. Alternatively, groups (to which the health care providers are occasionally invited) may be arranged for the team's family members. Staff group and family group could be arranged to run at the same time of the week, so that the ability to combine the groups is built into the design.

A method for dealing with this situation, other than through groups, is to assure staff that they are free to request a consultation whenever needed. In order for this to be an effective method of dealing with health care provider and family stress, this should not be seen as therapy, should be viewed as routine, and be readily accessible. Clearly, if stress becomes severe, referral for therapy should be considered, and this too should be viewed as normal, given the work setting. We have found that when therapy is needed, it is imperative to include the family in order to avoid isolation and to ensure that both family and health care provider receive support and understanding from the people they care most about and who care most about them.

We have been discussing support systems for health care providers themselves and their families. The same principles apply when considering using the patient's support systems. The mobilization of these systems can help prevent burnout of the health care professional, as well as providing effective support for the patient. The patient's natural support system consists (as described in Chapter 2) of those people who care most about the patient, are involved with him or her on a daily, weekly, or otherwise regular basis, and are going to be there for him or her throughout time. The better understanding they have of the patient's situation and the more they are involved in the care of the patient, the less the health care provider has to carry the full burden. If health care providers fail to involve the natural support system, and try to undertake heroic caretaking themselves, they will burn out with rapidity.

Community agencies, either HIV agencies, or agencies embedded in the particular community served, can be extremely important adjuncts to the natural support system through groups, hotlines, and case managers. When patients and their families are not accessing the local community agency, it may help for the professional to encourage it. Or, if local community agencies do not exist, it may be helpful to participate in their formation. (The formation of community agencies is described in Chapter 9.) Church congregations can also be constant sources of support, as can employers and school settings (see Chapter 9).

The professional or artificial support system is frequently very complex in HIV care. In addition to the natural support system members, many professionals may be involved in the care of the same patient. If they all work in isolation, failing to communicate or not being aware of each other's existence, they may inadvertently end up working at cross purposes, all feeling excessively burdened and solely responsible for the well-being of the patient. Unfortunately, and with the best of intentions, this may be a recipe for disaster. Not only is the health care professional likely to become overburdened, but the patient and family are unlikely to get what they need. We have seen cases in which each member of a family is being served by a different professional, not communicating with each other and not even being aware of the existence of other providers

In some cases, this assumes grave proportions, with the professionals replacing family members, or other natural support system members, in an attempt to provide adequate care. This substitution, or surrogacy, is unrealistic in the long term. The professional cannot, and is not really willing, to make the kind of commitment that only family and natural support system can make. In the attempt, the professional is bound to be exhausted while also disrupting the support system that needs to be there for the patient or client. This is a no-win situation for all. Rather, the professional who mobilizes and strengthens the relationship of the client to the natural support system, has time and energy left over for dealing with many difficult and demanding clients.

Unfortunately, even knowing and understanding these principles does not always protect the professional. It is remarkably easy to assume that "We know best," or to misinterpret a family member's early horror at the diagnosis. "He (or she) doesn't really care, how could I involve him (or her) in the management." It is also easy to assume that there are too many obstacles to working with the family. For an extensive list of initial excuses or resistances, and how these can be handled, please refer to Chapter 8.

If health care providers are convinced that the natural support system is not available, or that other professionals are not as good for the patient as they are, they run the risk of attempting to be all things to all people. Their own needs, and that of their own families, will tend to be neglected. Burnout becomes inevitable. They may then also be responsible for the failure of the patient's natural support system. In alienating them or failing to mobilize them when needed, health care providers encourage the dependence of the patient upon them alone, hence working harder toward their own burnout—and the ultimate failure of the treatment. This does no favor to health care providers, or to patients.

Collaboration and teamwork are the solution. Regular discussion between professionals and natural support system members can be very helpful and ensure that no one individual is carrying more than his or her load. It also ensures that the patient is receiving the best possible care, since the team can negotiate who is best to deal with each aspect. Negotiation is, however, a critical component of sharing the load in this way. A team leader needs to be assigned, and goals and tasks for the management of different situations need to be clearly allocated. If this does not happen, failure of treatment can occur through the confusion and disintegration of the organization. In fact, if the teamwork is not properly managed, the resultant failure can reinforce the professional's initial view, "Only I can deal with this. . . ."

*Clear Definition of Roles and Boundaries.* Living with your own peers, who may disagree with you or not respect the specific role that your particular profession may play in the management of the patient, can lead to difficulty for both you and the patient. In order to create effective teamwork, professionals sharing a case from different perspectives not only need to be acquainted with each other's strengths and special skills, but also must be ready to respect them. In order for this to happen, we need to take responsibility for educating others about our role, while learning as much as we can about theirs. The mental health provider needs to respect the more physical skills of his or her counterparts, be ready to live with complications created by certain medications, and be prepared to bypass mental health needs in the face of a medical emergency. Respect for one's colleagues in other fields is paramount, even if their agenda does not appear to make immediate sense.

Unless we ourselves respect our colleagues, we will not deserve respect and will be rendered incompetent when we try to allocate tasks. There will be times when other colleagues feel that time spent in talking to patients and their families is time ill spent in the face of the illness. Be tolerant, and they will gradually come to respect your talents. We have found that in the face of challenge and criticism of this kind, it is better to employ the oriental philosophy of "wu wei" (going with the system, rather than opposing it). Setting oneself up as the only expert is doomed to failure. Where possible, clarify boundaries explicitly, making certain that each member of the professional group is in agreement both with tasks and boundaries.

Clarifying boundaries with AIDS patients can present some problems because they are usually multiply diagnosed. For example, when sexuality needs to be dealt with, which specialty should be assigned which tasks? Is the patient comfortable going to his or her family doctor about how a condom should be used, or getting advice on how to inform a partner about HIV positivity? Should patients be sent to STD clinics where staff are well informed about such issues, and will patients be willing to go to an STD clinic? Should the local community AIDS agency be assigned the task, and how does one persuade patients to follow through with any of these recommendations? Knowing one's colleagues and their strengths enriches one's capacity to refer one's clients and patients to the appropriate service.

In Kevin's case, his infectious disease physician was experiencing a great deal of difficulty in handling the emotional and family situation. Kevin was becoming a difficult patient, demanding a great deal of the physician's time.

When the physician assigned his clinic nurse to manage Kevin's problems, the only effect was to transfer the time and demand to the clinic staff. As Kevin became even more difficult (not surprising, since his needs were not being met and he was being treated more and more like a nuisance), the physician made a referral to a younger psychiatric colleague whom he knew well. The psychiatrist, at the first office visit, learned that the physician had promised Kevin that he would be given a prescription for valium. Of course, the outcome of this collegial interaction was that the psychiatrist was annoyed with the infectious disease physician for infringing on her area of expertise and made a mental note to discuss the matter with him. This kind of system dynamics around referral and professional boundaries is to be avoided, and can be, if we learn to respect each other and establish clear rules around task allocation and clinical and professional boundaries.

*Setting Realistic Goals.* One of the most important tasks of health care is setting goals that are realistic within the total context. Goals can be biased, reflecting the health care provider's own particular value judgments. They can be naive, because they are seen exclusively from the perspective of the medical care institution. Goals can be overly ambitious, not taking into account the limitations imposed by the realities of the patient's life and circumstances and demanding far more than can be given over the long term. They may be too demanding of the health care professional and not demanding enough of the natural support system. Goals may not reflect the inherent trade-offs that are part of any complex system or disease, and, as a result, may actually do more damage than good. They can be short sighted or too short-term, not taking into account the chronicity of HIV disease. Goals can lack clarity, resulting in confusion that undermines the original intentions.

When the health care provider sets goals that reflect his or her bias, ambition, or naivete, and not the needs or reality of the patient and his or her family, the provider may be acting as a crusader, an advocate, a pioneer, or a political activist. This unilateral goal-setting can isolate the provider from the team and can result in a conviction that it is the world against the professional. The provider can become embattled or take on the role of a savior, resulting in inevitable failure and letting down the patient and the family. Constant frustration and failure always lead to burnout.

When goals are limited, either by not taking the context into account, ignoring the other components of the system (social or medical), or not taking the possible length of the illness into account, the professional is again setting himself or herself up for failure and the enmity of others working with the patient. In the case of a young woman with AIDS who presented for emergency treatment, the medical team decided that her social environment was inadequate. Thinking that she would die soon, they decided to admit her to hospital without consulting any member of her natural support system. The team had judged her family and social relationships to be "bad" for her and "responsible for her AIDS," and therefore set about isolating her from them in order "to protect her" and "to make her last days comfortable and safe." The woman gradually got better, her pneumonia remitted, and it became apparent that she was not about to die. By that time, however, she had become completely isolated from her social support setting and there was nowhere for her to go. Nine months later she was still in the hospital, and the team was wondering where it went wrong.

Goals therefore need to be clear, realistic, unbiased, and shared by professional and natural support systems. Meetings should be held at which the current situation and needs are clearly explored and appropriate goal-setting negotiated until all members of the system are in agreement. Goals should then be prioritized and goal-related tasks assigned to the most appropriate person. More details on goal-setting will be given in Chapter 8.

*Taking Care of Self.* We have talked above about the importance of support groups and the involvement of the health care provider's own family, as well as the need for team support. How can we as individuals take care of ourselves? The standard work stress relievers are really important. Probably the most effective is the use of humor and play. Gallows humor is widely recognized in the health care field and studies have shown that humor is a very effective tool for dealing with emotional and physical crises. In fact, humor is seen as a good indicator of improvement in psychiatric illness. Having people laugh each time they enter your office can do wonders for lifting your spirits and theirs. Play is a natural outgrowth of looking at the funny side of life. Don't be too shy to play with your colleagues, your clients, and their families. Healthy humor and play are not disrespectful or hurtful, but are in fact, healing. More formal play, such as athletic activities or dancing, are also important stress relievers. Organize a pick-up team of volleyball, or bring a dance tape to work.

Having an aesthetic and comfortable work space can also make a great deal of difference in the way you feel when you arrive in the morning. This is not always easy to achieve—regard it as a challenge. Simple things such as comfortable chairs, good lighting, and ventilation are necessities.

Most health care providers have a natural support system and individuals they can talk to about a particularly rough day. If you do not have people that you can trust at this level, try to establish some new relationships, either within or outside your work setting. Make sure that their phone numbers are readily available for a brief call when needed. Make a lunch hour appointment to get out of the work environment—other people regard lunch breaks as normal. If the work setting does not provide a support group, you could always arrange a mini group of your own.

Self-esteem is a basic human requirement. Health care professionals have multiple ways to reinforce self-esteem, such as the cure of the patient. But, working with AIDS makes that more difficult. The health care provider has to remember that there are two components to health care—curing and caring—and that comfort care is as important as curing the patient by returning the patient to baseline.

Happiness in one's work is also a necessity. Not that it can be there constantly, but a level of satisfaction and pride in what one does and happy moments with patients and colleagues who recognize one's special contribution and hard effort are required. Remember to thank your colleagues, praise your employer/employee, notice the effort undertaken by others. Celebrate each other's achievements, and even birthdays and holidays, when appropriate.

Working with AIDS cases, it is sometimes really difficult to be happy; it may even be inappropriate. A "Pollyanna" attitude will not suffice for dealing with grief and loss. These, too, need to be attended to. In our own hospital, the chief chaplain (A. Tartaglia, D. Min.) has organized regular memorial services so that the staff can come together and pray for our critically ill cases and grieve for those who have died. Meeting with the families of one's clients or patients who have died can be very helpful both to us and to them. We have found that celebrating the life and achievements of the patients we have lost really helps us and the families.

"Claiming the Gift."[23] As many people working in the field of AIDS have discovered, along with their patients, there can actually be very positive experiences in the midst of HIV disease.[23,26] The health care provider may forget this in the process of dealing with a difficult case, and needs to remind him or herself of it. HIV disease can result in a great deal of growth for the patient and his or her family; paradoxically, it may be one of the most meaningful periods of their lives. Facing chronic illness and death together may provide them with an opportunity to resolve long-standing enmities and problems, allowing them to grow both as individuals and as a family.

We have had numerous cases where the patient has expressed this sentiment. One Puerto Rican couple, Carmen and Pedro, who discovered they had AIDS after they were recovering from drug addiction, described this time as the"happiest time" of their lives. They said this despite his cytomegaloviral (CMV) retinitis and pneumocystis pneumonia and her genital thrush and skin lesions. Kevin, whom we talked about earlier, made the same statement as a speaker at an AIDS conference at St. Mary's Hospital in Rochester, New York in 1988. In the case of Paul, who had been separated from his family to the point of cut-off, the therapist* had persuaded him that his family should be given the opportunity to heal the relationships in time to say goodbye. Much to his surprise, the family meeting

---

*Therapist, G. Horsley, M.S.N., M.S.; Supervisor J. Landau-Stanton, M.B., Ch.B., D.P.M.

went well, and both he and his parents thanked God for the HIV disease that had brought them back together. In the case of Emily, she attributed her continuing recovery from drug abuse to her HIV disease. She had been in recovery on and off for several years and was convinced that she was headed for a relapse when she discovered that she and her baby were HIV positive. Realizing that time might be brief, she embarked on a path of committed recovery and self-development. Her story will be given in greater detail in Chapter 8.

All of these patients confirm that there is a gift that could be claimed, perhaps with some help, in the process of HIV disease. The health care professional who keeps his or her eye on this goal, as well as on the often hopeless goal of saving life, may have taken one of the most important steps toward avoiding burnout.

## REFERENCES

1. (1991). Update: Transmisson of HIV infection during invasive dental procedures. *MMWR* 40 (23): 377–381.
2. (Aug. 7, 1990). TB is now back with a vengeance. *The Medical Post.* p. 15.
3. Clements, C., Landau-Stanton, J., Horsley, G., Romano, J. (1989). *Dr. Romano Remembers*, Videotape. University of Rochester, Department of Psychiatry Audiovisual Center.
4. Fields, L. (October 2, 1990). From the plague to AIDS: What have we learned. *The Medical Post.*
5. Griepp, A., Landau-Stanton, J. (1989). *You Need Not Be Afraid*. Edited Videotape. University of Rochester, Department of Psychiatry Audiovisual Center.
6. Rosenbaum, E.E. (1988). *The Doctor.* New York: Ivy Books.
7. Greenson, R.R. (1974). The theory of psychoanalytic technique. In S. Arieti (Ed.) *American Handbook of Psychiatry, Vol. 1.* (pp. 764–788). New York: Basic Books.
8. Kubler-Ross, E. (1969). *On Death and Dying,* New York: Macmillan.
9. Parkes, C. (1982). *Bereavement: Studies of Grief in Adult Life,* New York: International University Press.
10. Clements, C.D. (April 19, 1988). Sometimes a policeman's lot is not a very happy one especially in a confrontation between values and duty. *The Medical Post.*
11. Freud, S. (1959). Three essays on the theory of sexuality. In J. Strackey (Ed. and Trans.), *Collected Works of Freud* (pp. 125–243). London: Hogarth.
12. Money, J. (1988). *Gay, Straight and Inbetween: The Sexology of Erotic Orientation.* New York: Oxford University Press.
13. LeVay, S. (1991). A difference in hypothalamic structure between heterosexual and homosexual men. *Science,* 253(5023), 1034–1037.
14. 1982). Vatican Council II (Declaration on certain problems of sexual ethics. In A. Flannery (Ed. and Trans.), *Vatican Collection* (pp. 486–499). Grand Rapids, MI: Eerdmans.

15. Markowitz, L.M. (1991). Homosexuality: Are we still in the dark? *The Family Therapy Networker.* 15 (1): 27–35.
16. Morris, D. (1967). *The Naked Ape: A Zoologist's Study of the Human Animal.* New York: McGraw Hill.
17. Ardrey, R. (1967). *The Territorial Imperative.* New York: Atheneum.
18. Goodall, J. (1986) *The Chimpanzees of Gombe:* Patterns of Behavior. Cambridge, Mass.: Belknap Press.
19. Fossey, D. (1983). *Gorillas in the Mist.* Boston: Houghton Mifflin.
20. Imber-Black, E. (1988). *Families and Larger Systems.* New York: Guilford Press.
21. Berger, M., Jurkovic, G.J, and Associates. (1984). *Practicing Family Therapy in Diverse Settings.* San Francisco: Jossey-Bass.
22. Wynne, L., Weber, T., McDaniel, S. (Eds.) (1985). *Systems Consultation: A New Perspective for Family Therapy.* New York: Guilford Press.
23. Winiarski, M.G. (1991). *AIDS-Related Psychotherapy.* New York: Pergamon Press.
24. Griepp, A. (1988). *The Neuropsychiatric Management of AIDS.* Edited Videotape. University of Rochester, Department of Psychiatry Audiovisual Center.
25. Miller, R., Bor, R. (1989). *AIDS: A Guide to Clinical Counseling.* London: Science Press.
26. Walker, G. (1991). *In the Midst of Winter; Systemic Therapy with Families, Couples, and Individuals with AIDS Infection.* New York: Norton.

# CHAPTER 5

# Staying Abreast of HIV Disease

Even as we consider the current state of knowledge about HIV disease, it will be described in new or modified ways; it will have spread into new populations and the pandemic will either have become an emergency worldwide or we will have succeeded in checking its spread; new treatments and experimental vaccines will be developed; and new policy decisions will be required. That is the historical story of any new disease. How can the health care professional keep up?

This chapter is an attempt to supply some tools for staying abreast of a new and changing disease. HIV isn't the first such disease, nor will it be the last. Dementia praecox (the early psychiatric diagnosis of a multiplicity of psychoses) was rediagnosed as schizophrenia in some and as tertiary syphilis in other patients when syphilis was discovered as a new disease. The late onset effects of polio have just recently been recognized. New viruses such as Ebola fever and Hantaan virus hemorrhagic fever are on the horizon. Where once conventional wisdom said retroviruses did not cause human disease, we now know that the retrovirus, HTLV-I, causes leukemia and lymphoma and is blood-transmitted. Our understanding of cancer is growing and changing with our understanding of the complex functions of oncoviruses, tumor necrosis factor, and other mechanisms to switch cell growth on and off. Many forms of previously lethal cancer and lymphoma can now be effectively treated. HIV disease isn't unique; it is *very predictable* if we think historically and systemically.

One of the great achievements in Shilts's book is his insight that the HIV story should be a chronological account (therefore historical and systemic), starting in Kinshasa, Zaire in 1976 with the Scandinavian surgeon, Dr. Grethe Rask, who died of PCP on December 12, 1977, and ending temporarily (with the completion of Shilts's book), in 1987, with Dr. Don Francis going to the World Health Organization to study AIDS in Africa.[1] Looking at his history carefully (Table 5-A), it is easy to see the change and progression of our knowledge about HIV disease and the mistakes that were made by thinking that our information was complete and that HIV disease was a static reality.

133

Another book that emphasized the importance of the historic and systemic view is Grmek's book on the history of AIDS, a look at how this modern pandemic originated and spread.[2] His book discusses several probable early cases of AIDS, including the English sailor who died in 1959. He argues that HIV-2 existed much before the current AIDS pandemic of HIV-1 and he links both viruses to an evolutionary scheme of retroviruses, extending the connections of HIV far back in time. He also develops the concept of "pathocenosis," which states that any single disease like HIV disease must be understood in its relation to all other diseases in the same population. His hypothesis is that our success in preventing the common infectious diseases gave slow viruses such as HIV the time to grow, and that modern 20th century life gave slow viruses the conditions they needed to thrive and spread. The virulent strain of an old virus, HIV-1, was, therefore, more easily transmitted because of less restricted sexual behavior, high-speed travel, widespread use of transfusions and blood products, and increased use of intravenous drugs.

Social history and medical history converged to make some slow virus pandemic highly probable. HIV-1 was the first to take advantage of those conditions. The description, transmission, and spread of the slow viruses is a new field, with information growing and changing in response to the growing and changing dangers to human health.

Both Shilts's book and Grmek's book point to HIV disease as a moving progression of information and developments that will be difficult to keep abreast of, and that will require constant updating and changing. That can be disconcerting for anyone, but particularly for health care professionals who are looked to as experts and problem-solvers. It is also difficult for patients because they erroneously want and expect certainty from professionals. It is difficult for professionals because they cannot give that guarantee or firm prediction and because they can feel threatened by the possibilities of mistakes. At the same time, it is challenging and exciting, as more and more is learned about a new disease, and it is gratifying when new interventions become possible and help can be given. It is also really possible to stay abreast, as a good ship can successfully ride the waves.

**TABLE 5-A**
**A Summary of Shilts's History of HIV Disease**

| 1976 | Kinshasa, Zaire | Scandinavian surgeon develops AIDS but is not diagnosed; 39 nurses, 2 doctors die of Ebola fever. |
|------|-----------------|-----------------------------------------------------|
| 1980 | San Francisco | Conference of gay physicians notes extreme rise in venereal diseases, Hepatitis B, enteric diseases, CMV and Epstein-Barr viruses; and beginnings of immune problems such as Kaposi's sarcoma (KS). |

| 1980 | Fire Island | Increase in KS, enteric and wasting diseases, toxoplasmosis, PCP and candidiasis in gay community. |
|------|-------------|--------------------------------------------------|
| 1980 | Kinshasa | Cases of cryptococcus in General Hospital. |
| 1980 | Paris | Reports of PCP, toxoplasmosis, aggressive KS in Central Africa. |
| 1980 | United States | Physician tests T-cells of young male patient with PCP and candidiasis, finds no helper cells. |
| | | 55 young men diagnosed with opportunistic infections in US; |
| | | 10 young men diagnosed with opportunistic infections in Europe. |
| 1981 | United States | Physicians see CMV and PCP pattern. |
| | | In New York City, Haitian patient diagnosed with candidiasis and tuberculosis; also patient diagnosed with drug addiction and PCP. |
| | | CDC fills 4 orders for pentamidine in 8 weeks. |
| | | CDC is informed of KS in San Francisco. |
| | | In June, CDC's MMWR publishes the first report of an epidemic of PCP. |
| | | CDC virologist postulates a retrovirus may be involved, with a long incubation period. |
| | | In Toronto, Gaetan Dugas contacts NYU about his illness, but continues his sexual practices. |
| | | CDC interviews all PCP patients and one physician thinks Hepatitis B may be a model for this new disease, suggesting looking for PCP in hemophiliacs. |
| | | National Cancer Institute test of 15 apparently healthy gay men shows that half have abnormal immune systems. |
| | | University of California at San Francisco has a young baby with immune dysfunction who had transfusions for Rh factor, and the 47 year old blood donor has lymphadenopathy and retina problems. |
| | | Albert Einstein Medical School, pediatric cases from 1979 of immune deficiency are confirmed. Drug addict mother with symptoms has child with symptoms, but the American Academy of Pediatrics refuses paper for a conference presentation. |
| | | CDC physician feels blood banks should be put on alert. |
| 1981 | United States | New York City gay community attacks writer Larry Kramer (also a member of the gay community) for homophobia and anti-eroticism. |

| 1982 | United States | Elderly hemophiliac dies of PCP. |
| | | New York's St. Luke's hospital tests gay men, finds 4 of 5 have serious depletion of T-helper cells. |
| | | Haitians continue to be diagnosed with toxoplasmosis in increasing numbers; drug addicts diagnosed with PCP. |
| | | Physician diagnoses an infant with AIDS contracted through transfusions. |
| | | AIDS is rampant among New Jersey addicts, and there are dozens of New Jersey pediatric AIDS cases. |
| | | CDC holds press conference on MMWR transfusion case. |
| | | Gaetan Dugas still goes to gay bath houses for sex. |
| | | Gay leaders oppose criticizing promiscuity. |
| Jan. 4 1983 | United States | Heads of blood banks oppose screening; FDA does not act. |
| | | For-profit blood banks begin screening because Hemophilia Association is demanding it. |
| March 3 1983 | United States | U.S. Public Health Service requests risk groups to refrain from blood donation. |
| March 4 1983 | United States | Guidelines on screening blood donors. |
| March 7 1983 | United States | Larry Kramer's article published on AIDS deaths, "1,112 and Counting." |
| | | Physician at NYU AIDS Conference claims transfusion evidence is lacking, inferential. |
| | | San Francisco epidemiology study suppressed by gay leaders. |
| | | Pasteur Institute publishes finding possible virus as cause. |
| March 1983 | United States | Belgium reports outbreak of AIDS in Rwanda and Zaire. |
| | | Lancet documents the Danish Surgeon case as an AIDS case. |
| | | Stanford begins doing helper-suppressor screening of donors. |
| | | Dr. Silverman (SF Public Health Director) opposes closing bathhouses or requiring posted warnings for tourists during the Gay Freedom Day Parade. Mayor insists warnings be posted. |

| March 1983 | United States | Dr. Montagnier learns his virus isn't an HTLV and is told about lentiviruses in animals. |
| | | A grandmother transfused in 1980 dies of AIDS. |
| | | First case of AIDS in the wife of a hemophiliac. |
| | | At the Cold Springs Harbor AIDS Conference, Dr. Montagnier is moved to the end of the schedule, Dr. Gallo is given prominence for the virus being an HTLV (HTLV-III). |
| | | Statistician figures incubation period of virus: 6 months to 11 years. |
| March 1984 | United States | San Francisco blood banks begin testing. |
| | | Antibody testing shows HIV arrives in San Francisco about 1976–1977. |
| | | Pasteur Institute tests in Zaire, finds 250 cases of AIDS per million, compared to 16 per million in U.S. |
| March 1984 | United States | Dr. Essex's theory: HIV was dormant in a small area of Central Africa for thousands of years, then moved to cities during modern migration, then to Europe and Haiti, then to U.S. |
| Oct. 9 1984 | San Francisco | Dr. Silverman has press conference to close San Francisco bathhouses. SF AIDS Foundation objects. By now, 2/3 of the San Francisco men who later became HIV positive were already infected with the virus. |
| 1985 | United States | Army researcher documents heterosexual transmission |
| | | Physician reveals 2 cases in San Francisco prostitutes. |
| | | Lambda Legal Defense Fund threatens to legally block HIV testing over issues of confidentiality. |
| | | Alternate test sites are funded. |
| | | San Francisco Irwin Memorial Blood Bank gets its first HIV test kits. |
| March 1985 | United States | New York City Health Commissioner orders that no lab in the city can do the HIV tests, except for research purposes. |
| | | A random sample of Parisians finds 1 in 200 are HIV positive and estimates hospitals are infecting 50 Parisians a week through blood transfusions. Blood banks in France require blood testing after the study is reported. |
| April 1985 | United States | Dr. Francis is called a fascist for recommending voluntary HIV testing. |

| April 1985 | United States | HIV incubation data finally made public. |
| July 30, 1985 | 'United States | Rock Hudson's AIDS made public. |
| 1986 | United States | Dr. C. Everett Koop, Surgeon General, asked to prepare a report on AIDS. |
| 1987 | United States | Dr. Francis goes to WHO to research African AIDS |

## A YEAR IN THE LIFE OF HIV DISEASE
## JANUARY 1991 THROUGH DECEMBER 1991

As this book was being prepared, continuing research constantly expanded our knowledge of HIV disease and reinforced what some AIDS experts have observed, that some information abut HIV is out of date six months after it is published. For that reason, we want to give the reader a sense of what was happening in the field of HIV during a specific period of time, a slice of HIV knowledge from January through December 1991. The reader can compare changes and additions since that time, and get a full grasp of the importance of staying abreast of knowledge of HIV disease.

**TABLE 5-B**
**A Year in the Life of HIV Disease: January, 1991 Through December, 1991**

| | |
|---|---|
| Jan. 1991 | The CDC reports possible HIV transmission during dental procedures to two other patients of Dr. Acer. Previous disbelief among dentists of such transmission (Aug–Sept 1990 survey) begins to moderate. |
| | In New York City, AIDS becomes the leading cause of death for women aged 20–40. |
| | Administrators of Johns Hopkins Hospital advised 2,000 women patients that a well-known breast cancer specialist, Dr. Rudolph Almaraz, who treated them, had died of AIDS. |
| March 1991 | Medical ethicist says this is not time for an AIDS backlash.[3] |
| | The CDC is dismayed that, in spite of an educational campaign about the risks of multiple partners, the number of sexually active teenage women continues to climb. |
| | Researchers at the Institut Pasteur confer partial protection against HIV for up to 6 months in vaccinated chimps using gp 120 antigen, followed by injections with peptides. The chimps were challenged with repeated injections of pure virus. It remains to be shown whether the vaccine would give protection against injections of infected cells or infection through the genital route.[4] |
| | Dr. Alfred Sabin questions vaccine testing with only free virus. Chimps and monkeys need to be challenged with infected cells as well, to test for lasting immunity. |

Dr. Shyh-Ching Lo reports that coinfection with *mycoplasma fermentans* enhances the ability of HIV-1 to cause cytopathic effects on T-cells, a coinfecton may be involved in the development of AIDS.[5]

April 1991   The projections made by WHO's Delphi projection (15–20 million infected by 1999) will be reached by mid-1990.[6]

So far, HIV appears not to have taken hold in a significant way in Eastern Europe. North Africa and the Middle East are relatively unaffected.

In Western Europe and the U.S., AIDS seems to be spreading primarily in certain sub-populations.

U.S. State Department's interagency working group on AIDS predicts by the year 2015, overall infection rates in urban areas in Africa will be 16 percent, infection rates in adults in their 30s will be 40 percent, and sub-Saharan African population could be reduced by as much as 50 million by the AIDS epidemic.

Nearly half of African AIDS patients have active tuberculosis.

WHO's James Chin says that with all the uncertainties about the way HIV is transmitted, predicting more than five years into the future about AIDS is very tricky.[6]

U.S. Agency for International Development spends $80 million on AIDS prevention education this year, but Jeff Harris says it's a drop in the bucket compared to what's needed to have a major impact on the HIV epidemic spread.[6]

Condom use in Kinshasa, Zaire has reached 8–10 percent of adult males.[6]

15–20 percent of the African workforce could die of AIDS. There could be 10 million orphans in the next decade.[6]

Dr. Michael Merson of WHO estimates 8–10 million individuals worldwide are HIV +. In sub-Saharan Africa, there are 700,000 AIDS cases and 6 million adults with the virus. Also, 500,000 infants are infected. Dr. James Curran of the CDC calls the estimated number of people infected with HIV "very frightening." There are an estimated 500,000 people HIV + in Asia and Southeast Asia, most in India and Thailand, and these are conservative estimates. Thai health officials estimate the number of infections between 200,000–300,000 in Thailand alone. In large Indian cities such as Bombay and Madras, HIV is increasing among prostitutes, with prevalence as high as 20 percent.[6]

WHO reports some of the highest rates of HIV infection are found in the Caribbean. In Haiti, one in 10 pregnant women is HIV +. PAHO estimates one million Latin Americans are HIV +. Dr. William Blattner of the NCI notes infection rates in Jamaica and Trinidad, despite "very informed and appropriate" approaches to education and intervention, are shooting up: "One is faced with the reality to my mind that we can't hold this problem in check with just prevention campaigns. There's an urgent need for an effective vaccine, and we're not there yet."[6]

| | |
|---|---|
| April 1991 | Using saliva to test for HIV has many advantages and is reliable.[7] |
| April 1991 through July 1991 | More than 170,000 individuals had been reported to the CDC as having AIDS. Reconstruction and future trends of AIDS in the U.S. indicate AIDS may plateau during the next five years. The number of individuals with advanced HIV disease is expected to increase 40 percent by 1995. Demands on the U.S. health care system will remain enormous.[8] |

French researcher stops the testing of a vaccinia virus vaccine for HIV after adverse reactions to vaccinia.

|  |  |
|---|---|
| May 1991 | There are several protocols testing new antibiotics to prevent MAI infection. |

Candida esophagitis is the most common AIDS-defining diagnosis in women. Other opportunistic infections are candida vaginitis, squamous intraepithelial neoplasia caused by HPV (papilloma virus), cervical disease, pelvic inflammatory disease, genital ulcers (may be a primary manifestation of HIV), other STDs. The burden of HIV disease is shifting away from white males to minority women.[9]

Martin Van Der Maaten of the Agriculture Department's National Animal Disease Center reports a relative of HIV in U.S. cattle, but says it does not pose a threat to human health. Researchers do not know how bovine immunodeficiency virus (BIV)—four percent of Southern and Southwest cattle are positive—is spread, although Van Der Maaten says it may be transmitted through blood, perhaps insect vectors, or during minor surgical procedures and vaccinations. Several government studies on BIV done by him and colleagues were released by Jeremy Rifkin. HIV and BIV are members of the lentivirus family which includes Feline and Simian immunodeficiency viruses.

|  |  |
|---|---|
| June 1991 | Drs. Robert Gallo and Mikulas Popovic, who gave the first molecular characterization of HIV, receive the report of NIH's Office of Scientific Integrity on its investigation of their possible scientific misconduct. |

Barbara Webb, 65, a former Florida high school teacher of the year, is crusading nationally for mandatory HIV testing for health professionals. Lawyers for the estate of dentist Dr. David Acer asked for a gag order because of lawsuits filed by Webb and another patient, Richard Driskill, against Dr. Acer for transmitting HIV to them. Webb said she will continue giving interviews.

Long Island Dentist Philip Feldman dies of AIDS. Two former employees charge he rarely used protective gloves or a mask because he thought people were paranoid and it was ridiculous to put on gloves, and that his instruments were not sterilized properly. His assistants are angry because he denied having HIV disease, although he knew since 1985. He told them he had tested negative. Scores of his patients called the NYS Health Department special hotline.

June 1991   University of Texas students were tested anonymously for HIV (one percent were positive) as part of the first nationwide attempt to determine HIV infection rate for U.S. college students. There was a fivefold increase over a 1988 study.

CDC cumulative totals of AIDS cases:

Adults/Adolescents = 179,694
Male = 161,493
Female = 18,201
Pediatric = 3,140

July 1991   AIDS prevention researchers in San Francisco are alarmed because two studies report young gay men are engaging in high-risk sexual activities that could produce a new surge of HIV infections.[10]

Canadian scientists develop a PCR test for newborns that can use routine heelstick samples on filter paper and detect HIV as early as 1 week after birth.

Dr. Albert Lowenfels reports that the risk of a known HIV+ surgeon infecting a patient is one in 48,000.

The Seventh International AIDS Conference was held in Florence, Italy.

The Eighth International Conference on AIDS was cancelled for Boston next May because of threats of violence by AIDS activists over a compromise to lift travel restrictions but not immigration restrictions.

An underground needle exchange program for IV drug users in San Francisco is helping to prevent the spread of HIV without promoting drug use.[11]

A very promising new drug for AIDS, RO 24-7429, will not be developed by its owner, Hoffman-La Roche. The company is trying to license it to another company. It will focus on DDC and an anti-HIV-protease drug further along the development pipeline. The antiviral AIDS drugs that companies have in the pipeline are ddI, DDC, Fluorothymidine, 4 (which are all Nucleoside Reverse Transcriptase Inhibitors), Azidothymidine, L-Drugs, BI-R6-587, TIBO (which are all Non-Nucleoside), Protease Inhibitors, Myristoylation Inhibitors, "Uniroyal Jr.", Hypericin and CD4-PE 40.

The most consistent estimates of the probability of conversion to AIDS after seropositivity are: 0.02 within two years of conversion, 0.25-0.35 within seven years, and 0.50 within 10 years.[8]

Therapies may lengthen the incubation period. Estimated cumulative HIV infections in the U.S. by April 1990 was within a plausible range of 850,000–1,205,000.

July 1991    Dr. Albert Sabin, at an International workshop on the Classification of Guillain-Barre Syndrome (GBS) said there has been thousands of cases of "acute flaccid paralysis" in Latin America in the last three years. Almost none of 7,000 cases of this puzzling condition reported to the Pan American Health Organization from 1987–1990 are polio. Hundreds of cases of a crippling and paralyzing disease in Northern China also are not classic polio. A diagnosis of GBS is also not confirmed. The Chinese government invited Dr. Guy McKhann and his Johns Hopkins colleagues to examine 40 children. They found the disease was not GBS, but something medically new.[12]

A San Francisco Study says the risk of getting AIDS from blood transfusions, whose testing for seroconversion misses those infected who haven't seroconverted but are infected, is one in 61,171.

The CDC says as many as 128 Americans have been infected with HIV by their dentists or surgeons, based on statistical formulas comparing the number of HIV+ dentists and surgeons to the number of invasive procedures: 1. Estimated 1,248 dentists HIV+ may have infected between 10 and 100 patients during tooth extractions, oral surgery or other procedure during the 10 year-old AIDS epidemic. 2. Estimated 336 HIV+ surgeons may have infected 3–28 surgery patients.

Dr. Harold Jaffe, CDC, identifies the dental handpiece as the possible source of blood contamination and HIV transmission. David Lewis' study shows that internal parts of the dental handpiece can be coated with blood, saliva and tooth fragments. Lewis says the pieces should be heat-sterilized.

The U.S. Senate voted 81 to 18 to impose prison terms and fines on HIV+ health care workers who do invasive procedures without telling patients they are HIV+. The Senate also passed, 99–0, a measure to lead to HIV testing for all health care workers. AIDS activists reacted strongly, calling it an absolute outrage.

Dr. Neal Rzepkowski, an emergency room physician who practiced for 6 years after testing HIV+, revealed his HIV status but says he didn't infect any patients. The president of Brooks Memorial Hospital in Dunkirk, New York, said there is almost no chance Dr. Rzepkowski infected any of the 4,100 patients he treated there. Four hospitals where Dr. Rzepkowski worked sent letters to patients informing them. Dr. Rzepkowski said he learned in 1985 that he was HIV+ but continued practicing because he knew it was unlikely he would infect anyone. Hospitals fielded hundreds of calls from worried patients and set up special hotlines. One Buffalo hospital received 300 calls in 24 hours.

July 1991  Kimberly Bergalis, the first patient of Dr. Acer's who developed AIDS and the case that pointed to dentist-to-patient transmission, says in what may be her last public words "Who do I blame? Do I blame myself? I sure don't. I never used IV drugs, never slept with anyone, and never had a blood transfusion. I blame Dr. Acer and every single one of those bastards. Anyone who knew Dr. Acer was infected and had full-blown AIDS and stood by not doing a damn thing about it. You are just as guilty as he was. You've ruined my life and my family's."

The CDC issued new guidelines for health care workers shortly before Dr. Rzepkowski took a leave. The guidelines recommend that HIV+ health care workers not perform "exposure-prone" procedures unless they inform patients and receive permission from a panel of medical experts.

Dr. Feldman's patients experience fear, discrimination, and family stress. One mother of a five-year-old won't treat a sore on his foot for fear she'll infect him. She's afraid to touch her son. An industrial hygienist says his friends have fled. They don't even telephone. A father won't allow his daughter to kiss him on the lips until his test results come back.

Patients felt better after talking to a counselor at two special clinics set up by the NYSDOH, but said their fears soon returned. 650 went to the clinics. Many had dreams about AIDS and all worried about infecting people they love. Gail Strouse files a class-action suit against the dentist's estate, saying: "Sometimes I lie in bed and think stupid things like I shouldn't have sex because it's bad enough the twins will lose me at an early age. But if I give it to him, they'll lose him as well. I firmly believe I don't have it, but I don't know."

Although the CD4 molecule is the principle cell receptor for HIV, several cell lines without CD4 (nervous system, liver) can be infected by HIV. These findings indicate there are different modes of virus entry, galactosyl ceramide being one[13]

August 1990  AIDS is the leading cause of adult death in the West African City of Abidjan, Ivory Coast. From a study of the city's two largest morgues, 41 percent of males and 32 percent of females had been HIV+. 15 percent of adult male and 13 percent of adult female annual deaths are due to AIDS. The first AIDS cases were recognized in 1985.[14]

August 1990–1991  In South Africa, the number of HIV+ cases is doubling every 8 1/2 months. WHO estimates that 180,000 blacks in South Africa are HIV+ and will increase to 446,000 by 1992. TB is on the rise and sanatoriums that were closed for decades are reopening. It is estimated that three percent of all blacks, five percent of those attending prenatal clinics, 14 percent of mine workers and 17 percent of all males with STD's will carry the virus by the end of 1991. In Zambia, 70 percent of would-be blood donors test positive, 85 percent of Nairobi, Kenya prostitutes are HIV positive, and Zambia's general population may be 20–30 percent HIV positive.[15]

August 1991    Shortly after a person is infected with HIV, the virus reaches the nervous system. University of Pennsylvania scientists claim to have found the gateway—a protein on the surface of specialized nerve cells to which the virus attaches.

AIDS is posing a legal minefield for health care workers.

Dr. Perry Smith, head of AIDS epidemiology for the NYSDOH participates in a special meeting of state health officials, medical specialty associations, hospital groups and other representatives of health workers on developing guidelines for health care workers with HIV.

A majority of physicians and nurses favor mandatory HIV testing of health care workers, a study done by the Agency for Health Care Policy and Research Reports.[16]

Hoffmann-La Roche, after acquiring rights to commercialize PCR technology in 1989 from Cetus Corp., begins to develop PCR as a standard tool for testing and research. It will seek FDA approval for test kits for AIDS in newborns, chlamydia and Lyme disease in 1991.

Fall 1991    The CDC supplies its list of exposure-prone procedures.

Sept. 1991    Researcher Simon Le Vay of the Salk Institute reports that male homosexuals have a smaller area of the hypothalamus, the third interstitial nucleus, than male heterosexuals. The size is identical to that area in female brains.[17]

A committee of physicians appointed by the Red Cross to investigate blood-collection procedures at its Portland Center after FDA inspection found fault with its procedures, said the local blood supply was safe but recommended tightening screening of donors nationwide by using fingerprinting or drivers licenses to confirm donor identities.

British economist Robert Whelan advised his government to cut funding of AIDS research and education, arguing such funding takes money away from other diseases (e.g. heart disease and cancer) from which a much greater number of people die. He recommended an 80% cut.[18]

The drug 3 Thiocytidine (3TC) has been approved for clinical trials in Canada and the U.S.

U.S. President George Bush, at a press conference, called for behavior change to halt HIV infection and contrasted AIDS with cancer, which he said did not involve behavior choices.

The New York State AIDS Institute adds a teaching module on Tuberculosis to its AIDS education and prevention training.

The government of Uganda, which has the highest number of reported AIDS cases in Africa, ordered state-run media to stop announcements about condoms and their use in preventing AIDS. Islamic and Christian leaders argue that promoting condom use encourages promiscuity.

Sept. 1991 The congressional panel which had invited Kimberly Bergalis to testify about her infection with HIV by Dr. Acer postpones the hearing date. Miss Bergalis, who is near death, is described by her father and another HIV-infected patient of Dr. Acer's as having stayed alive for the hearing. Her family is furious about what they call AIDS politics and say they will no longer allow her to testify, even if she is alive by the date of the new hearing.

The only member of the president's advisory commission who had AIDS (contracted from a blood transfusion) died. She was 33.

Kimberly Bergalis does finally testify before congress at the end of September for 30 seconds.

A new hepatitis which can destroy a healthy person's liver in a matter of days, fulminant liver failure (FLF) is identified and linked to either a paramyxovirus or togavirus.

Oct. 1991 Two studies presented at the American Society for Microbiology reported an alarming and sharp increase in HIV infection among poor adolescents. Blood samples taken from adolescents in the emergency room of Washington Children's Hospital showed an HIV infection rate of .4 percent in 1987, rising to 1.3 percent in 1991. Blood tests done on U.S. Job Corps. recruits showed the rate of infection in females had doubled from 1988 to 1990.

Oct. 4, 1991 The governor of Illinois signed the most sweeping AIDS notification law, requiring health care providers who are HIV+ to inform patients who have undergone invasive procedures that they are at risk, or the state will so notify. Patients who are HIV+ must also notify health care providers who may have been exposed. The AIDS Foundation of Chicago and the Illinois ACLU oppose the law.

Oct. 8, 1991 The New York State Department of Health recommended against testing health care workers for HIV and against limiting the practice of all infected doctors and dentists, putting state officials at odds with the Centers for Disease Control recommendations on universal restrictions.

Oct. 9, 1991 The FDA approves ddI.

Oct. 1991 The American Dental Association voted to oppose mandatory HIV testing of health care workers.

Michel Lucans, inspector general of health affairs for France, reported that in 1985 health authorities knowingly authorized transfusions of HIV-contaminated blood, and delayed requiring heat treatment or screening for blood products used by hemophiliacs. The French Association of Hemophiliacs estimates that 1,200 of 3,500 hemophiliacs in France carry HIV and 200 have died of AIDS. On Oct. 22, Dr. Michel Garretta, former director of the National Blood Transfusion Center, was criminally charged with failing to warn recipients about blood products he knew were contaminated with HIV during the years 1984 and 1985.

Nov. 1991    A Buffalo TV station reported that a children's hospital anesthesiologist died of AIDS. The hospital set up a special telephone line to answer questions from parents and patients.

Nov. 3, 1991    New York State joins Florida, Maine, Michigan, Montana, Oklahoma, Rhode Island and others who require testing of potential donors of skin, corneas, heart valves, tendons and other nonvital human tissue for HIV before transplantation. The state Health Department issued emergency regulations to hospitals and independent companies that deal in body parts or operate human tissue banks. This adds tissue banks to regulations already governing semen, breast-milk, bone-marrow banks, and whole organs like hearts, livers and kidneys.

Nov. 5, 1991    The CDC holds a special session to develop a specific list of "exposure-prone" procedures that health care professionals who have HIV infection should refrain from doing. The American Dental Association opposes such a list, preferring "universal precautions" education, but the American Medical Association is willing to be part of the process. The American College of Surgeons opposes the CDC guidelines because the risk to patients seems very low, not justifying costly responses such as mandatory testing and limiting procedures.

Nov. 1991    A study by the Amsterdam Municipal Public Health Service (1985 to present) of 359 intravenous drug users found that free needle exchange and free methadone maintenance may slow HIV infection but does not prevent the spread of HIV. After five years, 33 subjects (10 percent) are now HIV positive.

A survey finds that six percent of Thailand's military recruits are HIV positive. In India, 10 percent of men attending STD clinics are HIV positive and other surveys indicate HIV is spreading rapidly and is larger than the epidemic in Thailand. Myanmar (Burma) is becoming severely infected and the Philippines and Indonesia may be next.

WHO recently estimated there may be 250 million new cases of STDs by all pathogens worldwide this year, showing the continuing potential for HIV spread.

Nov. 7, 1991    Basketball superstar Magic Johnson tests positive for HIV and will end his career on advice of his physicians, announcing his retirement during a press conference today.

Nov. 13, 1991    The 44th Annual Meeting of the American Association of Blood Banks discussed ways of protecting the blood supply and blood banks are preparing to use a new combination test for HIV-1 and HIV-2.

Veterans of the Persian Gulf War were requested not to donate blood because of possible infection with *Leichmania tropica* during their tour of duty. This is a precautionary move since health officials are not sure the disease is transmitted through blood transfusions.

Nov. 18, 1991    New York State begins testing all prison inmates and employees for TB to try to stop the spread of the resistant TB strain which has killed 13 prisoners and 1 prison guard. All the inmates who died were HIV positive, and the guard had cancer. Officials hope to test the 90,000 prisoners and employees by the end of the year. Employees are being tested first because of risk of spread to the community. There were 84 confirmed cases of active TB (infectious) in the prison system this year with 34 deaths, 13 of those from the drug-resistant strain. The State Health Department will track all infectious individuals and isolate them, but although some state prisons have isolation rooms that are pressurized and equipped with air filters and germicidal lights, not all meet the Department's standards. Although there is a strong TB/HIV link, state law prohibits mandatory mass screening. TB has increased 31 percent in New York from 1989–1990; 38 percent from 1990–1991. In New York City, one in four TB cases are caused by the drug-resistant strain, with a mortality rate of 72–89 percent.

Nov. 19, 1991    Dr. Kevin de Cock, head of an AIDS program in Ivory Coast, Africa, says: "AIDS is winning."

Nov. 1991    Magic Johnson accepts appointment to the President's National Commission on AIDS.

Dec. 1991    By the end of the year, AIDS will be the 5th leading cause of death among women of reproductive age in the U.S.[19]

In 1991, AIDS research accounts for 9.7 percent of NIH's $8.3 billion budget.

The CDC abandons plans to list medical and dental procedures that HIV-infected health care professionals should not perform. Instead, the CDC proposes general recommendations and case-by-case decisions to evaluate whether such professionals could safely perform the procedure.

A Gallup Youth Survey conducted since "Magic" Johnson announced he was HIV+ showed teenage awareness that AIDS can be contracted from heterosexual sex, rose from 94 percent to 97 percent, and from homosexual sex from 89 percent to 93 percent. However, behavior change was mixed, with 23 percent saying they have changed behavior, 11 percent thinking about changing, 11 percent saying behavior had not changed, and 55 percent saying they did not need to change.

Dec. 3, 1991    Drug-resistant strains of TB, concentrated among HIV+ individuals, continue to spread in many states of the U.S., with 50 workers infected at one New York hospital. The CDC says there are serious deficiencies in hospital procedures and public policies for control of TB.

Dec. 8, 1991    Kimberly Bergalis, the first documented case of HIV infection of a patient by a health care professional, died this morning of AIDS. She was 23 years old.

Dec. 15, 1991   Nigerians are beginning to talk more openly about birth control and AIDS, touching traditional views about women, privacy, sexuality and responsibility. Announcements on TV about condom use are carried after 10 p.m. Health minister, Olikoye Ransome-Kuti has begun a public education and counseling campaign, but because of a belief that homosexuality occurs only in the western world, his program has not addressed homosexuals. Approximately 600,000 Nigerians are estimated to be HIV + .[20]

Dec. 18, 1991   Carmelo Beltran died of AIDS after years of serving as an AIDS educator, and working with outreach programs to the Hispanic community, the urban churches, substance abuse community, and the Rochester community at large. He was also a major educational contributor to our AIDS Training Program.

Dec. 31, 1991   The CDC plans to change its AIDS case definition by January 1, 1992, were postponed to April 1, 1992. The change will add to the existing definition all HIV-infected individuals whose CD4 cells fall below 200/cubic mm. This addition will triple the current number of U.S. AIDS cases. The CD4 test may not be available to developing countries by that time.

## NEW DISEASE AND NEW INFORMATION

There is a natural process to the accumulation of understanding about a new disease. Health care professionals can expect three typical steps in this process:

1. *Some data and conclusions will be confirmed over time.* For example, there is now no argument that HIV can be transmitted through blood and other body cells. We know part of the mechanism involved in the virus entering cell lines, integrating into the cell DNA, replicating itself, and killing the cell. We are beginning to learn about the latency of the virus and what might trigger the eventual development of AIDS. We have recognized AIDS dementia as primary. Early treatment does improve health and prolong survival.

2. *Although some conclusions will prove correct over time, others will be demonstrated to be inaccurate or false.* HIV was not a member of the HTLV family of viruses. AIDS was more than a gay plague. HIV could be transmitted through medical procedures, from blood transfusions to organ transplantation to dental extractions, and Kimberly Bergalis did not lie about how she became infected.

3. *There will be unpleasant surprises.* New diseases have a way of giving us nasty surprises, particularly when we try to achieve premature closure or base consensus on assumptions. AIDS dementia was such an unpleasant surprise, although it shouldn't have been. Pediatric AIDS was a tragic surprise, and shouldn't have been. There will be more such surprises before the course of HIV disease is run, such as the

report of the Eighth International Conference on AIDS, that an AIDS-like illness, for which patients test HIV-1, HIV-2 negative has been known by the CDC since 1989. Health care professionals should be aware of the defensive reactions that this process will generate, so they can help themselves and their patients or clients understand and cope with these natural developmental steps of any new disease. This is not HIV disease-specific. If the new pediatric paralysis illness now found in Latin America and China (described in Table 5-B) turns out to be a new infectious disease, this same process will be repeated with it, as it will with every new disease.[12]

### Typical Defensive Responses

Health care professionals will be able to recognize some typical defensive mechanisms in themselves, patients, other experts, and the general public:

*"Kill the Messenger."* When the Kimberly Bergalis case delivered new data to the CDC, it represented troubling information and a message no one wanted to hear—that HIV might be transmitted iatrogenically more easily than had been thought. At first, Miss Bergalis' statement that she had never had sexual intercourse was treated skeptically, partly as scientific skepticism, but also partly as a firm conviction that all persons who fell into an "Other" category of HIV transmission were really concealing the risk-behaviors that transmit HIV. Miss Bergalis' two boyfriends were tested; even her father was tested, she claimed, to rule out the possibility of incest.

The firm assumption that HIV + persons must be lying when they deny homosexuality, injection drug use, or multiple sex partners can make it difficult for such individuals to report their infection and contributes to the self-protective secrecy surrounding HIV disease. No one readily accepts having his or her truthfulness and integrity doubted and many would be traumatized to have their sexual behaviors depicted in the way Miss Bergalis' behaviors were. Not only was she ill with HIV disease, but now she had the added burden of being publicly depicted in hurtful ways. Even when tests showed that her dentist was the probable source of infection, and even when four other patients were shown to have been infected by the same dentist, the anger directed at the bearer of bad news was apparent.

Good people who had dealt compassionately with many AIDS patients, who had been active in gaining public support and sympathy for AIDS patients, still reacted with hostility to Kimberly Bergalis for being the messenger with bad news. They resented her public appearances and the public support she received. They felt too much attention was being given to this young woman and that too much was being made of her illness when there were so many ill people (read: she doesn't need compassion and care; only typical AIDS patients do). Such anger can be understood only as a product of our fear at hearing the message that a health care provider with AIDS had infected, in ways we did not anticipate, five of his patients.

The dentist, Dr. Acer, himself came under posthumous attack as an expression of this same mechanism. Rather than believe or conclude that recommended CDC universal precautions might not be sufficient to prevent transmission, and noting that no such other multiple transmissions from health care workers had been documented, some experts began suggesting that Dr. Acer may have deliberately infected his patients.[21] There is no evidence that he was negligent in using precautions, and certainly no evidence that he deliberately injected virus into his patients. The possibility cannot be absolutely ruled out, since no possibility can be absolutely ruled out, but the CDC final report confirms Dr. Acer's then-adequate infection control measures. The public speculation that he chose to infect his patients is a "kill the messenger" response that could lead to even more devastating conclusions than attributing infection to a failure of universal precautions. Any HIV+ health care worker could then be seen as a person who could choose to infect patients or clients with HIV, either because of malice and anger, or because of AIDS dementia's early effects.

The same mechanism occurred early in the AIDS epidemic, when members of the gay community tried to bring the message of a lethal disease spreading quietly through gay communities in New York City and San Francisco. That terrifying message generated the same anger at the messengers that happened with Miss Bergalis. Those who tried to carry the message were accused of homophobia, antieroticism, or disloyalty by their own community's newspapers.[1]

The same mechanism also operated among health care professionals. When Dr. Neal Rzepkowski, an emergency room physician in Upstate New York, revealed that he had continued to practice for six years after learning that he was HIV+, patients of the hospitals in which he worked became very concerned and anxious. Free testing was offered to all patients who wished it, but any patients who tested positive and became messengers of unwanted and troubling information were at risk for the "kill the messenger" response. A Chautauqua County health official was quoted by the press as saying that tests on all Dr. Rzepkowski's patients might well turn up some people with HIV infection, but this would not necessarily mean the infection came from the physician. This, in fact, is technically true, but any patient who tested positive would have not only the terrible burden of a positive HIV test, but the burden of proof to show they had not become infected through socially unacceptable behaviors such as injection drug use or promiscuity.

There are two main dangers with this defensive mechanism. It can impede the communication of very important information, which in HIV disease can mean further spread of infection and death. It can also impede compassion and the cohesion of the human community, which in HIV disease means withholding the support that ill individuals need.

*"Cling to Conventional Wisdom."* Conventional or common wisdom may be comforting, and therapists know how uncomfortable individuals can feel about uncertainty and ambiguity. However, conventional wisdom is often not wise, and holding too closely to a current consensus may bring a false sense of security or control. HIV disease has a history of such clinging to what should not really be seen as certain. Shortly before HIV disease became known, the common wisdom among experts was that human retroviruses did not cause disease. Dr. Robert Gallo questioned the wisdom of that consensus and his research showed that the retrovirus, HTLV-I, did in fact cause leukemia. Unfortunately, he did not continue to question expert wisdom about the AIDS virus. If he had, he might not have convinced American researchers that the AIDS virus was yet another human T-lymphocyte virus, HTLV-III, thus inadvertently setting American research off in the wrong direction. The French researchers, however, not committed to the HTLV consensus as Gallo was, looked at other possible virus families and found the lentivirus that finally became known as HIV.

For all the pediatric clinicians who kept trying to point to the infants and children who were dying of an acquired immune deficiency, conventional wisdom must have been especially frustrating. Conventional wisdom assumed, without any reliable hypotheses, that babies and children could not get AIDS, since it was transmitted only through sexual intercourse, and that pediatric cases must be the genetic form of immune deficiency. Few, as a result, attended to the risks to children that HIV disease presented. Conventional wisdom may be comforting in the short term, but its consequences can eventually be devastating. In HIV disease, we should have learned that clinging to such "wisdom" is exactly the wrong thing to do with a new disease, but we keep repeating the mistake of that defense mechanism over and over again. Health care professionals with special understanding of better ways to deal with uncertainty can make an important contribution here, but only if we first deal with it ourselves.

*"Deny the New Data/Deny All Data."* Mental health professionals know the power of denial mechanisms. Denial can have both positive and negative effects; it is important for health care providers to distinguish between the two. Denial is ubiquitous in medical care; it can be found in couples going through genetic counseling, in families trying to protect the family system, in individuals with a poor medical prognosis, in young homosexuals who believe AIDS is a disease of older homosexuals, and in AIDS patients who try to believe in the beneficial effects of unproven methods or alternative "cures."

Probably the most famous denial in the continuing story of HIV disease was that of Gaetan Dugas, the Canadian airline steward who is sometimes called Patient Zero, although there really were many anonymous Patient Zeros in the beginning of the AIDS epidemic in the U.S.[1] Dugas developed Kaposi's Sarcoma but refused to believe he would die of "gay cancer," until the very end. In his ambivalence and denial, he alternately both accepted and refused to accept that this "gay cancer" could be spread by sexual activities. He used the essential probability of scientific evidence to rationalize that even medical scientists had not absolutely proved that sexual behaviors spread "gay cancer." This allowed him to continue his sexual activities with multiple and often anonymous sexual partners across the country, including frequent visits to gay bathhouses He kept insisting, at times, that this disease was not transmitted through sex. Concurrently, he is reported to have said to sexual partners after sex that he had gay cancer and now they did too.[1]

These inconsistencies are typical of denial mechanisms. Denial is difficult to maintain, so the fragmenting of information and beliefs easily occurs, and an integrated view of reality may not be possible. Denial is easier to maintain with a new disease, since information is constantly changing and some previous conclusions will prove to be wrong. With a new infectious disease, denial can pose some benefit or some risk to the individual who needs to use this mechanism, but it will also pose health risk for the wider community. From a public health perspective, such denial could be seen as a defense mechanism that needs to be confronted and changed. From the perspective of an individual health care provider, the decision whether to confront denial is more problematic.

It is easier, however, to examine the patient's defenses than to consider one's own defenses. The health care provider is not immune from the need for defenses or from applying denial to HIV disease. Revising one's opinion and accepting new data can be difficult and uncomfortable. It is more comfortable, for example, to deny the probability that health care workers could transmit HIV to their patients in "exposure-prone procedures" (the CDC term). Many professionals during the Dr. Acer investigation (the Bergalis dentist), the Dr. Feldman report (the Long Island dentist), or the Dr. Rzepkowski report (the emergency room physician in Upstate New York) used the same mechanism as Gaetan Dugas. They characterized scientific fact as needing to be absolutely proved, refusing to accept high probability as scientific knowledge. They characterized tests developed through biotechnology, which are routine and reasonably standardized, as "experimental" and without sufficient sensitivity and specificity. They used statistics of quite low risk to conclude that therefore there was *no* risk.

A hospital administrator from Upstate New York argued: "The key point is, there is no risk. My own children have been treated in the emergency room in the past year, and I don't even want to know if Dr. Rzepkowski treated them. I'm not worried." Dr. Rzepkowski himself denied any risk to his patients, saying he kept practicing because he knew it was unlikely he would infect anyone, and somehow "unlikely" came to mean "not possible." In this way, denial can involve minimizing the risk or equating minimal risk with no risk.

The spokesman for the New York State Department of Health described Dr. Rzepkowski as very seldom performing invasive procedures. The same spokesman, in describing the Long Island dentist who concealed his AIDS and denied to his staff that he had HIV disease, said there was no evidence that the dentist had transmitted HIV to any of his patients—even though the patients had just been informed and had still not been tested—since nobody had tested positive. Three of the hospitals in whose emergency rooms Dr. Rzepkowski practiced did not notify patients of their potential risk, nor did one hospital where he worked in an outpatient clinic.

Health care professionals, as experts in health science, have a special responsibility to be aware of denial mechanisms on their own part with regard to new data. The protective effect of denial functions for professionals as well as for their patients, but professionals have an obligation to be aware of those needs and to meet them in ways that do not compromise either their expertise or their patients. It always takes time to overcome the resistance that new data can be expected to generate. That is a common phenomenon in science. But in the case of an infectious disease like HIV disease, time is a critical factor in dealing with the problem. It is necessary to stay abreast of accurate and unrestricted research, even when that research is disturbing or violates what we dearly want to believe. This is difficult for all of us. The urgency of HIV disease requires an uncommon effort.

*"Convert to political or moral 'correctness.'"* In an effort to find stability and comforting belief, information about HIV disease (or any new disease or experience) can be politicized or moralized, to the detriment of its accuracy. A politically or morally correct point of view results, which censors information or restricts the flow of certain data. There is usually no unanimity in this "correctness," but there can be either two polarized camps or a power-consensus for one view. Either process can interfere with our understanding of HIV disease and with scientific progress.

Condoms are a good example of the conversion of data into polarized "correct" views. It is perceived by many that religious views about the immorality of condom use or the political standpoint that families, not schools, should control sex education are moral and political statements that may not encompass the realities of HIV disease. The public health concern is that the dangers of spread of HIV are so great to both the individual and the community that health goals may need to take precedence over moral and political beliefs and that a compromise must be reached. When life is at stake, other values may be altered. The descriptive anthropology of sexual behavior also indicates that abstinence outside of marriage, whose practice could be increased with enormous social pressure, will not work in enough contexts to assure public health. The history of syphilis is a good example of the inadequacy of this approach.[22]

However, it is not as generally perceived that the advocacy of condom use and condom availability to all individuals, including dispensing of condoms in schools, is also a politicized and moralized position about HIV infection. In fact, it is the other pole. A great deal of faith has been placed in condoms as the solution that allows safe sex (removing the need for abstinence) and stops the spread of HIV. From this pole, it is politically correct to advocate sex education and condom use with adolescents, with patients, and with residents of third world countries as the effective means of preventing the spread of HIV disease.

The descriptive realities of anthropology, economics, contraception, and virology do not support such political and moral beliefs from this pole either. Condom failure occurs when condoms are used for contraception, so what was originally described as "safe sex" needed to be changed to "safer sex," which means that the probability of HIV infection is reduced but does not approach zero. Condom use is also not consistent, since sexual behavior is rarely as rational as Decision Theory. Again, the probability of infection is reduced, but over time can approach a risk level that informed individuals might be reluctant to take. Condom use in third world countries can be too impractical. The cost of a year's supply is far above the budgets of both individuals and countries. Distribution can be economically and geographically impossible.

Politicizing and moralizing can make it very difficult for health care professionals to evaluate information as it develops, or to avoid receiving only "politically and morally correct" data. So, although this mechanism can give short-term comfort and certainty, it rapidly becomes an impediment to understanding HIV disease. Health care professionals can encounter this problem on a personal level, as the discussion over HIV testing, and specifically testing of health care workers, increases and moves into the political arena. The problem with political correctness is that its position is purely political and does not convey genuine scientific or empirical conclusions. What may be politically "correct" can allow biological disaster; it may certainly interfere with health care professionals being accurate with their patients or clients, or even accessible to new information about HIV disease.

## REALITY TESTING WITH HIV DISEASE: A MODEL FOR DEALING WITH NEW SITUATIONS

What follows will hopefully be a guide and provide practical assistance to health care providers on ways of staying up to date on information about

HIV disease and the means for assessing the reliability of data when one isn't a specialist in neuropsychiatry, virology, epidemiology, immunology, biostatistics, or any of the other fields of knowledge involved in HIV disease.

1. *Approach the informational aspects of HIV disease as a mystery story, with you as the detective.* This may sound cold and unfeeling, and it would be if this method were applied to patients where human interaction should be occurring. But the method is being applied to HIV knowledge, not to people with HIV disease. Such an investigative and probing perspective can give the health care provider access to the knowledge he or she needs to create a strong background from which best to help the patient. Such a perspective will also help you avoid denial and politicizing, and allow you to welcome all the messengers with additional news about HIV disease. It can distance you from preconceived ideas and beliefs. It can make you comfortable with uncertainty and probability, and it can help you appreciate the hard, ongoing task of HIV research.

2. *Do not limit sources of information.* Information about HIV disease comes from multiple sources: Gay Men's Health Crisis, Centers for Disease Control, the U.S. Surgeon General, World Health Organization, National Institute of Allergy and Infectious Diseases, National Cancer Institute, International Coordinating Council on Cancer, NIMH National Demonstration Grants, the American Medical Association, AIDS Educational and Training Centers, plays, films, television hotlines, community agencies, news stories, journals, books (both lay and professional), celebrity spokesmen, AIDS Treatment News, Project Inform, People with HIV/AIDS Action Coalition, Women's AIDS Network, American Psychological Association, American Psychiatric Association, ACT UP, independent researchers, the Pasteur Institute—no list can be exhaustive.

   Not all the information will be consistent. Some will be wrong. Some will disguise other purposes. Some will be preliminary research. Some will come from questionable sources. But no matter what the source, it is very important not to close off any sources of information prematurely. It is better to collect a full range of views before separating out what is valid and what is not. You may feel you are too busy and need just one reliable source, but that narrows your view considerably. Your patients or clients will come in with many things they've heard from sources you've closed off and aren't aware of. It's easier to work with them and their issues if you are at least somewhat aware of the sources of their information.

3. *Consider the reliability of sources from a scientific, not authoritarian, standard, and consider the mission of the information source.* Sources are not infallible authorities, but investigators like you, who have more expertise and experience than you do with HIV disease. But that doesn't

mean they can't be wrong. In fact, public policy agencies or sources identified as official AIDS experts may be too conservative in interpreting new data precisely because they are viewed as authoritative and feel a strong responsibility to have almost absolute certainty before they release information or make an interpretation. Experts speaking for agencies or institutions will be particularly conservative because of their perceived responsibility. Experts speaking for activist groups may select information to advance their particular mission.

Information from unreliable sources in the past is likely to again be unreliable, but need not be. Spread out for yourself the full range of HIV disease information, from least to most reliable, and know why you ranked it that way. Your patients will bring in questions and statements that will not only run the full gamut of your range, but will extend beyond it. If you're prepared, you can talk to them about that wide range and what you've found most reliable for yourself. This will help you keep abreast of your patients or clients, as well as of HIV disease.

4. *Always keep in mind that HIV knowledge is probable, not absolute.* You and your patients may wish it were absolute, certain, but that is not the reality of HIV disease. We know, for example, that the retrovirus HIV is an important factor in the collapse of the immune system, but we're not sure how that occurs. The mechanism of destruction of CD4 cells in itself is not fully understood and may or may not be the full explanation for immune system collapse. Co-factors, once dismissed as not important, are now assuming importance. Other pathogens, such as the retrovirus, human intracisternal virus, may cause illness indistinguishable from AIDS, although the research is still questionable.

5. *Make a referral list of information sources you can access for assistance.* Help is available for health care professionals and a referral list can help you access the specific information you need at a particular time. The following exercise is an abbreviated referral list outline that you can continue to fill in as you build experience with the sources you find especially helpful to you.

**TABLE 5-C**
**Your Resource List for HIV Infection**

---

**LOCAL INFORMATIONAL RESOURCE LIST**

Fill in:

Your local AIDS library

Your local AIDS agency or local community agency

Other local community agencies with HIV+ clients

Your local hospital's infection control expert

Your medical AIDS Center and AIDS Clinic

Your county AIDS agency

Your State AIDS agency

Your regional Education and Training Center (The Health Resources and Services Administration of the U.S. Public Health Service lists sites)

NATIONAL RESOURCE LIST[23]

American Foundation for AIDS Research
1515 Broadway, Suite 3601
New York, NY 10036-8901

Gay Men's Health Crisis
129 W. 20th Street
New York, NY 10011-0022

Project Inform
347 Dolores Street, Suite 301
San Francisco, CA 94110
Hotline: 1-800-822-7422

American Psychiatric Association
AIDS Steering Committee
1400 K. Street N.W.
Washington, DC 20005

American Psychological Association
1200 17th Street N.W.
Washington, DC 20036

Centers For Disease Control
National AIDS Hotline
1-800-342-AIDS; in Spanish 1-800-344-SIDA
Statistics: (404) 330-3020, (404) 330-3021, (404) 330-3022
1600 Clifton Road North East
Atlanta, GA 30333

Pediatric AIDS Hotline
(212) 430-3333

National Institute of Allergy and Infectious Diseases
Division of AIDS
National Institute of Health
Clinical Trials: 1-800-TRIALS-A

National Institute of Drug Abuse
1-800-662-HELP

National Research Center on Women and AIDS
2000 P Street N.W.
Washington, DC 20036

Agency for Health Care Policy and Research
2101 East Jefferson Street
Room 600
Rockville, MD 20852

National Hemophilia Foundation
110 Greene Street, Room 406
New York, NY 10012

National Institutes of Health
Publications and Information Branch
18-12 Parklawn Building
Rockville, MD 20857

National AIDS Information Clearing House
U.S. Department of Health and Human Services
Public Health Service, CDC
P.O. Box 6003
Rockville, MD 20850

Minority Task Force on AIDS
95 St. Nicholas Avenue
New York, NY 10026

The American Medical Association
515 North State Street
Chicago, IL 60610

Association of Nurses in AIDS Care
704 Stony Hill Road, Suite 106
Yardley, PA 19067
The World Health Organization
Global Program on AIDS
1211 Geneva 27
Switzerland
Add any others you find helpful:

**LOCAL REFERRAL, CONSULTATION AND SUPPORT LIST**

Fill in:

Your own growing referral and consultation network:

Your own support network of colleagues:

**JOURNALS AND NEWSLETTERS**

*AIDS*
*CDC Morbidity and Mortality Weekly Report*
*AIDS Clinical Care*
*Journal of Acquired Immune Deficiency Syndrome*
*CDC AIDS Weekly*
*Health Education Quarterly*
*AIDS Education and Prevention*
*AIDS Treatment News*
*Project Inform Perspective*
*Psychology and AIDS Exchange*
*Family Systems Medicine*
*Science*
*The New England Journal of Medicine*
*Nature*
*Journal of Infectious Diseases*
*Lancet*
*American Journal of Psychiatry*

*The Medical Post*
*Community and Preventive Psychiatry*
*Family Process*
*Journal of Marital and Family Therapy*
*British Medical Journal*
*Sistemas Familiares*
*International Journal of S.T.D. and AIDS*
*Journal of the American Medical Association*
*American Journal of Public Health*
*Infection Control and Epidemiology*
*AIDS and Public Policy Journal*

Add any others that are a good source for you (include those in your own
   specialty):

**FAVORITE BOOKS ON AIDS**

Fill in: The AIDS Knowledge Base

**CONTINUING MEDICAL EDUCATION**

Fill in: (your local schedules, etc.)

6. *Avoid premature consensus.* By now it is clear that a new disease argues
   against premature consensus. Lack of consensus is not an evil or an
   indication of lack of knowledge. It is a creative part of the process of
   understanding new diseases like HIV. Neither the patient nor the
   health care provider is served by premature consensus. Keep learning
   about HIV disease and don't assume the consensus position is the correct one. It can give you a false sense of security and control.
7. *Separate or categorize information.* Here is a suggested scheme for order-
   ing the information you have about HIV disease. In the following exercise, place the statements about HIV disease into the most appropriate
   category.

## TABLE 5-D
## Categories

A.  *Long-Term Confirmed Information* (still probable, but subject to less change)
B.  *The Preferred Interpretation at this Time* (the best hypotheses given the available current data)
C.  *Tentative and Practical Working Data*
D.  *Cutting-Edge Research*
E.  *Theories That Are Being Developed*
F.  *Information That Is Probably Wrong*

Where would you place:*

1.  Dr. Lo's work on *mycoplasma fermentans* indicates a co-factor.
2.  ELISA/Western Blot HIV testing for blood donations is required to prevent blood transmission of HIV.
3.  The risk of physician-to-patient transmission of AIDS is quite low.
4.  HIV disease is a sexually transmitted disease.
5.  Early treatment with AZT is beneficial.
6.  HIV is not transmitted through casual contact.
7.  A Belle Glade, Florida study indicated a mosquito vector for HIV.
8.  Dental handpiece for drills and other equipment may be a mechanism for HIV transmission.
9.  Aerosolized blood can transmit HIV.
10. Closed mouth kissing will not transmit HIV.

*There is no right answer. Each category is to some extent arguable, and what this exercise is more likely to show is your own meaning of confirmed, probable, working, experimental, theoretical, and incorrect information. What we have done is indicate how, given our experience with HIV disease, we might classify the current information. You may feel more or less sure of some statements than we do. The important thing is to think in terms of a range of categories for the data you receive. Understand yourself and how you evaluate such data.

*Answers (as of 1992):* 1-D, 2-B, 3-C, 4-A, 5-C, 6-B, 7-F, 8-E, 9-B, 10-C.

8.  *Expect new information and new conclusions.* Don't let HIV disease surprise you. Expect and anticipate new data and new theories. We are still in an early phase of this disease and should not assume we know enough to give definitive answers or reach completeness. Premature closure is as risky in HIV disease as in therapy.
9.  *Work at handling the discomfort of uncertainty.* Health care providers share with their patients this ongoing task. As uncomfortable as uncertainty is, it is a standard feature of everything you do and is not limited to HIV disease. You are already competent in handling the stress of uncertainty and being able to adapt to new information and events. Use that competence with HIV disease as part of your normal practice and you will find that keeping up with this unfolding disease becomes part of your routine response in your own specialty.

## NORMALIZING A NEW DISEASE

By completing your own resource list, you have initiated some important steps for integrating HIV disease into the mainstream of the medical care system. You have started to build lists of your consultation, referral, and support resources. An integrated network of specialists is a basic structure for delivering quality care. Not even an experienced diagnostician can comfortably manage an infectious disease like Ebola fever, a genetic disease like Wilson's, an autoimmune disease like systemic lupus erythematosis, or psychiatric diseases like somatization disorder without considerable help from a strong referral network. HIV disease is simply one more addition to that list, albeit a very dangerous one (though little more dangerous than Ebola fever). Any clinician or counselor will routinely depend on such consultation and referral networks as part of good practice. The important thing is to have good networks—networks that are competent, caring when dealing with patients, and committed to maintaining good contact and feedback with all involved.

In a regional survey of physicians done some years ago by one of the authors (Clements), some of the questions involved referrals to the large medical center by physicians in outlying towns and rural communities.[24] One of the most consistent comments was that the referring physician was cut off by the specialist, who took over the care of the patient and often did not even generate a report back to the referring physician. That physician was then completely uninformed about what had happened to the patient and was deprived of what he or she should have learned from the referral network to be able to provide ongoing care after the patient was discharged by the specialist. A good network should keep all its members informed and included. This is also crucial for continuity of care, which is essential to quality of care. Good referral networks for HIV disease should maintain this standard.

With the special needs and risks of HIV disease, an alternative model is to develop on-site specialty clinics for HIV patients. There are both problems and benefits inherent in this model. Staff are highly committed, but they are also highly susceptible to burnout, unless staff are seconded to the service on a part-time basis and have ready access to mainstream networks. In order to provide all the services available in the larger medical care community, such models must be comprehensively staffed and invest in considerable technology and facilities.

A disadvantage of the model is that it does separate HIV disease from mainstream medical care, although this was also done with tuberculosis sanitoriums and is now done with cancer centers. Patients going to such centers run some risk of stigmatization, but at the same time they may be more accepted and feel more comfortable being with others who intimately understand their problems. Infection control poses less of a problem in such specialized settings, with highly experienced staff and patients whose problems are clearly identified. Treatment is highly specialized and plugged into cutting-edge research, with experimental protocols readily available to patients and funded through the research protocols. There will always be trade-offs between the mainstream care model and the specialty center model.

Another model is the community care model, which can be the source of referrals to either a specialty center or mainstream medical care. Operations can be integrated if two major risks are avoided: (1) the community care model may use the major centers to "dump" HIV patients, refusing to accept any responsibility for care, or (2) the major centers may "appropriate" HIV patients from community health care providers and fail to integrate care, making community providers reluctant to use the center's resources. This separates them from the expertise they need.

These are, of course, normal problems in health care, not idiosyncratic to HIV disease. As we've said before, one of the themes of this book is that HIV disease is a normal event in medicine. Similar events have happened before; similar events will happen again. What the attention to HIV disease can achieve, if used positively, is to throw a spotlight on *generic* problems in the health care field. Every question or issue that HIV disease raises is a general question or issue in health care. This is a new disease, but disease isn't new.

Finally, HIV disease gives us the opportunity to learn together, health care professional with patient or client. There is a good deal of popular literature from the gay community (e.g. the Q Journal)[25] documenting how involved members of that community have been in learning about their disease. The same response is seen in couples carrying the genes for one of the genetic diseases or in parents who have a child with a severe or life-threatening disease. These patients and families become lay experts in the signs, symptoms, and course of the disease. They also keep abreast of new research and new hypotheses in the field—sometimes forming groups for information sharing and support.

That healthy curiosity is a mechanism for coping with the blind chance that gave them the disease. Learning is therapeutic for many patients, even in the presence of denial mechanisms. If the health care professional engages this learning process, rather than feeling defensive about it, both the patient or client and the professional can increase their understanding of HIV disease and of how HIV-infected individuals cope and create their own life stories from the HIV disease experience. Staying abreast of HIV disease becomes more than learning the etiology and natural history of the disease. It becomes a learning process about the individual histories of people who have HIV disease or are at risk of contracting it.

Learning together is really the theme of the remainder of this book, starting with medical experience and ending with ethical and policy decisions.

## REFERENCES

1. Shilts, R. (1987). *And the Band Played On: Politics, People, and the AIDS Epidemic.* New York: St. Martin's Press.
2. Grmek, M.D. (1990). R.C. Maulitz, J. Duffin (Trans.), *History of AIDS: Emergence and Origin of a Modern Pandemic.* Princeton, NJ: Princeton University Press.
3. Murphy, T.F. (1991). No time for an AIDS backlash. *Hastings Center Report, 21*(2): 7–11.
4. (1991). *The Medical Post, 27*(9): p. 28.
5. Lo, S., Tsai, S., Benish, J.R., Wai-Kuo Shih, J., Wear, D.J., Wong, D.M. (1991). Enhancement of HIV-I cytocidal effects in CD4 lymphocytes by the AIDS-associated mycoplasma. *Science, 251*:1074–1076.
6. Palca, J. (1991). The sobering geography of AIDS. *Science, 252*: 372–373.
7. Major, C.J. (1991). Comparison of saliva and blood for Human Immunodeficiency Virus prevalence testing. *Journal of Infectious Diseases, 163*: 699–702.
8. Brookmeyer, R. (1991). Reconstruction and future trends of the AIDS epidemic in the United States. *Science, 253*: 37–42.
9. Minhoff, H., DeHovitz, J.A. (1991). HIV infection in women. *AIDS Clinical Care, 3*(5): 33–35.
10. (1991). *The Medical Post,27*(26): p. 26
11. (1991). *The Medical Post, 27*(26): p. 27.
12. Gibbons, A. (1991). New "China Syndrome" puzzle. *Science, 253*: 26.
13. Harouse, J.M., Bhat, S., Spitalnik, S.L., Laughlin, M., Stefano, K., Silberberg, D.H., Gonzalez-Scarano, F. (1991). Inhibition of entry of HIV-I in Neural cell lines by antibodies against galactosyl ceramide. *Science, 253*: 320–323.
14. DeCock, K.M., Baerere, B., Diaby, L., LaFontaine, M., Gnaore, E., Porter, A., Pantobe, D., LaFontant, G.C., Dags-Akribi, A., Elte, M., Odehouri, K., Heyward, W.L. (1990). AIDS-the leading cause of adult death in the West African city of Abidjan, Ivory Coast. *Science, 249*: 793–796.
15. Hyman, J. (Aug. 19, 1990). Ravages of AIDS cross all boundaries in South Africa. *Democrat and Chronicle*, p. 6A.
16. (1991). *American Association of Homes for the Aging, 6*(8): p. 12.
17. Le Vay, S. (1991). A difference in hypothalamic structure between heterosexual and homosexual men. *Science, 253*(5023): 1034–1037.
18. (1991). *The Medical Post, 27*(29): p. 8.
19. Chu, S.Y. et al. (1990). Impact of the Human Immunodeficiency Virus epidemic on mortality of women of reproductive age, United States. *JAMA, 264*: 225–229.
20. AIDS taboo eases in Nigeria in face of overwhelming plague. *Democrat and Chronicle.* December 15, 1991, p. 9A.

21. Sellers, T. (March 12, 1991). Did Florida dentist deliberately infect patient with AIDS, Canadian wonders. *The Medical Post*, p. 45.
22. Brandt, A.M. (1988). The syphilis epidemic and its relation to AIDS. *Science, 239*: 375–380.
23. Winiarski, M.G. (1991). *AIDS-Related Psychotherapy*. New York: Pergamon Press.
24. Sorenson, A., Clements, C.D., Parker, R. (1981). Treatment of psychological problems by non-psychiatrist foreign medical school graduates. *New York State Journal of Medicine, 81* (12): 1802–1805.
25. Reed, P. (1991). *The Q Journal: A Treatment Diary*. Berkeley, California: Celestial Arts.

# PART II

## Biopsychosocial Intervention: Clinical Management

# PART II

## Biopsychosocial Intervention: Clinical Management

# CHAPTER 6

---

# Epidemiology, Transmission, and Medical Management

## EPIDEMIOLOGY

In the last chapter, projections were given for the spread of HIV across the world. Although these numbers appear precisely quantified, there is considerable uncertainty in the estimates of past and current infection rates both in the United States and internationally. Brookmeyer discussed some of those difficulties for the United States.[1] He pointed out that, while we can obtain statistical estimates of historical infection rates of AIDS based on incidence data and the incubation period, this approach has a number of sources of uncertainty. Two other statistical approaches, epidemic models of HIV transmission and surveys of HIV prevalence, are used to improve the statistical estimates. A final approach, called back calculation, employs AIDS incidence and incubation period distribution to reconstruct historical infection rates that are assumed to have occurred in order to explain the observed pattern of AIDS diagnosis.

All four of the approaches described above have inherent problems and the reader should remember that AIDS numbers and projections are not as certain as they appear. The first approach depends on the choice of the mathematical function, and can produce questionable results. The second depends on AIDS cases, and not HIV prevalence or incidence; even AIDS incidence (one of the most reliable sources for monitoring the epidemic) is subject to delays in reporting, underreporting, and changes in the definition of AIDS. Also, estimates of HIV prevalence are biased because of unknown size of risk groups and lack of response to surveys. The third approach requires assumptions about groups at risk, about the probability of HIV infection per contact, about the number of high-risk behaviors of an individual, about behavior change over time, about incubation-period distribution, and about estimating initial HIV prevalence. The fourth approach is also uncertain because of lack of knowledge about incubation-period distribution, because of the effects of therapy that can alter incuba-

169

tion period, and because of errors in AIDS incidence data. Recent infections will not be reflected in AIDS incidence data because of the long incubation period.

With all of those caveats, Brookmeyer himself tried to estimate recent trends in the United States and to develop projections of advanced HIV disease and AIDS incidence.[1] His results suggested what the World Health Organization has also suggested, that overall HIV infection rates in the United States have declined since the peak in the 1980s. He warns, however, that we can't determine whether this trend is still continuing, and a second-wave epidemic cannot be ruled out. AIDS incidence may plateau in the next five years, but this plateau would be due not only to a decline in the underlying infection rate, but to therapies that can delay AIDS diagnosis. In spite of this apparent plateau, advanced-stage HIV disease will grow by about 40 percent in the next five years, meaning that future demands on the health care system for treatment and care will remain huge.[1]

The World Health Organization's Delphi projection on HIV infection (15 to 20 million infected by 1999) will be reached by the mid-1990s.[2] The United States Interagency Working Group on AIDS predicts that by the year 2015, overall infection rates in urban areas in Africa will be 16 percent. The Hudson Institute predicts that, at a rate of 30,000 new infections per year, there will be 14.5 million infected persons in the United States by the year 2002.[3] This estimate appears high, given the current CDC estimate of one million current infections in the United States.[3]

The World Health Organization, as indicated in Chapter 5, has reported that HIV disease has not yet taken significant hold in Eastern Europe, while North Africa and the Middle East are relatively unaffected. Eight to ten million individuals are estimated to be HIV positive worldwide. Sub-Saharan Africa has 700,000 AIDS cases, six million adults with the virus, and 500,000 infants who are HIV positive. In South Africa, the rate of HIV cases is doubling every eight-and-a-half months. Conservative estimates for Asia, with most cases being in India and Thailand, are 500,000 infected with HIV. However, HIV is spreading rapidly in Asia and Southeast Asia. Greater detail of the specific distribution was given in Chapter 5. Some of the highest rates of HIV infection are in the Caribbean, with one in 10 pregnant women in Haiti being HIV positive. Estimates are that at least one million Latin Americans have the virus.

The Centers for Disease Control in the United States are the basis for studies of seroprevalence in this country. Glasner and Kaslow have given seroprevalence data for homosexual men, intravenous drug abusers, hemophiliacs, heterosexuals, female prostitutes, and the general population.[4] According to them, the prevalence rate of infection in large cohorts of homosexual and bisexual men, excluding San Francisco and New York, ranged from 20 to 50 percent in 1984. They also state that the rate of spread in these homosexual communities has declined steadily in recent years. The prevalence rates in intravenous drug users (as mentioned in Chapter 3) vary geographically, ranging from 50 to 60 percent in some studies, zero to 70 percent in others. Hemophiliacs, according to Glasner and Kaslow, have fairly uniform rates throughout the country. Hemophilia A patients have rates around 70 percent with hemophilia B at rates of 35 percent.

Glasner and Kaslow also state that prevalence rates are low in the general heterosexual population of the United States although, as we indicated in Chapter 3, rates can be high for women in inner cities. The CDC also estimated in a nationwide study that the seroprevalence in female prostitutes ranged from zero in Las Vegas to 57 percent in Newark/Jersey City/Paterson, New Jersey. According to Glasner and Kaslow, up to mid-1988, prevalence in the general population remained low. They based their findings on the monitoring of blood donors and military recruits. During 1985 to 1987, 0.043 percent of first-time blood donors were seropositive. A study of military recruits showed a 0.15 percent prevalence.

In Chapter 5, we described some methods for staying abreast of the epidemiology and for achieving some level of comfort in the face of the uncertainty that is typical of a new disease.

## HIV INFECTION AND AIDS

When AIDS first became recognized as a new illness, the CDC had the task of attempting to set up definitions for the disease. At first, these definitions were based on commonly occurring infections and they still remain primarily syndromic. The CDC, as of January 1, 1992, proposed revising its definition to include the criterion of a less than 200/cubic mm CD4 cell count. As an example of the changing consensus in this field, the CDC revises its definition of AIDS on an ongoing basis. Indicator diseases that have been used as defining criteria include the following:[5,6]

Without laboratory evidence:
   Candidiasis of esophagus, trachea, bronchi and lungs
   Cryptoccocosis outside the lung
   Cryptosporidial diarrhea for more than a month
   Cytomegalovirus of liver, spleen, lymph nodes
   Herpes simplex causing skin ulcers for more than one month, pneumonia, bronchitis or esophagitis
   Kaposi's sarcoma in patients less than 60 years of age
   Lymphoma of the brain in patients less than 60 years old
   Lymphoid interstitial pneumonia or pulmonary lymphoid
      hyperplasia affecting a child younger than 13 years of age
   Disseminated *mycobacteria avium*

Pneumocystis pneumonia
Progressive multifocal leukoencephalopathy
Toxoplasmic encephalitis

With laboratory evidence:
Multiple or recurrent bacterial infections
Disseminated coccidiomycosis
HIV encephalopathy (AIDS dementia)
Disseminated histoplasmosis
Isosporal diarrhea for more than a month
Kaposi's sarcoma at any age
Lymphoma of brain at any age
Non-Hodgkin's lymphoma of B cell or unknown phenotype
Disseminated mycobacterial infections
Diseases caused by *M. tuberculosis*
Recurrent salmonella (non-typhoidal) septicemia
Severe wasting (slim disease)

As our knowledge of the disease increases, these lists change considerably over time, and vary depending on the country. In the United States, for example, they originally did not include the typical diseases of women. Some of the diseases reported in women include:[7]

Candida vaginitis, even with normal CD4 counts
Sqamous intraepithelial neoplasia (human papilloma virus)
Cervical disease
Pelvic inflammatory disease
Genital ulcers
Other STD's which may be resistant to therapy

In addition to infections occurring in women that were not included in the early definitions of AIDS in the United States, one of the primary infections resulting from HIV was not initially included, AIDS dementia complex. There may be a number of central nervous system diseases in which HIV results in a primary infection of the central nervous system, such as: aseptic meningitis, peripheral neuropathy, and AIDS dementia complex. The neurological picture will be further discussed in Chapter 7. On an international level, the defining opportunistic infections will also vary. In Brazil the most common infection is not pneumocystis pneumonia or Kaposi's sarcoma, as in the United States, but rather toxoplasmosis. In Africa, in addition to a high rate of Kaposi's sarcoma, tropical diseases uncommon in the United States or Central Europe are associated with HIV infection. In Australia, a report identified two equestrians who had AIDS and were treated for a rare disease usually found in horses, *rhodococcus equi*. "Such organisms, found in birds, deer, cats and fish and seldom causing disease in humans, will appear when there has been profound damage to the immune system," said Graeme Stewart, president of the Australian Society of HIV Medicine.[8]

The CDC criteria were developed for surveillance and are useful in research and epidemiology. For clinicians, HIV disease may appear to be a continuum, ranging from HIV infection through serious end-stage disease. Individuals will vary in how fast they move along this continuum. Researchers at the University of Nebraska Medical Center reported that they found predominantly unintegrated viral DNA in the T-lymphocytes of asymptomatic HIV-infected patients and that these cells were inactive. Stevenson hypothesizes that HIV is limited in its ability to overwhelm and destroy T-lymphocytes by the limited number of T-lymphocytes that allow virus integration and replication. The question to be answered is why the nondividing, quiescent T-lymphocyte does not allow virus DNA integration. In patients with symptomatic HIV infection, T-lymphocytes have integrated HIV DNA.[9] Stevenson's study was an *in vivo* rather than culture-based study.

We have previously mentioned a Puerto Rican couple, Carmen and Pedro. Pedro appeared to be progressing to the terminal stage of HIV disease, while his wife, Carmen, appeared to be relatively asymptomatic. In fact, the AIDS community agency had raised money to send Pedro to Puerto Rico in order to fulfill one of his last wishes before he died. On the other hand, his wife, who appeared far healthier, suddenly became critically ill and died one year later, while he was still very ill, but alive. Carmen died in July of 1991. Pedro, weighing only 83 pounds and having lost all immune function months earlier, died in December of 1991. Pedro maintained his goal of educating others about the disease up to the moment of his death. In fact, his last newspaper interview was given a few days prior to his death and the media were allowed to share the details of his death with the public.

Another example of the unpredictability and erratic course of the disease is that of a young woman whom we mentioned in Chapter 4. The emergency staff had decided that she was almost terminal and should be allowed to die in hospital since she was out of touch with all social supports. She has not yet died and has ended up spending many months in the psychiatric ward of the hospital. Stevenson concluded: "The take-home message . . . is that we really have to now more carefully look at what's going on in the infected individual . . . at least to address questions of latency and persistence and disease progression."[9]

Some researchers maintain that the full story of this virus may be complicated by co-factors. Both Dr. Montagnier and Dr. Lo have found co-infection with *mycoplasma fermentans*, which enhances the capacity of HIV to kill cells. The theory is that this mycoplasma may be heavily involved in the development of AIDS.[10] Also, although the CD4 molecule is the principal cell receptor for HIV in the immune system, neural cell lines may have a receptor called galactosyl ceramide, which some researchers feel could be the route for entry into the central nervous system.[11]

The CD4 cells are not the only immune system cells infected by HIV. The immune system also consists of monocytes, or macrophages when outside the bloodstream. Macrophages are ubiquitous in body tissue and interact with lymphocytes. "During these interactions, foreign antigens are presented by macrophages to helper lymphocytes, in a manner that causes the lymphocyte to promote vigorous antibody production, or cell-mediated toxicity . . . "[5] Macrophages may be among the first victims of the human immunodeficiency virus and might theoretically serve as a reservoir for the virus.

In other words, our understanding of the process of HIV infection is still unfolding, as is our knowledge of the detailed functioning of the immune system. Understanding the immune system has become more urgent since more than 31 cases of an AIDS-like illness have been reported. ELISA/ Western Blot, PCR, and direct virus culture tests were all negative for HIV-1 and HIV-2 in the CDC cases, but in some others, blood samples were negative but urine samples were HIV positive.*

## HIV INFECTION

It is commonly stated in public AIDS education and prevention that AIDS can be transmitted only through contact or exchange of "bodily fluids." This can be subject to a great deal of misunderstanding. It is, perhaps, better to specify the contact or exchange, since "bodily fluids" can mean many things to many people, and since definitive proof of infection from specific fluids is lacking.

HIV infection is associated with sexual intercourse; the virus has been isolated from seminal fluid and pre-ejaculatory fluid, as well as vaginal and cervical secretion.[12] There is some evidence that anal intercourse is a particularly effective behavioral mode of transmission. HIV transmission may be male to male, male to female, female to male,[13] or female to female.[14] Researchers have reported that HIV may be transmitted through fellatio and cunnilingus.[15] Scientists cannot yet demonstrate whether the virus in these cases may have entered the body through openings in the mouth or whether it can enter the bloodstream through the digestive tract.

The implications of kissing as a means of acquiring HIV infection are still being argued. HIV is found in saliva. However, most experts still advise

---

*Tom Spira, CDC; David Scott, University of Rochester School of Medicine.

that superficial (lip contact) kissing is unlikely to transmit the virus. However, deep (or French) kissing is not recommended (see Chapter 4). Another possible transmission route through saliva is human bites. In Europe there are two suspect cases, as yet unproven, and the possibility cannot be ruled out.

Injection drug use is another mode of transmission, discussed in some detail in Chapter 4. Here the fluid referred to is minute quantities of blood remaining on the works or in the water used to clean the works or to dilute the drug. However, there are other ways in which needles pose a risk that do not involve cocaine or heroin use. Tattooing, ear piercing, acupuncture, or the sports use of steroids and other adjuncts may also be a means of transmission, again, generally hypothesized to be through blood.

In Chapter 4 we discussed the possiblities of infection by blood transfusion, and in Chapter 5 carried this a little further. Testing of blood for HIV began in 1984, so until that time blood transfusion was a significant source of infection. Since 1985, tested blood has been relatively safe, although the window period between infection and seroconversion still poses some problem. Blood may also be a source of infection through needle sticks and other sharp instruments (sharps). Although we tend to think of fluid as liquid, blood also can present a problem when it is aerosolized, as discussed in Chapter 4. Laboratory workers and blood technicians as well as research scientists join health care workers in being at risk through this probable mode of transmission.

In Chapter 3 we discussed the risk to hemophiliacs who require clotting factor, which can be made by pooling thousands of units of blood plasma. As we mentioned, since the introduction of heat treatment and blood screening with ELISA/Western Blot tests in 1985, hemophiliacs are far less at risk. Some researchers put the figures of infection of hemophiliacs with HIV, acquired prior to heat treatment and screening, as high as 98 percent.[16] Production of clotting factor by recombinant DNA techniques is about to become commercially available and would entirely obviate the risk.

Another fluid that needs to be kept in mind as a possible means of HIV transmission is amniotic fluid and the placental exchange between fetus and pregnant woman. As we discussed in Chapter 3, it appears that babies have a 16-33 percent chance of acquiring HIV infection from an infected mother, either in utero or while traversing the vaginal birth canal. In addition, as discussed in Chapter 3, breast milk may be capable of transmitting HIV. A case from Russia has also been reported in which a nursing mother appears to have acquired HIV from her infant, who had probably been infected by a contaminated needle in the hospital.

It is possible that the virus may also be transmitted across mucous membranes, for example, mouth, rectum, vagina, eyes, and nose. This mode of transmission would appear not to need fluid as a vector, but might occur by the virus passing directly across the mucous membrane. Therefore, it is possible that the modes of transmission by fluid described above may also be accompanied by the additional dangers of infection across the mucosa. Any biotic material may be a potential hazard. Organ transplantation may also spread the virus, as described earlier in Chapter 3. The capacity for urine and feces to transmit HIV is also questionable. A case has been reported of a grandparent becoming HIV positive, perhaps because diapers of a grandchild with AIDS were changed without the use of gloves. This case has not been substantiated, but the possibility of this route of transmission needs to be considered.

The CDC has a special category of AIDS exposure category called "Other/ Undetermined" in their listing of both adult and pediatric statistics. As of April, 1992, there was a total of 8,283 AIDS cases in this category for adults and adolescents, plus 90 for those under 13 years of age. This undetermined category refers to AIDS patients whose mode of exposure is unknown. It can include patients under investigation by the CDC, patients who died before mode of exposure was determined, patients who were lost to follow-up, patients who refused interview, and patients whose mode of exposure remained undetermined even after investigation.

Into this unknown category can fall our fears, our yet-to-be discovered knowledge, and our biases. How to differentiate among our fears and hysteria, our prejudices, and the possibility of a new route of transmission is a problem that has not yet been resolved. People have been concerned about some of the following: insect vectors, food and utensil contamination, toilet seats, airborne transmission, touch, sweat.[17] There is no scientific evidence establishing any of these routes of transmission as real risks and it is important to inform clients and patients of this. In addition, the health care professional may want to avoid the use of the term "casual contact" since it is too vague to be of much use. It is better to specify exactly what contact the person has in mind when describing an interaction that has caused him or her to fear that HIV might have been transmitted.

How did the individual cases we mention in this book become infected with HIV? This question cannot be answered with certainty, but some tentative conclusions can be reached. Mary was the first patient we talked about; she probably became infected through sexual intercourse with an unknown partner, someone whose HIV status she had not determined. This occurred during a brief period of her life following her husband's death, when she was lonely, visiting bars, and picking up strangers to help her feel less isolated and depressed. She increased her exposure risk by having multiple sexual partners.

Helene became infected while attempting to follow her cultural tradition of having intercourse with an older experienced man. Since the elders of her family were not available to select the appropriate person, she made her own selection, not dreaming that he would be HIV positive. We doubt that the family would have insisted on HIV screening; however, their selection might well have been a person at lower risk. Both Helene and Mary, therefore, were probable cases of male-to-female heterosexual transmission through vaginal intercourse. What mechanism produced the infection cannot, however, be conclusively demonstrated.

Kevin, on the other hand, was a sexually active homosexual, involved in a committed, monogamous relationship with Bill. Unknown to either of them, during the period of his promiscuity prior to their relationship, Kevin had probably been infected with HIV by a casual partner. By the time Kevin discovered that he was HIV positive, Bill had also been infected. Their route of transmission was probably anal intercourse and male-to-male. In Paul's case, the transmission was also probably male-to-male and through anal intercourse. Julian, who will be discussed in Chapter 8, was also homosexual and may have acquired his infection from his partner. Again, the "bodily fluid" or specific behavior that produced the HIV infection again cannot be conclusively demonstrated.

In the case of Emily, her infection was probably acquired during heterosexual intercourse with a man who was an intravenous drug abuser and also bisexual. His infection could have been acquired either by needle transmission or in male-to-male transmission through sexual intercourse. Although Emily was a drug abuser, she had not used intravenous drugs, and this particular partner appeared to be the probable conveyer of the infection.

Carmen and Pedro, like Emily, were drug abusers. They were also Puerto Rican and lived in the inner city. They were, therefore, at multiple risk. In addition, unlike Emily, they were both addicted to the use of intravenous heroin and cocaine. Amy, discussed in Chapter 8, was married to Brian, also a cocaine user, and she herself used intravenous cocaine. All four of them had placed themselves at multiple risk of HIV infection and probably became infected with HIV via the use of contaminated needles or by having intercourse with each other once the other had become infected by a contaminated needle.

Finally, Latisha, an inner city African-American woman mentioned in Chapter 4, probably became infected from a blood transfusion given because she had lost a great deal of blood during the delivery of her baby. Another case of HIV infection around the context of the birth of a baby was that of Mike, Emily's son, who probably acquired the infection from his mother, either in utero, or during delivery, or through breast-feeding.

The above cases illustrate the typical probable modes of HIV transmission.

## TESTING FOR HIV

Let us now explore how each of the above cases went through the process of being tested for HIV infection.

Mary had multiple symptoms of AIDS, but had no idea what they meant or that it would be a good idea for her to be tested for HIV infection. Her physician also did not recognize the significance of her symptoms or the need for testing. It was only when she was hospitalized for intractable pneumonia that the hospital physician realized, upon the diagnosis of pneumocystis pneumonia, concomitant with her other symptoms, that HIV testing was indicated. Mary was shocked at the results of the test and required extensive post-test counseling and psychotherapy.

Helene, on the other hand, suspected that she might be HIV positive when she first noticed that she had genital warts. She was a well-educated woman, who had read extensively about AIDS and was aware that coming from Haiti she was at special risk. She sought out testing soon after her symptoms began. Her response to the positive test was a sense of fear and shame, combined with the feeling that she was dirty and undesirable. Post-test counseling for her was also important, but insufficient to alleviate her emotional difficulties. She was referred for psychotherapy.

Kevin found out he was HIV positive prior to developing any symptoms of ARC or AIDS. Three months later, however, he had his first episode of pneumocystis pneumonia. Bill, his lover, was tested after finding out Kevin's results and was also positive. This created a great deal of anxiety for them both, as well as for Kevin's mother.

Emily did not consider herself really at risk for HIV infection, and denied many of her early symptoms, such as night sweats and lymphadenopathy. Her drug abuse was not intravenous and she was unaware that her former lover had been bisexual in addition to his intravenous drug abuse. He had not informed her that his HIV test was positive. Her family doctor, prior to the pregnancy, had not requested that she be tested, despite her symptoms. And, during the pregnancy, her obstetrician also failed to see the signs that indicated that HIV testing should be done. It was only after the delivery of her baby, Mike, when both she and he were suffering from fairly serious symptoms, that she herself insisted on being tested. At that stage, her primary doctor still felt that the test was unnecessary and Emily went to a different physician to be tested. She described the wait for the results as extremely difficult, aggravated by her concerns about her baby. When Emily's test came back positive, Mike was also tested and found to be infected as well.

In all these cases, the patients had begun to have symptoms prior to being tested. One hopes, however, that one's clients and patients will be tested routinely, and therefore well before their symptoms begin since early treatment may increase the period between seroconversion and the onset of ARC and AIDS.

Pedro, who was asymptomatic, agreed to be tested only after his wife, Carmen, discovered that she was HIV positive. When he tested positive too, he had no idea whether his infection had been acquired by his own intravenous drug abuse or from sexual intercourse with his wife. The couple managed to cope with the positive test results, relying extensively on their religion and their church community, as well as on the local community AIDS agency.

In contrast to these individuals, who realized that HIV testing was the right decision for them, there are people with such strong needs to deny the appropriateness or necessity of testing, that they do not see testing as an option.

Gino, whose dilemma we will explore further in Chapter 8, refused to be tested even when his wife, Maria, was found to be HIV positive. Both the couple and their extended families were deeply religious Italian Catholics. Gino knew, since he was forbidden by his religion to practice safer sex with condom use, that his risk of infection was extremely high. However, in light of his and the family's insistence on the couple's procreating to fulfil both their religious mandate and the cultural tradition of their heritage, he refused adamantly to be tested. He felt that a positive test would increase Maria's doubts about the appropriateness of her risking a pregnancy. As long as he remained ignorant of his HIV status, he felt he could assure her that he would be around to raise the child if she died, and if the child survived.

All the above cases, except baby Mike, were tested by the ELISA/Western Blot test for antibody to HIV. Mike was tested using virus culture. The following are some potential diagnostic tests:

*ELISA/Western Blot Test.* These sequential tests are readily available, relatively inexpensive, efficient, highly sensitive, and specific. These are the tests most commonly used and available at all official test sites. They test for antibody and will pick up only those individuals who have seroconverted. Generally, individuals seroconvert within 3–6 months of infection, but there may be a longer delay in some cases. The ELISA is a very sensitive test that is performed first. It is specific in high-risk populations, less specific in low-risk populations since it produces a number of false positives.

If an individual has two positive ELISA tests, the blood is then tested by the Western Blot method. The Western Blot is an excellent confirmatory test and there are almost no false positive Western Blot tests (except for laboratory error). In most test sites, the delay between testing and receiving the results is approximately 4–6 weeks. HIV testing for antibodies in saliva rather than blood is being developed as a possible replacement for tests requiring the drawing of blood.[18] For developing countries, it is more cost effective and may be useful. Some researchers claim that it may be as accurate as the use of blood.[18]

*Direct culture of the virus.* Although this is not readily available due to its high cost and the lack of experts and facilities, it is reliable and is important for determining the HIV status of young babies who appear to be HIV positive. It is dependent, however, on the level of virus present, and may therefore give a false negative and should be used in combination with the ELISA/Western Blot test. Since it may take 18 months, or more, for maternal antibodies to clear, direct culture may give an earlier indication of the baby's own HIV status. This test may take from four to 28 days to obtain results. Our own AIDS Center does 500 such tests per year. In combination with the ELISA/Western Blot test, virus culture might be helpful for other cases if it were available, since it might reduce the lengthy wait for seroconversion. Particularly for rape victims, for health care professionals who have experienced needle sticks or other exposure, and for others who are at risk in their employment, a combined virus culture and ELISA/Western Blot might give earlier reassurance.

*Polymerase Chain Reaction Test (PCR).* This is a very sensitive test that allows for detection of very small amounts of nucleic acid. The test, however, is not well standardized and errors in interpretation are not uncommon. At present, this test is used only in research settings, but Hoffman-Roche has applied to the Federal Drug Administration (FDA) for approval of a PCR test kit for general use in HIV testing. The PCR test is routinely used in research on genetic diseases and has led to such advances as the identification of the cystic fibrosis gene. It is possible that this test may become significant in determining the presence of HIV.

*P24 Antigen Testing.* Freely circulating P24 protein can be detected in persons infected with HIV before seroconversion. However, it appears possible that fewer than 20 percent of patients with HIV infection have P24 circulating in their blood, while only 60 percent of individuals who die with AIDS ever have P24 detectable in their serum. For this reason, testing for P24 is not sufficiently reliable for use on its own.

*Clinical Assessment.* Using the CDC criteria, a clinician may determine an individual's HIV status without an HIV test.

Despite the accuracy of the commonly used ELISA/Western Blot test, problems still arise due to the lengthy wait for seroconversion and definitive answer on HIV positivity. This lengthy wait can be extremely difficult for patients and clients, since they may feel that they have been at risk during a particular episode and need to be tested at intervals prior to being certain whether they were infected or not. It is also difficult for the family, since the individual may fear infecting spouse, lover, or children, and may feel obliged to change his or her behavior. In addition, the delay between receiving the test and hearing the result may be as long as 4–6 weeks. This tends to be an extremely anxiety-provoking time for both client and family.

The popular press is constantly reporting potential new developments. One of these reports concerns the development of a new test by the Toshiba Corporation that may detect the AIDS virus as well as the nucleic acid of other pathogens involved in human diseases.[19] Toshiba hopes that this test might turn out to be more accurate than existing tests such as the ELISA/Western Blot and eliminate the wait for the window period since it would be able to detect the presence of the virus directly. They hope that results could be produced in only one hour, as opposed to the common one-month wait for results of the ELISA/Western Blot test.

Toshiba also has plans to use their new method, if successful, to construct a sensor that could automatically diagnose patients with infectious diseases such as HIV. The new method may allow physicians to handle testing more safely and efficiently in their own hospitals, rather than requiring special medical laboratories. The test was presented at the Japan Society of Chemistry Convention on September 22nd, 1991. According to Toshiba, if their early work proves successful, the sensor would take at least five years to develop.[19]

Clients who are in touch with others who have been tested tend to know that the earlier the result comes in, the more likely it is to be negative. Therefore, if the weeks stretch on, clients become progressively more anxious. Also, there is general awareness that physicians tend to call about a negative test result, but to ask for a personal appointment in the case of a positive one. Thus, even if the physician intends to discuss the positive result very gently and thoroughly with his patient, the phone call from the receptionist requesting an urgent office visit frequently precipitates the very panic that the physician is trying to avoid. In view of the anxiety of being told to have an HIV test, waiting for the results, and hearing them, pre- and post-test counseling is an important facet of HIV testing.

## PRE- AND POST-TEST COUNSELING

Health care providers can view pre- and post-test counseling in two ways: either as one more item on a checklist that has to be completed in a formal manner, usually because it is required by state law, or as an important part of the management of HIV risk and/or infection, an integral part of the relationship between the health care provider and the client. The second alternative is clearly the best because it involves quality of care and trust rather than defensive medicine performed by rote to meet obligations outside of the clinical relationship.

Among the first questions to be asked in pre-test counseling are: "Why now?" "What has brought you here today?" "What makes you concerned that you might be HIV positive?" There are many motivators that bring clients and patients to seek HIV testing. Some patients or clients are already reasonably sure that they are infected. They have begun to experience symptoms, as in Emily's case, or know that a sexual partner is HIV positive, as in Kevin and Bill's case. Many have read widely about the disease, keep up with it through the media, and discuss its implications with their friends and family. These individuals are in some ways better prepared to receive a positive result. However, ready as their clients may appear to be, health care providers should be careful not to underestimate the emotional impact of confirmation of their fears. Health care providers should also not be misled into thinking that these better-informed clients are in less need of receiving counseling, up-to-date factual information about HIV disease, and support services. Although some of the issues may have been worked out before the client sees the professional, there may still be important areas to explore.

Some individuals may have suddenly been informed by their physician, substance abuse counselor, or other health care provider that an HIV test should be done. Others may have been sent by a concerned spouse or lover. Still others, who are hospitalized, may be told that an HIV test is indicated. These people are all confronted with an unexpected need to consider an HIV test with results that are potentially very frightening, since it is common knowledge that AIDS is a chronic and fatal disease. Even if they were aware that they themselves are part of a high-risk group, they may not have been emotionally ready to be tested. Some of these people may not even have considered the possibility that they might ever need to be tested. For example, Mary did not really consider herself at risk for HIV; and Helene, in fulfilling her cultural and family obligation, had no idea that she might be putting her life at risk.

Health care providers who need to be tested form a special group of their own. In some ways, their needs around the testing situation are even more delicate than those of the general population. It is easy for pre- and post-test counselors to forget that health care providers are people too, that they experience the same hopes and fears and that, in their private lives, they may be at the same risks as their patients. Health care providers may acquire the virus in the same ways as other people, while also being subject to emergency needs for HIV testing because of needle sticks or other occupational hazards. It is also important not to assume that the professional is completely knowledgable about the virus or has the emotional resources to deal with the testing situation and the results. Health care providers are also subject to the VIP syndrome, which can result in either overmanagement or undermanagement of their problems.[20]

One of our AIDS Training Program educators, a phlebotomist by training, who worked part-time drawing bloods, experienced a needle stick during the course of duty. She immediately requested an HIV test, despite realizing that it had no chance of immediate accuracy because of the window period that might extend for six months (or more). The clinician on duty assured her that a test was not indicated, then, or ever, since she didn't think that the patient whose blood had been drawn was HIV positive. The AIDS educator, knowing full well that without a test the clinician could not be sure of the patient's HIV status, still insisted on being tested. No counseling was provided; in fact she was not even asked whether she would like to be counseled despite the New York State requirements. It was assumed that as an AIDS educator she was fully informed, and that being informed of the facts would give her immunity to the emotional consequences of HIV testing. Counseling was indicated and would have lessened her anxiety, thus enabling her to access her vast fund of knowledge.

In addition to health care professionals, other professionals also run the risk of accidental transmission of HIV and may need to be tested on an emergency basis. These include emergency medical technicians, police, firefighters, first aid workers, patient transport staff, funeral directors, hospice and hospital volunteers, and others who have contact with people who might be infected.

The "worried well" should also be considered as a category in its own right when HIV testing and counseling are discussed. Their concerns should always be taken seriously, since they are no less at risk of being positive than is the general population. Even if their current request seems overstated and they do not appear upon careful questioning to have been involved in any high-risk situations, they may nonetheless be HIV positive, and should be given careful and thoughtful consideration. It is important to take them seriously and to understand what is fueling their concern. This group can present difficulties for health care providers, testing one's patience and tolerance to the extreme. Many of them request testing on a frequent, if not constant, basis; it becomes really challenging to the health care provider to remain considerate and empathic. If the requests persist, it is worth considering referral to therapy if you yourself are not a therapist (as discussed in Chapter 3). The fear of the "worried well" should be validated and their HIV status checked, as one would with any other client or patient.

Another category of individuals needing pre- and post-test counseling consists of those ordered for testing by their employers, the courts, or an insurance company. These people are not easy to counsel. They are reluctant to be tested; nevertheless, they share the same concerns as others needing to be tested. They may be resentful and are usually ill-prepared for testing, making pre-test counseling difficult. They are also highly unlikely to have brought anyone with them at post-test counseling to support them in the event of a positive test result.

It is helpful to establish early on in the counseling session which category people belong to, since it makes a great difference in the approach that is likely to be most effective. Other important questions to be asked, if one is going to maintain a systemic approach to the problem, are: "Who came with you for this appointment or test?" "Who is important to you?" "Who can be a support for you?" "Whom should you tell about the HIV test?" It is very helpful to involve other members of the client's natural support system as early as possible; including them in the counseling session expedites this process provided the client is agreeable. It is important to remember that, in addition to the person's fears for him or herself, he or she will also have fears about infecting other people, or about dangers of contact with the important people in his or her life. Also, there may be a fear of losing significant relationships or concerns about trying to form new ones.

Emily was really worried that she would spend the rest of her life alone with her baby, without a partner, because she knew how important it was to be honest with potential lovers about her HIV status. She was also concerned about the danger of infecting other members of her family and friends, as well as their children. Other clients, unlike Emily, need to be told about the importance of protecting others by informing significant and intimate associates about their HIV status. It is not uncommon for people to feel that, regardless of their own HIV status, others should take responsibility for their own behavior and that it is not their personal obligation to inform others of their HIV status.

What do you do in post-test counseling if the client has no intention of informing spouse, family, or sexual partners about his or her positive HIV status? This question has to be answered on a case-by-case basis. There is an obligation, sometimes written into law, to inform the sexual partners of an HIV-positive patient that they have been placed at risk. Generally, the requirement is to maintain the confidentiality of your patient, but frequently in these circumstances people automatically know to whom you are referring. Confidentiality is not an absolute requirement and can be breached for very important reasons. Just as it is permitted for confidentiality to be breached when people are placed at risk by a psychiatric patient who may be homicidal or violent, our ethical responsibility extends beyond our immediate patient or client. However, if it is likely that the sexual partner is already infected, the emphasis should be on bringing that partner in for testing and treatment, rather than on merely informing him or her of risk.

At the same time, discussion about whom to tell should emphasize a certain degree of discretion; the whole community need not be informed by the patient. The counselor needs to work with the individual on making decisions about whom it is appropriate to inform and how best to do so.

International public health policy has traditionally taken care of epidemics and pandemics by a process known as mandatory notification. In Chapter 1 we discussed the political arena into which HIV infection entered. The embroglio that ensued has limited our ability to formulate an effective public health policy. The pandemic continues to spread worldwide, with responses ranging from laissez-faire to "leper colony." HIV infection, despite being one of the sexually transmitted diseases, is not treated like syphilis or gonorrhea, which require immediate notification of public health authorities and all sexual contacts. Politics are not the only culprit for this decision; the window period before seroconversion makes tracing of a potential multiplicity of contacts extremely difficult and costly. The economic cost of testing also constrains traditional public health responses. Thus, the CDC-proposed recommendation that all hospital patients be encouraged to have HIV testing has been criticized because of the cost. For those providing post-test counseling, the question of notification is a medical, legal, and ethical question that must be addressed.

After post-test counseling, the counselor should be sure that the individual, if positive, is immediately linked up with support networks. These can include family (traditional, nontraditional, or both), community HIV agency, church community, friends and neighbors, and family doctor. We have found it useful to routinely request that individuals bring someone they are close to with them to the post-test counseling session to ensure that they do not leave the office alone and unsupported.

Another set of questions includes: "What do you know about HIV disease?" "What are you afraid of?" "Have you ever thought about being HIV positive?" "Have you ever talked about HIV disease with anyone?" "What will you do if the test is positive?" It is important to ascertain what knowledge the person already has and not overestimate how much is known. The blanks in knowledge need to be filled in. It is also important to be aware of the level of denial and the reasons for it, since some denial may be protective and healthy. Fears have to be addressed realistically, while anxiety should be expected and dealt with respectfully. It is helpful to remember that anxiety is normal and that we all use defense mechanisms to survive.

Sometimes health care providers forget how they themselves might react under similar circumstances since the constant emotional stress and routine of their jobs may render them unempathic. Use the physician's tool to avoid this: "What if this were a member of my family?" "What if this were me?" "What if this were my lover? my child? my parent?" Some of the more common fears are: Fear of losing a job, or not being hired; being ostracized or isolated;

losing a lover; not getting health insurance or becoming economically deprived; becoming incapacitated; not being able to have children; becoming unattractive, or even demented; and finally, the fear of death, including not living to raise the children or not being able to support the family.

One should also guard against being overemotional or overidentified with the patient, since one's own feelings can blind one to his or her specific needs. The fact that many of these people are at a similar stage of their personal development or family life cycle stage makes it difficult to remain objective at times. It is important to keep one's own resources intact in order to help the client most effectively.

Patients may become severely anxious, depressed, or even suicidal at post-test counseling if the results are positive. They may even deny the importance of a positive HIV test and be unrealistic about the need to take action or receive treatment. The counselor needs to attempt to keep the individual in contact with some part of the health care system, in addition to ensuring referral to formal counseling or therapy whenever possible. Referral to the emergency room may be indicated in the case of suicidality. The post-test counselor should be certain not to leave the individual alone until specific plans for management are in place and a responsible person has taken over. If the post-test counselor is a qualified therapist, then these issues may be dealt with immediately in session. We will discuss the therapeutic management of such problem reactions in Chapter 8.

For a negative test result, the counselor needs to concentrate on risk reduction and organizing further testing as needed. HIV-positive clients also need counseling on risk reduction, since they need to be assured that they are not placing loved ones at unnecessary risk. Wherever possible, counselors should ascertain that clients do have a primary health care provider who will be able to continue the counseling process as needed. If the client or patient gives permission, and most do, it is useful to talk to the primary care provider in order to share the outcome of both the test result and the counseling session.

## TREATMENT AND MANAGEMENT

We have indicated earlier that HIV disease needs to be seen as an ongoing process, starting with infection, and finally culminating with an AIDS-defining disease. HIV disease can be unpredictable, with patients moving toward the end stage of the spectrum and then recovering to an earlier, healthier state, only to become critically ill once more. This cycle can repeat many times, and is both physically and emotionally wearing on patient and family. The perception of AIDS has changed over the past few years from an acute and rapidly fatal disease to a chronic, but eventually terminal disease.

Whether this perception is accurate is open to question. Some argue that HIV-positive patients are living longer due to early diagnosis and early treatment (shortly after a positive HIV test result) with drugs that were initially administered only to the acutely ill patient. These antiviral drugs, including azidothymidine (AZT) and dideoxyinosine (ddI), may keep CD4 counts from becoming dangerously low over a longer period of time. Others could argue that living longer is an artifact of earlier detection of HIV infection.

Whatever the answer, it is important to remember that HIV disease is also a primary central nervous system infection and that neurological symptoms and AIDS dementia remain a treatment problem. The course of HIV infection is characterized by its attack on the immune system and the multiple opportunistic infections that result from the reduction in immune function. The treatment of opportunistic infections has become more aggressive and possibly more effective, perhaps constituting another factor in AIDS becoming a chronic progressive disease.

In the case of Mary, her first symptoms were fever, cough, and loss of weight. When Mary eventually got to the hospital, the diagnosis of pneumocystis pneumonia (PCP) was made. This common opportunistic infection is a chronic pneumonia, caused by a parasite, pneumocystis carinii, that commonly starts with fever of undetermined origin (FUO) and then builds up over many months with accelerating fever, shortness of breath, and cough. Diagnosis is made from the history and confirmed by the laboratory examination of sputum. However, with early prophylaxis, either inhalation therapy with pentamidine or the administration of trimethaprine sulphasoxazole (bactrim or septran) pills, it is more difficult to make the diagnosis.

None of the patients we talked about in this book developed tuberculosis, but TB is, in fact, one of the most rapidly growing opportunistic infections in the United States, particularly in the lower socioeconomic areas of major cities such as Los Angeles and New York. TB is caused by a mycobacterium and is becoming a major health threat not only in Sub-Saharan Africa, but in the U.S. and other developed countries. Reichman reported that the rate of TB infection in the U.S. increased five percent in 1989, with a 10 percent increase in New York City and a 35 percent rise in Newark.[21] TB may also manifest itself differently in AIDS patients, as extrapulmonary TB (pericarditis, osteomyelitis, brain abscesses, TB of the wrist, ankles, intestines, and testes), rendering the TB skin test less reliable.[21] Reichman also reported a 20–30 percent TB infection rate among I.V. drug users in New York City and an estimated 6,600 new cases each year. The New York State AIDS Institute reports that 5 percent of the state's AIDS cases are dually diagnosed with active TB (highly infectious).[22] In New York City 50 percent of TB/AIDS cases are intravenous drug users and 82 percent are minorities.

An individual with active TB is likely to manifest chronic cough, fatigue, weakness, weight loss, fever, and blood in the sputum. Extrapulmonary TB may not be as easily transmitted as pulmonary TB. Untreated TB is a serious illness that often results in death. The AIDS Institute estimates that seven percent of TB/AIDS cases per year develop Active TB. Given a person with Active TB, 29 percent of close contacts and 15 percent of not-close contacts become infected. In New York City, the contact infection rate for TB/AIDS was 21 percent. Health care professionals who do medical procedures such as aerosolized pentamidine treatment, bronchoscopy, or sputum induction are at increased risk for TB. The CDC guidelines for preventing TB transmission in health care settings recommend screening of the following people:

Contacts of individuals with Active TB, individuals with HIV infection or risk of HIV infection, individuals with diabetes and some cancers, intravenous drug users, alcoholics, prisoners, the elderly, the homeless, inner-city residents, and immigrants from areas with high prevalence of TB. Health care personnel also need to be screened.

Isolation, ultraviolet lights, rooms with negative air pressure, and prompt control of outbreaks are all infection control recommendations. In addition, the U.S. government has developed a strategic plan for the elimination of TB from the U.S. that consists of providing TB preventive education to all HIV service providers so that they will refer individuals at risk for TB screening tests. The government estimates that 10–15 million persons have TB infection. TB is generally treated with Pyrazinamide and Ethambutol.

In the case of Kevin, he developed Kaposi's sarcoma (KS). This neoplasm appears to occur at a higher rate in the homosexual population, even without HIV infection.[23] The most troublesome symptom of KS is the disfiguring, purplish lesion on the skin, commonly on the face. It can also affect internal organs and the mouth. KS became so well known and easily recognized during the early days of AIDS that people with easily visible KS were discriminated against, whether the cause was HIV infection or not. Patients with KS need special counseling in dealing with such a prominent badge (or brand) of the illness. KS is treated with chemotherapy, immunotherapy with interferon, radiation, cryosurgery, and cosmetology. Both chemotherapy and interferon therapy can produce severe side effects similar to those experienced by other cancer patients.

Other neoplastic conditions seen in HIV cases are non-Hodgkin's lymphoma and, specifically in women, squamous intraepithelial neoplasia associated with human papilloma virus (HPV). HPV is a sexually transmitted disease, common among sexually active women. The general rate of abnormal pap smears in HIV+ women is greater than in HIV- women, and the characteristics of cervical disease may vary with HIV positivity.

Pelvic inflammatory disease (PID) is also associated with sexually transmitted diseases and is a major public health problem in the United States, affecting one million women annually.[7] Its possible sequelae include infertility, chronic pelvic pain, and ectopic pregnancy. Researchers at San Francisco General Hospital reported a high rate of HIV infection among women with PID. Data from Brooklyn showed a 13.6 percent prevalence of HIV infection among women hospitalized with PID as compared to a 2.0 percent seroprevalence without PID.

In the case of Pedro, infection with cytomegalovirus (CMV), one of the disseminated opportunistic infections associated with HIV disease, resulted in his losing the sight of one eye from cytomegalovirus retinitis. CMV is caused by a herpes virus and can become a persistent management problem for patients. CMV can also affect the gastrointestinal tract and cause esophagitis, gastritis and ileitis. It can affect the central nervous system, causing encephalitis, or the lungs, causing pneumonia. The physician has to monitor CMV retinitis carefully, particularly when CD4 counts are below 200. An opthalmologist can make the diagnosis of CMV retinitis; the diagnosis of other CMV diseases is more difficult because CMV is so ubiquitous.

Other disseminated conditions caused by herpes viruses are herpes simplex and herpes zoster. Herpes simplex causes vesicles, ulcers, and fever. Ulcers can occur in the mouth, genital, or rectal areas. Esophagitis may be a symptom, as well as acute encephalitis. Genital ulcers in women can be the result of herpes simplex, but may also be found without it in HIV-positive women. These latter ulcers are often resistant to treatment. Treatment for herpes simplex includes Acyclovir and Foscarnet. Herpes zoster, or shingles (the same virus that causes chicken pox in children), is a painful localized rash with vesicles, that may disseminate to the lungs, liver, and central nervous system. One of Emily's symptoms was shingles, which led to her being tested and diagnosed as HIV positive. Treatment for herpes zoster is the same as for herpes simplex, Acyclovir and Foscarnet.

Finally, mycobacterium avium intracellular (MAI) is also a disseminated condition caused by a bacterium, resulting in malaise, fevers, night sweats, weight loss, and diarrhea. It may disseminate to lungs, bone marrow, blood, liver, and other organs. Some patients present with high fevers (104–105 degrees Farenheit) of unknown origin (FUO) and physicians may mistakenly think that there is another, non-HIV, bloodstream infection. Patients are often treated before laboratory diagnosis, because blood culture may not be positive for up to a month. Treatment requires a number of drugs, four of which are oral. Unfortunately, the best drug so far appears to be an intravenous one, Amikacin.

Mike developed an opportunistic infection to which children are particularly prone, oral thrush, or candidiasis, caused by the fungus candida. Women also can get candida vaginitis. If thrush proves resistant to standard treatment, or recurs, HIV should be excluded. Oral candidiasis presents as a white coating in the mouth, which can be removed by scraping, unlike another HIV opportunistic infection, hairy leukoplakia, which cannot be removed by scraping. Thrush may also present as candidial esophagitis, which can be difficult to treat.

Two other fairly common oral conditions are HIV gingivitis and HIV periodontitis. These may result in irritated gums and soft tissue necrosis, which can lead to loss of teeth and the need for ongoing dental treatment. Dentists may be the first to make the provisional diagnosis of HIV infection from these symptoms.

Opportunistic infections of the central nervous system, such as chronic meningitis, or cryptococcal meningitis, tend to be very serious and will be discussed in Chapter 7. Another central nervous system infection, the most common opportunistic infection in Brazil but less common elsewhere, is toxoplasmosis. This is caused by a protozoan, toxoplasma, and is suspected when patients present with headache, fever, and stroke-like symptoms.

Finally, one of the most serious central nervous system infections is progressive multifocal leukoencephalopathy. This manifests as multiple lesions in the brain, which result in progressive mental deterioration; there is, as yet, no treatment.

We have described only the opportunistic infections most common in the United States. Such infections vary from country to country, so it is important for health care professionals to develop a list of those commonly found in their area. Health care providers may now appreciate the complexity of HIV treatment and the effects that treatment can be anticipated to have on their patients. There are no magic bullets, but early recognition and diagnosis may lead to more effective management.

Sabin, with extensive experience in the development of vaccines, has urged us to be cautious in our expectations of an effective vaccine.[24] Will there eventually be a safe vaccine to protect against HIV infection? Research centers continue to test the safety of experimental vaccines and the World Health Organization is developing facilities in Central Africa, Asia, and South America for performing large-scale tests of efficacy and safety. In the meanwhile, the pandemic continues to spread, and a vaccine may be the most realistic hope of stopping it.

## REFERENCES

1. Brookmeyer, R. (1991). Reconstruction and future trends of the AIDS epidemic in the United States. *Science*, 253: 37–42.

2. Palca, J. (1991). The sobering geography of AIDS. *Science*, 252: 372–373.

3. Winiarski, M.G. (1991). *AIDS-Related Psychotherapy.* New York: Pergamon Press.

4. Glasner, P.D., Kaslow, R.A. (1990). The epidemiology of Human Immunodeficiency Virus Infection. *Journal of Consulting and Clinical Psychology, 58(1):* 13–21.
5. McCutchan, J.A. (1990). Virology, immunology, and clinical course of HIV infection. *Journal of Consulting and Clinical Psychology, 58(1):* 5–12.
6. Osmond, D. (1990). Definitions and codes for HIV infection and AIDS. In P.T. Cohen, M.A. Sande, P.A. Volberding (Eds.). *The AIDS Knowledge Base.* Waltham, Massachusetts: The Medical Publishing Group.
7. Minhoff, H., Dehovitz, J.A. (1991). HIV infection in women. *AIDS Clinical Care,* 3 (5): 33–35.
8. Animal infections in AIDS patients. *The Medical Post,* 27 (40): 21.
9. Murray, T. New research yields insights into latency of AIDS. *The Medical Post,* 27 (40): 30.
10. Lo, S., Tsai, S., Benick, J.R., Wai-Kuo Shih, J., Wear, D.J., Wong, D.M. (1991). Enhancement of HIV-1 cytocidal effects in CD4 lymphocytes by the AIDS-associated mycoplasma. *Science,* 251: 1074–1076.
11. Harouse, J.M., Bhat, S., Spitalnik, S.L., Laughlin, M., Stefano, K., Silberberg, D.H., Gonzalez-Scarano, F. (1991). Inhibition of entry of HIV-1 in neural cell lines by antibodies against galactosyl ceramide. *Science,* 253: 320–323.
12. Wofsky, C.D., Cohen, J.B., Hauer, L.B., Padian, N.S., Michaelis, B.A., Evans, L.A., Levy, J.A. (1986). Isolation of AIDS-associated retrovirus from genital secretions of women with antibodies to the virus. *Lancet,* 1: 527–529.
13. Zuger, A., Steigbigel, N.H. (1990). Heterosexual transmission of human immunodeficiency virus infection. *AIDS Updates,* 3: 1.
14. Marmer, M., Weiss, L.R., Lyden, M., Weiss, S.H., Saxinger, W.C., Spira, T.J., Feorino, P.M. (1986). Possible female-to-female transmission of human immunodeficiency virus. *Annals of Internal Medicine,* 105: 969.
15. Spitzer, P.G., Weiner, N.J. (1989). Transmission of HIV infection from a woman to a man by oral sex. *New England Journal of Medicine,* 320: 251.
16. Blake, J. (1990). *Risky Times: How to be AIDS-Smart and Stay Healthy.* New York: Workman Publishing.
17. Booth, W. (July 24, 1987). AIDS and insects. *Science,* 2: 355–356.
18. Major, C.J., Reed, S.E., Coates, R.A., et al. (1991). Comparison of saliva and blood for Human Immunodeficiency Virus prevalence testing. *Journal of Infectious Diseases,* 163: 699– 702.
19. *Democrat & Chronicle,* September 14, 1991, p. 1A.
20. Clements, C.D. (1990). When patient's a VIP, special care may mean less care. *The Medical Post,* 26(3): 34.
21. (August 7, 1990). TB is now back with a vengeance. *The Medical Post,* p. 15.
22. New York State AIDS Institute. (1991). *AIDS Preventive Education Manual.*
23. (Nov. 27, 1990). Kaposi's/AIDS riddle: Is there another STD? *The Medical Post,* p. 5.
24. Sabin, A.B. (1991). Effectiveness of AIDS vaccines. *Science,* 251: 1161.

# CHAPTER 7

# The Neuropsychiatric Aspects of HIV Infection and Patient Care

## A. Griepp, J. Landau-Stanton, C.D. Clements

By 1990, there was clear and convincing evidence of the involvement of the HIV virus in the brains and nervous systems of patients who were infected with HIV. Neurologic behavioral and cognitive changes have been well described by Navia, Jordan, and Price[1] and other groups. HIV has tropism for brain tissue, fostering the development of neuropsychiatric abnormalities.[2] There is evidence that the virus lives in the macrophages of the brain, although questions still remain as to when exactly the virus enters the brain, the exact mechanism of viral passage through the blood-brain barrier, and what the mechanisms are that cause activation of the virus in the central nervous system.

It is still unclear exactly how the virus causes neural damage. Yet, it is obvious, by the neurologic manifestations and imaging of the brains on Magnetic Resonance Imaging (MRI)[3] and Computed Tomographic (CT) Scan, as well as in viewing brains on post mortem,[4] that brain damage is quite extensive in this disease, and that virtually no neural cell line is left untouched (with some relative sparing of the neurons themselves).

Primary infection of the brain by HIV is one of four general categories of intracranial central nervous system disorders found in HIV + patients: (1) Primary infection of the brain by HIV; (2) Opportunistic infections by parasitic, fungal, viral and bacterial organisms; (3) Central nervous system neoplasms; and (4) Complications of systemic disorders such as cerebral infarction from vasculitis, and metabolic encephalopathies.[5]

In addition to intracranial disorders, spinal cord disorders and disorders of the peripheral nerves make up two large groups of central nervous system diseases.[5] The spinal cord disorders include vacuolar myelopathy and acute myelopathies. Peripheral neuropathies include distal symmetric polyneuropathy (DSPN), inflammatory neuropathies, lumbo-sacral polyradiculopathy, and rare neuropathies such as sensory ataxia. The clinical symptoms of these peripheral neuropathies include painful burning sensation in the feet, toes, and fingers, as well as decreased sensitivity to touch and a feeling of numbness or tingling when the sensory nervous system is involved. In motor neuropathies, motoric weakness and involvement of bladder and bowel seriously impair the patient.

Despite the discomfort of these conditions, treatment options are limited. In the case of DSPN, there is no effective treatment to alter the clinical course. There is likewise no treatment, with the exception of plasmaphoresis, for inflammatory neuropathies. For the lumbo-sacral polyradiculopathy, although a few patients initially improved after treatment with gancyclovir, weakness rapidly progresses to complete paralysis and death.[5]

While systemic treatment of the disease through use of antiretrovirals is widely practiced, there is currently no brain prophylaxis paralleling the aerosolized pentamidine used to prevent pneumocystis carinii pneumonia (PCP) infections of the lungs. As patients continue to live longer and to have better treatment for their early opportunistic infections, there is more time for the development of neurologic, brain, and behavior manifestations of HIV. Patients and their families are confronted with the need to derive a multitude of strategies, some for when the patient is healthy but worried about CNS problems, others for when dementia and peripheral neurologic problems truly exist.

These facts present frightening and important challenges for the mental health professional caring for someone with HIV disease. How does one, as a therapist, maintain a flexible and therapeutic posture in working with a patient in insight-oriented therapy while he or she is asymptomatic and healthy, and then switch to a more focused behavioral or supportive mode when cognitive function no longer allows insightful work? How can a brief goal-oriented family treatment aimed at living with HIV make the transition to preparing for dementia and death? What happens to a therapy group when some of the group members become demented? How does one help individuals and families prepare for a dementing illness that occurs in young people? What role should medications play in treatment?

These neuropsychiatric questions can most usefully be addressed by our looking at some examples of patients and their families and learning from the lessons that they have taught caregivers.

## CLINICAL EXAMPLES

### Tim's Case and Neuropsychiatric Diagnosis

Tim was a 35-year-old stockbroker from the West Coast, who returned to his parents' home in rural upstate New York after receiving a diagnosis of HIV. He had left home at the age of 18 and had lived on his own on the West Coast for the past 17 years to protect his family from living with his homosexuality. By Christmas time of 1985, he had fallen into a fairly severe depression. He made an attempt to take an overdose of pills and was hospitalized in a psychiatric unit.

Shortly after this suicide attempt, he began to share with friends and, eventually, family members, that during that fall he had tested HIV+. Within a few months, he was stricken with a bout of pneumocystis pneumonia in which he nearly died.

His parents flew to the West Coast and stayed with him daily at the hospital. In view of his weak state and his inability to return to work, it was agreed that Tim would return to upstate New York to live with his family.

All went well for about three weeks, and then Tim's mother, a 65-year-old homemaker, began to notice that something seemed unusual about Tim. While the family style was not to discuss problems at great length, Tim seemed unusually elated and happy, given the severity of his life circumstances. He began to chatter about idle topics in an incessant fashion and with a fair amount of pressure. He became careless about finances, not worrying about the fact that he had no income to support his lengthy and frequent long-distance phone calls to friends on the West Coast. The family began to become nervous about leaving money or credit cards around, since Tim would take the money or randomly use the credit cards to purchase things that were advertised on TV or by mail. At times Tim appeared to be sleepless, but since he had little to do to expend his energy and took frequent catnaps, he thought his sleeplessness was probably because he simply wasn't tired. Initially, the family was able to maintain a negotiated but delicate balance.

Suddenly, this changed. Tim took a family credit card and car keys and drove himself to the airport, purchasing a ticket to the West Coast. His friends were surprised to see Tim back without prior arrangement, but welcomed him and arranged a place for him to stay. For several days, Tim's parents both brooded over how Tim could have done this to them and worried about his health.

Several days later, Tim's parents began to receive phone calls from friends in the West who were concerned about him. Friends reported: "Tim is spending money like a drunken sailor. How could he afford to buy a new car when he doesn't have a job?" "I never knew Tim to be such a "partier" and drinker, but he seems to be out partying and drinking almost every night. "Wait 'til you see what he's done to his hair!" The last call, from one of Tim's best friends, was the most serious: "I think you'd better come out here. Tim is really getting himself in trouble, and I think he needs his parents. He got drunk and in a fight and got himself arrested last night."

Anxiously, Tim's parents got on the first available plane to the West Coast. Not only had he lost a significant amount of weight, but he was dressed in an extremely flamboyant manner that they had never seen before. The most shocking feature of his appearance was his bleached-blond Mohawk. His parents felt that he would be safer with them and were able to convince him, with the help of his friends, that he needed to come back home, and he did so. He became increasingly angry and irritable with his parents. "How could you bring me back here? I have no life here! If I'm going to die, let me stay where I have a life." Finally, in desperation, his parents brought Tim to his medical doctor, who quickly realized that the situation was not a straightforward medical problem. Tim was sent to the Psychiatric Emergency Department for evaluation.

When Tim arrived in the Psychiatric Emergency Department, he was really quite something to behold. An extremely thin man, he was wearing clothes that were many sizes too big, belted with several thick cloth belts. Amid the remnants of his blond spiked hair, substantial portions of dark roots were showing. He was restless, constantly pacing, demanding to smoke, and speaking incessantly. He needed constant structuring to return to his room and to remain seated. He was accompanied by his parents, his father appearing concerned and his mother tearful, through much of the interview. "There is nothing wrong with me," Tim maintained. "I don't know why they're so upset."

His mental status examination demonstrated that there was something neuropsychiatrically wrong. He was irritable, with increased motor activity. He was restless at times and his gait appeared a little unsteady. His language processing appeared to be receptively and expressively intact. However, since he was so busy chattering, wandering from subject to subject, and not paying attention to the questions that were asked, it was very difficult to assess how much he really did understand. His speech was pressured and mumbling, but was understandable. His formal thought processes were quite disordered. He was rambling and tangential. He exhibited flight of ideas, answering only partially in a well-associated fashion and then derailing to some unrelated topic. His thought content focused on his desire to return to the West Coast and how everyone was picking on him and limiting his spending money.

He began talking about the three 6s and 9s, but was unclear what these represented— yet he repeated this series to himself several times. He described his mood and affect as "fine," though he was alternately irritable and silly. He denied auditory or visual hallucinations, suicidality, or homicidality. His cognitive status showed some deficits. He knew his name and the city he was in; he did not know the hospital he was in or the date. It took two tries to get him to recall three items; after five minutes he remembered one of the three items. His concentration and attention were so poor that he had extreme difficulties with digit span and serial 7s.

Tim's accelerated mood, his deteriorated physical state, and his parents' physical exhaustion as a result of his erratic behavior led to the decision to admit him to the psychiatric ward for a work-up. Tim's loving parents required reassurance from staff members that it was really all right for them to leave.

From a neuropsychiatric point of view, this patient represented a very interesting diagnostic challenge. His behavior and cognitive status were both severely disturbed. This disturbance appeared to have developed gradually over a period of at least 6–7 months. As is frequently the case, there was limited collateral information available at the time of assessment. It would have been helpful to have had a discharge summary from the prior psychiatric admission or information from a reliable close companion.

In order to arrive at a thorough differential diagnosis, a broad systems assessment can be helpful. Only the people in Tim's natural support network could present an accurate picture of his baseline personality, cognitive status, drug use, and general behavioral patterns. They would also be able to detail any stress that he had experienced. At the time of admission, he himself was not a reliable historian. In a case like Tim's, the people who had an opportunity to observe his deterioration over time were his close friends on the West Coast. Telephone calls can augment the information provided by the local family.

To diagnose and treat Tim appropriately, however, one must have more than collateral information from friends and family. HIV is a medical illness and a mental status change could signal the onset of infection, trauma, drug effect, metabolic abnormality, delirium, or dementia. Involving Tim's medical practitioner is absolutely essential in diagnosis. Take a minute to fill in the information you would need:

- What more do you wish you knew right now?
- Are there parts of the history that have been neglected?
- What medical concerns require immediate work-up versus those that can be gradually evaluated on an outpatient basis?

Tim's practitioner would be in a position to answer questions about the patient's recent condition, especially his immune status, medications, drug/alcohol history, allergies, and most recent mental status. This would help focus the diagnostic evaluation. In addition, the practitioner can add another important dimension, a baseline impression of the patient as a person and an objective view of the patient in his or her social context.

The care provider who knows the patient well can easily provide a more detailed history, which can save unnecessary repeat procedures (for example, the patient may have had a recent outpatient CT of the head if the practitioner had been noting mental status changes. This would render a repeat CT in the emergency room redundant). The primary physician may also know names and telephone numbers of family, friends, or agencies with first-hand information about previous personality and behavioral changes.

In an emergency room, it is always important to sort out true emergencies. Some of the problems that produce a change in mental status or precipitate agitated behavior, if untreated, quickly could result in death. Head trauma, space-occupying brain lesions, drug overdose or side effects, stroke, sepsis, severe electrolyte disturbance, or brain anoxia can all lead to deranged behavior, coma, or death. Less severe infections or metabolic disturbances may contribute to a mental status change, but may not require emergency attention or pose a catastrophic threat if not detected immediately. The evaluator has the burden of ascertaining which parts of a work-up are essential for correct diagnosis and patient survival, versus those which can be completed in a more comfortable and inexpensive setting.

Tim's medical status was of critical importance in the understanding of his behavioral change. One part of the history that was lacking was the current pattern of Tim's substance use. In the history, we had heard about possible abuse of alcohol, but there was no quantification or exploration of other possible intoxicants. Certainly, some of Tim's behavior could have been attributable to intoxication and/or to withdrawal if he was being separated from substances upon which he was dependent. It is important to be aware of local patterns of drug abuse when trying to piece together an adequate history. For example, cocaine or "crack" may be the drug of choice in one city, whereas "ice" or heroin may be more popular in another city or subculture. In the early 80s, "poppers" were extremely common in the gay community. Such knowledge is helpful in an emergency room setting where the type of intoxication or timing of withdrawal may be critically important, particularly when one is trying to understand the etiology of altered mental states.

There are medical abnormalities that need to be considered in all patients exhibiting a change in mental status, including those inflicted with HIV. The causes of delirium are many and can roughly be broken into categories represented by the acronym WHHHHIMP: Wernicke's, Hypertensive, Hypoglycemia, Hypoperfusion of the CNS, Hypoxia, Intracranial bleed, Meningitis, Poisons.[6] A careful physical examination and some screening laboratory tests, such as a complete blood count with differential urinalysis chemistry panel including electrolytes and calcium, can help in eliminating such problems in the differential diagnosis of altered mental status.

In the case of persons with HIV disease, tumors and opportunistic infections are more likely to be responsible for changes in mental status than they are in the HIV negative person. Approximately 31–65 percent of patients with HIV disease will have some form of neurologic abnormality through the course of their disease;[3] 50–90 percent of children with AIDS will have neurologic involvement,[7] and this percentage is likely to rise as patients' life spans are prolonged. Approximately 10 percent of patients' first manifestation of HIV disease is a neurologic or behavioral problem.

In the United States, the most common neurological opportunistic infection found in persons with HIV disease is cryptococcal meningitis. In other parts of the world, toxoplasmosis of the central nervous system is so common as to be the most frequent AIDS-defining opportunistic infection.[8] Progressive multifocal leukoencephalopathy,[9] as well as a variety of even less frequently occurring infections, such as herpes simplex encephalitis, cytomegalovirus encephalitis, nocardia, and even tuberculosis can be present in the brain and can affect mood, behavior, sensation, and motor skills. A careful neurological examination, MRI or CT scan, electroencephalogram (EEG), lumbar puncture, rapid plasma reagen test (RPR), toxoplasmosis titer, and the presence of cryptococcal antigen can provide valuable information in evaluating patients who are immunocompromised.

Infections are not the only source of difficulty for an HIV-infected person's central nervous system. There is an increased incidence of cancers, particularly of primary Central Nervous System (CNS) lymphoma, in persons who are HIV positive. In the case of any space-occupying lesion seen on a head CT scan, the possibility of a lymphoma needs to be considered.[10] Some groups would advocate strenuously for aggressive biopsy of brain lesions, although this is not common practice.

Even if Tim's central nervous system did not show signs of opportunistic infection or tumor and his body did not show general metabolic abnormality, there was a remaining source of possible brain damage—infection with the HIV virus itself. The virus is believed to be neurotropic in nature, living in macrophages and becoming activated at some point, usually manifesting later in the course of HIV illness. Early on during the acute infection, patients may experience an encephalitis related to their HIV infection. During the chronic stage, patients may experience a combination of cognitive, motor, and behavioral disturbances that have been characterized as the AIDS dementia complex (ADC).[11] ADC (also known as AIDS neurocognitive disorder, HIV encephalopathy, HIV subcortical dementia) is a phenomenon that is usually evident later in HIV infection, as the CD4 lymphocyte count begins to fall. It is categorized by changes in memory (slowing and loss of precision), mood (apathy or agitation), decreased concentration, and subsequent motor symptoms such as hyperreflexia, tremor, ataxic gait, impairment of rapid alternating movements, and dysarthic speech.

The diagnosis of AIDS dementia complex is both an ominous and important one. It is ominous in that there is currently no treatment that will specifically arrest the progress of the virus in the CNS, and because, in general, patients and their families despair when the word "dementia" is applied. It is an important diagnosis to make because, if made during the mild to moderate stages, it gives care providers, patients, and families some time to prepare and plan for the time ahead when the individual becomes less autonomous and less competent to participate in treatment decisions.

The diagnosis is usually one of exclusion made when certain clinical conditions are present and there is no other clear etiology for memory loss or motor or behavior problems. There are no true tests that are diagnostic for ADC and, even at times of severe impairment, cerebrospinal fluid (CSF) may not grow HIV virus in cultures.[12,13] Some data like brain atrophy on CT,[14] fornical enhancement on MRI,[15] and some characteristic abnormalities (difficulty with complex sequencing, reduced verbal fluency, impaired rapid movement with relative preservation of other verbal abilities) on neuropsychological tests (such as Trails A & B, Finger Tap, Wisconsin Card Sort) are associated with the diagnosis of ADC.[16]

Although no single instrument can lead to a conclusive diagnosis, neuropsychological testing in conjunction with neurological and psychiatric examination helps in making a definitive diagnosis. The following is a clinical neuropsychological battery developed by Rex Swanda, Ph.D., of New York University Medical Center, Bellevue Hospital:[17]

The WAIS-R
Digit Span from the WAIS-R
Shipley Institute of Living Scale intellectual quotient
Rey Auditory Verbal Learning Test
A Cancellation Test (scanning rows of numbers and indicating repeated numbers)
Finger-tapping from the Halstead-Reitan Neurological Battery
Grooved Pegboard
Trailmaking A and B (resembling connect-the-dot tasks)
Complex Figure Test (measures immediate and delayed recognition)
Benton Visual Retention Test
Word Fluency

Once medical reasons for behavior change are eliminated, there are still a large number of psychiatric possibilities. In the case of Tim, the Diagnostic and Statistical Manual of Mental Disorders (DSM) III-R Axis I differential diagnoses could include: Psychotic Disorder, NOS; Schizoaffective Disorder;

Brief Reactive Psychosis; Major Depression, Recurrent; Bipolar Disorder, Manic Phase; Organic Mood Disorder, Manic Phase; Adjustment Disorder with Mixed Disturbance of Emotions and Conduct. An Axis II diagnosis of Personality Disorder, NOS, must be explored as there are some patients with severe character pathology who are known to regress to psychotic behavior. Alcohol or Drug Delirium should also be considered in the differential diagnosis. In the case of symptoms of recent onset, it is wise to consider a broad-based psychiatric differential diagnosis. Narrowing down the differential diagnosis too quickly may close the door on therapeutic strategies that could be effective.

Let us consider Tim's differential diagnosis. For the sake of discussion, let us assume that delirium, intoxication/withdrawal, ADC, and other medical reasons have been eliminated. Though there is a history of a brief depressive episode, his current symptoms (excessive spending, pressured speech, acceleration, grandiosity) are not consistent with depression. These symptoms are much more in keeping with a diagnosis of bipolar disorder. The presence of a diagnosis of AIDS with low CD4 also suggests that the virus may have played some role in the CNS. This makes a diagnosis of organic mood syndrome, manic phase, the most probable contender.

Tim's psychotic state was too insidious in onset and too long-lasting to be a brief reactive psychosis. The time frame falls outside the 3–6 month limit for adjustment disorders. Schizoaffective disorder could not be eliminated at the time of assessment, but there had been no episodes of delusions in the absence of mood symptoms. Affective disorders had not yet been ruled out. While psychotic disorder, NOS, could not be ruled out, it looked as though more specific diagnostic possibilities existed. Given Tim's premorbid high level of function, personality disorder severe enough to regress to psychosis was unlikely.

Such a review of possibilities leaves organic mood disorder, manic, or bipolar disorder, manic, as the most likely choices. Which diagnosis one chooses will depend to some extent on the theoretical background of the clinician. A neuropsychiatrist is more likely to see this as an organic mood disorder, manic phase, and indeed there have been a number of papers noting manic presentations in people with AIDS.[18,19]

Treatment will proceed in largely the same manner with either diagnosis, relying on a combination of antipsychotic medication and lithium as the initial treatment.[20] The diagnosis of organic mood disorder assumes some neurological vulnerability, and medications used might need to be lower in dose or less anticholinergic (i.e. Nortriptyline instead of Amitriptyline; low-dose Haldol instead of Mellaril). The prognosis is also somewhat different, since patients with bipolar illness frequently have good recovery and a substantial period of wellness, whereas patients with organic mood disorder will suffer from the effects of the virus upon the nervous system, even after mania subsides. Kieburtz, Zettelmaier, et al. note that patients whose mania resolves reveal underlying and previously undetected ADC.[21]

It is important in considering both the psychiatric and physical etiologies of altered mental status in HIV+ patients to recognize the importance of examining the patient carefully after the manic phase is resolved.

People with AIDS are afflicted both with a virus that cannot be cured and with a deteriorating health picture. However, many of the symptoms that make living with the HIV virus difficult are treatable. In the United States in the early to mid eighties, pneumocystis pneumonia was the most common disease manifested by people with AIDS and it was usually virulent. People often died during a first or second episode in under a year. With the advent of AZT and aerosolized pentamidine, pneumocystis pneumonia is a much less common cause of death or disability for people with AIDS.

Similarly, there are a wide variety of central nervous system pathogens that can be treated. There is a high concurrence of HIV and multiple sexually transmitted diseases, with syphilis rates increasing rapidly in certain parts of the United States. Syphilis has long been known to produce mental status changes and it would be irresponsible to miss the opportunity to treat neurosyphilis in a patient experiencing mental status changes. Other agents such as toxoplasmosis or cryptococcal meningitis are also common and respond quite well to treatment.

Not only are such organic health problems amenable to treatment, but the field of psychiatry has a lengthy history of successful treatment of many mental illnesses. The use of psychotherapy and psychopharmacologic agents can help considerably to improve the quality of life of people with HIV. Even with diagnoses such as AIDS dementia complex or other conditions with poor prognosis, there is still a great deal that can be done to improve the quality and length of life of the patient with HIV.

### Todd's Case and the Importance of the Natural Support System

At the point that health care providers begin to feel that they have the least to offer, the natural support mechanism becomes critical to the preservation of the patient's day-to-day functioning. In Todd's case, the health care providers were able to assist in the mobilization of a highly effective family and community support system.

Todd had been diagnosed with an organic mood disorder, manic phase, and he also had full-blown HIV disease, AIDS. He had already been afflicted with pneumocystis pneumonia. His immune system was severely compromised. He had been admitted to a psychiatric hospital and during his hospitalization he was stabilized on a combination of small amounts of an antipsychotic medication and lithium. In the structured setting of the hospital, Todd did well given his deteriorated physical and mental state, but was still impulsive, intrusive, and in need of frequent supervision, particularly in the handling of cigarettes and matches. Todd's persistent wish was to leave the hospital. He was a man who enjoyed his career as a teacher of dance and had a group of artistic friends. He was the father of an adolescent son and wished to spend his last days with his family and friends enjoying life. Todd's spiritual development was also important to him and he spent much of his time pursuing church activities such as sacred dance and potluck suppers.

In order for Todd to feel well again, he needed to leave the hospital and resume a normal life. However, given the difficulty of his problems, Todd would be unlikely to succeed in this endeavor without the help of a natural support system. When Todd became insistent upon trying to make it on his own in an apartment, his family, although skeptical about his ability to do this, agreed to help him move. They visited many times during the week to see that he had adequate groceries and heat, and that he was not in any type of crisis.

Not only was the immediate local family an important support, but Todd cared deeply for his elderly mother. Additionally, Todd's sister helped arrange Todd's visitation with his adolescent son. Since his ex-wife was justifiably concerned about sending her 14-year-old son to spend an extended time with a man who was suffering from AIDS dementia, Todd's sister offered to have the child stay with her.

Todd also reached out to the local spiritual community and gained acceptance by a particular network of clergy who dedicated much of their time to working with people with HIV. In addition, he participated in activities at the local community-based organization for people with AIDS and this became a source of support. One further source of support was Todd's landlord.

Todd's landlord was also a gay man who felt empathy and compassion for Todd's difficult situation. Despite recognizing the risk of taking a person who had serious medical and psychiatric problems and was living on disability into his apartment building, he took this risk and became Todd's most consistent daily visitor.

Eventually, this intricate natural support system needed to arrange for Todd's admission to a nursing home, prior to his final hospitalization and death. They felt great satisfaction that they had been able to give Todd many weeks living life to the fullest.

It is important to remember that no matter how good, caring, or reliable the health care system is, it can never provide for a patient what the community, family, and friends can provide. No nursing staff member would or should have taken Todd into his or her home. No therapist could have kept him safe or brought him groceries. No day hospital program could provide the family love and compassion that Todd felt in his last weeks of life. When one is taking care of patients with complicated medical and psychiatric problems, it is easy to blame families for past cut-offs or problems, to view them as dysfunctional or somehow at fault. If this happens, therapists risk allying themselves with the patient alone and becoming adversarial to family members, to their concerns and wishes. This can be disastrous for the patient. The natural support system (family, friends, and community) is the best and most cost-effective agent for lasting change and should be involved from the beginning and through all care planning.

The earlier case of Tim illustrates how family support systems can be helpful to health care providers. In the hospital setting, Tim was a challenge. He was intrusive, used bad language, and sometimes appeared aggressive and angry toward eldery patients on the unit. All of this made the staff angry with him. His behavior on the inpatient unit required frequent limit-setting and reminders of rules. Over time, through participating in unit behavior plans, medication administration, and accessing the support of their extended family, the parents learned how to care for Tim in their home. The health care providers were able to work out a plan in which they periodically gave Tim's family some respite when they were exhausted by caring for him. This meant that the family and not the health care system provided Tim's long-term placement. This was a situation in which all benefited: the patient for being able to stay with his family, the family for feeling good about being able to be there for their son at a critical time, and the health care team for being able to have reasonable disposition plans for Tim and for having help in monitoring him during his brief stays on the unit.

### Roberto's Case and Problems of Placement

Roberto was a 50-year-old man from Puerto Rico who had lived in the United States for most of his adult life. He still had strong family connections to Puerto Rico and had brothers both there and in the United States. He was married to Belinda who, despite having one Puerto Rican parent, was very Americanized. Roberto had become HIV positive as a result of his drug use, while Belinda had acquired the virus through her sexual contacts with Roberto.

Their medical treatment was difficult, since Roberto periodically went out on drug sprees, which resulted in noncompliance with treatment and family chaos. Roberto began to show signs of cognitive impairment. He exhibited the classic signs of early HIV dementia, including confusion and cognitive slowing, balance problems and ataxic gait, forgetfulness and memory impairment, withdrawal and apathy, mood lability, difficulties in concentration, some dysarthric speech, and the inability to perform rapid alternating movements.[17] Belinda took care of him as long as she could, until his behavioral change resulted in a violent episode in the home that made her feel frightened for her safety. At that point, she brought him to the emergency department where she insisted that he be admitted.

Upon his admission to the psychiatric unit, it became clear to the staff that Roberto was very near the end of his life. He had profound wasting, was extremely apathetic and withdrawn, and exhibited late-stage symptoms of AIDS dementia.[17]

Belinda continued to attend college and became tearful and anxious whenever the staff mentioned her taking Roberto home. It was only upon referral to therapy that a careful investigation of their family and their culture revealed that assistance might be available from the natural support system. Belinda had never felt fully accepted by Roberto's family. She had always been different—not completely Puerto Rican, too American in her ways. Belinda was constantly torn between knowing that she could not care for Roberto alone, but that she should take him home if she cared for his family's opinion of her.

Finally, after several therapy sessions with Belinda and Roberto, the care team asked Roberto's brothers to come in. With Roberto's help, his brothers were able both to bless his marriage to Belinda and to praise Belinda for what she had been able to do in caring for their brother. With their support and blessing, Belinda felt freer to take the risk of trying to care for Roberto at home, even though she knew that his death was imminent. She took him home and he died within 72 hours of leaving the hospital. Both Belinda and Roberto's family felt good that his last hours had been in his own home with people who loved him. The brothers perceived that Belinda was not really a bad wife and they recognized her wisdom in calling them in to help her.

In this case, it is easy to see how significant cultural factors could have been missed. Care teams usually are stretched thin, with too many patients and too little time to know each patient well. In a case like Roberto's, where the care team realized that he was going to die soon, the impulse to discharge him despite Belinda's protests would generally prevail. It was only by exploration of the natural support system and cultural context of this demented patient that the real stumbling block was discovered. The central issue was Roberto's family's lack of support for Belinda when she needed it so desperately. By uncovering Belinda's fear of asking for their support and dealing with the cultural issues involved, the therapist was able to help the family resolve their difficulties.

Another component of treatment raised by Roberto's case was that of chemical dependency. Many patients who are HIV positive abuse chemicals or alcohol, whether that was the way they came in contact with the virus or not. For some patients, HIV positivity marks a signal for a drug spree, since they feel they have nothing more to lose. There are others for whom HIV positivity demonstrates the first real consequence of drug use and frightens them sufficiently to encourage them to change their ways. The case of Emily, described in Chapter 8, illustrates the latter response. From a neuropsychiatric perspective, it is important to understand how drugs and alcohol further cloud already impaired thinking and complicate the diagnosis of patients with central nervous system conditions. An acute withdrawal or intoxication can mimic psychosis, dementia, or mania. Active use of substances may also impede treatment with other psychopharmacologic agents and will often interfere with placement options for individuals who need placement in long-term care settings.

For these reasons, it is important to have patients who have such problems assessed by substance abuse counselors and, when appropriate, enrolled in programs to help them deal with their problems. It is important to remember that many patients may feel more comfortable if they attend a chemical dependence group or 12-step fellowship program with people like themselves, such as a young adult group, a gay men's group, a women's group, an ethnic group, or a hearing-impaired group. It is also important to remember that as patients' cognitive abilities decrease, their ability to tolerate confrontational group settings may also decrease. At such times, it may be more useful to search for an appropriately supportive group and/or to pair the client or patient with a sympathetic sponsor.

## CLINICAL MANAGEMENT

### Psychopharmacology

Medications are an important component of the treatment of patients with central nervous system manifestations of HIV disease. As noted before, it is always imperative that we rule out other central nervous system pathogens prior to attributing aberrant behavior to the HIV. Antiretrovirals like AZT can improve some mental status abnormalities in a previously untreated patient.[22] Once that has been achieved, there are some general rules of thumb that can be applied in the use of psychopharmacology.

It is useful to think about HIV-infected brains, particularly in the later stages of the disease, as being similar to the brains of elderly patients. Indeed, images of brains (CT scans) from young patients with advanced HIV disease resemble the atrophy seen in the brains of elderly patients. A general principle of psychopharmacology in the elderly is to expect that side effects of medications will be worse. This is true in HIV as well. For this reason, when using antidepressants, it is important to think about minimizing sedation, orthostatic hypotension, constipation, and other unpleasant side effects. It is important to obtain an electrocardiogram (EKG) before starting a tricyclic antidepressant, and, whenever possible, to use one that has relatively low anticholinergic side effects, such as nortriptyline or disipramine.

Clearly, there are patients who for a variety of reasons cannot tolerate these medications but do respond well to other categories of medications like fluoxetine. Fluoxetine dosing should be done carefully, as in the elderly, starting with a low divided dose such as 10 milligrams four times a day and gradually titrating upward. As in the elderly, the idea of starting low and going slow is helpful for most people with HIV disease.[23]

It is also helpful to have clearly identified target symptoms against which one can balance the side-effect profile and drug response. The target symptoms should be measurable and be expected to go away when depression lifts. For example, if a patient is extremely anemic and fatigued secondary to AZT-induced anemia (which may frequently require a transfusion), it would be unrealistic to list increased engergy as one of the target symptoms for an antidepressent. However, improved sleep or appetite may be very appropriate symptom targets.

Benzodiazepines are given at times, but need to be used with judicious concern. They seem to be most useful at some of the psychological junctions in the progression of HIV disease. Such important hallmark times in the disease are: a) when the person is first told that he or she is HIV positive, b) when waiting for a lover or partner's test to come back, or c) at the time of the first AIDS-defining illness. At such times, features of anxiety and panic predominate and benzodiazepines can be highly effective. (Over time, however, the anxiety may evolve into true depressive symptoms, at which time antidepressants are the drug of choice).

In low and time-limited doses, benzodiazepines can help keep people at a high level of functioning and should be considered while antidepressants are reaching adequate blood levels. However, they must be considered and used carefully for two reasons: First, just as in elderly patients, there can be some paradoxical response in brains that are damaged by HIV infection; instead of experiencing a calming effect, the patient may become more disinhibited and agitated. Secondly, given the complex number of medications that patients are on, as well as the propensity for drug and alcohol use and abuse shown by many of the patients, there are certainly some dangerous potentials for side effects when benzodiazepines are utilized.

Antipsychotics do become necessary at times in the treatment of people with HIV disease. In the case of Tim, the only way the family was able to maintain him in their home environment was by the use of some Trilafon at bedtime, which allowed him to have some sleep and be more relaxed. Specifically, patients who present with organic mood disorders, bipolar illnesses, or psychotic disorders may require some antipsychotic to help them maintain stable behavior and be able to live at home instead of in an institution. Again, caution needs to be taken since HIV may potentiate the side effects of antipsychotics. Patients may develop tardive dyskinesia more rapidly, have more dystonia and extrapyramidal symptoms, or suffer more from the hypotensive effects of antipsychotics.

Nonetheless, medications like Haldol, Thorazine, and Trilafon do have a role in the treatment of acutely agitated and disturbed individuals. Lithium can also be very useful in patients who present with a manic picture, though generally, due to the state of health of the individuals, the dose required to produce an effect may be somewhat lower than the usual 900 milligrams a day and many patients respond well at 450–600 milligrams. There are some clinicians who recommend the use of Ritalin for increasing energy and appetite; this may be beneficial in cases of severe apathy and anorexia. However, since this is usually a time when individuals are approaching death, the benefits of the Ritalin may be overlooked.

**Psychotherapy**

In addition to hospitalization, medication, and mobilization of family and natural systems support, the role of psychotherapy for patients should not be minimized. Patients have multiple issues to examine when they must face a terminal illness; a supportive context in which patients and their families can come to some peace with such problems and concerns is clearly helpful. This will be discussed in greater detail in Chapter 8. In helping patients and their families deal with the onset of dementia and behavioral disturbances, Boss's model for working with Alzheimer's patients and their families is directly applicable.[24] In addition, the psychoeducational approaches to schizophrenia[25,26,27] and the educational programs for families of alcoholics[28] may be adapted to HIV disease.

Group, individual, family, and multifamily group psychotherapy can be useful adjuncts to care. They can provide a forum in which patients and their families can identify with others, gain support, and learn new approaches for dealing with situations involved in coping with HIV. Because of the CNS manifestations of HIV, group therapy can become extremely challenging, particularly if one of the patients begins to dement. A decision to ask the patient to leave the group illustrates to the other patients that there are some forms of HIV disease that are unacceptable in the group. On the other hand, keeping the patient in the group is likely to result in disruption and heartbreak for other group members, or for family members in multifamily groups when they are exposed to watching another person become cognitively limited. Such decisions require frequent group discussion, processing, and talking about the issues up front.

As an adjunct to the above approaches, brief supportive individual therapy may be helpful during the early stages of neurologic involvement. Patients frequently need reassurance about their concerns for family members; one may need to meet alone with the patient to persuade him or her not to shut the family out in an attempt to protect loved ones. Patients may also feel more comfortable sharing initial concerns with the therapist in order to plan how to share them with family members.

Bonjean describes the interface of demented patient and caregiver in her work with Alzheimer's patients.[29] Many of the problems and principles of management that she identifies apply equally well to AIDS dementia patients and their families. She stresses that the patient's dementia creates a constant, stressful vigilance in the caregiver, since the caregiver has to handle the patient's depression, wandering, paranoia, incontinence, belligerence or assaultive behavior, or constant repeating of conversations and questions. In addition to the primary caregiver, secondary caregivers who do not live in the same household can also be affected. They have concerns and questions about the evolving care of the patient and also worry about giving emotional support to the primary caregiver. All caregivers may experience communication pattern changes, disrupted family structure, change in roles, grief for the loss of a loved one, and worry about contracting the disease.

Patients in the early stages of dementia should be included in family therapy sessions in order to allow them to talk about their preferences about care and take some of the burden away from other family members. As we mentioned earlier, patients and their families may need help in managing their feelings about the loss of cognitive and functional capacities. Family treatment prevents the isolation that often characterizes such loss of personhood and, finally, loss of life. Families also assist in the normalization of such losses, providing the patient with a level of support that would be inappropriate for the health care provider.

In both Alzheimer's dementia and AIDS dementia, the family and loved ones realize that there is no cure, and that they will have to stand by and watch while the patient "mentally declines into a state of gross deterioration with only the physical body as a reminder of who the person once was."[30] However, with AIDS dementia, the physical body also deteriorates and the loved one may be barely recognizable by the end, generating even deeper "feelings of despair, anger, helplessness and anguish."[30] Ware and Carper[30] suggest dealing with the family by thoroughly explaining the nature and progression of the disease, providing a tiny ray of hope for research progress, informing the family of various support groups in the community, and giving the family a sense of common cause and purpose. The family also needs to be helped in dealing with the stress and anger caused by the increasing dependency of the patient. Family members need to be counseled about neglecting their own activities and needs, and recognizing the normality of their reactions. They should be encouraged to draw upon community facilities such as respite care and hospices.

Not only does the patient need the support of the caregiver and the family, but family and friends should be mobilized to support the caregiver.[31] As the Zarits note, "Kahn has proposed that dementia is a 'biopsychosocial' phenomenon, and while the biological may not currently be modified, the psychological and social aspects are often amenable to intervention."[31] In addition to psychopharmacology and psychotherapy, practical skills may be shared with patient and support system to make dealing with dementia a little easier.

### Practical Skills in Dealing with Dementia or Delirium

If caregivers can learn to trace the sequences of frustrating behaviors, and develop a behavioral training program, they can construct practical techniques for managing the demented patient.[29] Winiarski lists such techniques for patients with AIDS dementia,[17] and the techniques suggested by Bonjean,[29] Ware and Carper,[30] and Zarit and Zarit[31] for Alzheimer's patients can also be adapted for this population. The following table integrates some of their suggested techniques with strategies that we have developed and found to be useful.

**TABLE 7-A**
**Practical Coping Strategies**

| | |
|---|---|
| Maintain consistency of environment in patient's living situation and relationships. | Keep patient close to home. Keep living quarters stable. Keep food, personal belongings, medications, etc. in the same place. Be sure patient has dentures, glasses, hearing aid in same place, and uses them. Maintain social patterns, e.g. visits on same day of week. Make a chart of where things are. Keep a light on in the bathroom. |
| Create a care team to help the caregiver and family cope. | Have regularly scheduled visits. Assign regular telephone checks. Assign family members and friends to call the patient. Provide emergency access to patient's home. Utilize personal care assistance in the home. |

| | |
|---|---|
| Create a reminder system. | Have patient carry a calendar and supervise the recording of all appointments. Use an oversize calendar posted in the bedroom. Mark calendar days with X's. |
| Reinforce memory strategies. | Use pictures, nonverbal aids such as arrows to bathroom. Utilize verbal or written cues for necessary activities of daily living. Reduce environmental stimulation. Maintain focus on one task at a time. Help patient keep a diary recording daily activities for easy recall. |
| Adapt technology and environment. | Buy a pillbox marked for the days of the week. Set the pillbox to beep, or use a clock or wristwatch with alarm or voice. Subscribe to a telephone service to make reminder calls. For motor neuropathies, buy special equipment. Use simple books with pictures (such as children's books) and magazines. |
| Reality orientation. | Have friends and visitors continue to identify themselves and orient the patient to time, place and circumstance. Speak slowly in simple sentences and stay with concrete phrases. When in doubt, ask patient to rephrase. Pause between sentences to allow patient to interact. |
| Maintain an emotionally and physically safe environment. | Monitor the patient's condition. Call the physician if changes occur. Remove or lock up any dangerous objects. When in doubt, call the medical hotline or go to the emergency room. When possible, include the patient in care planning. Once deficits are severe, do not talk about them in his or her presence. Do not talk to patient as if he or she were a child. Encourage patient to feel a sense of worth and confidence. |

|  | Deal with patient's feelings as if he or she were not impaired, but do not get into arguments; rather, change the subject. |
|---|---|
| Maintain a realistic outlook on support. | Recognize caregiver will become fatigued, irritable, angry, fantasize escape, or need respite. Ensure that caregiver seeks respite and takes necessary time off. Help caregiver realize the normality of his or her reactions. Help caregiver and family seek community groups. Suggest caregiver take time alone, go for a walk, have a separate room available. |
| Assist in problem-solving. | If patient is awake at night and sleeping in the day, adjust sleeping pattern and if necessary, check sleeping medication. Help caregiver and family members learn to change their responses by recognizing the function of the patient's behavior. Help caregivers design simple tasks for family and friends. |

## REFERENCES

1. Navia, B.A., Jordan, B.O., Price, R.W. (1986). The AIDS dementia complex: I. Clinical features. *Annals of Neurology,* 19: 517–524.

2. Fauci, A.S. (1988). The Human Immunodeficiency Virus: Infectivity and mechanisms of pathogenesis. *Science,* 239: 617–622.

3. Levy, R.M., Bredesen, D.E., Rosenblum, M.L. (1985). Neurological manifestations of the acquired immunodeficiency syndrome (AIDS): Experience at UCSF and review of the literature. *Journal of Neurosurgery,* 62: 475–495.

4. Petito, C.K., Cho, E.S., Lehman, W., Navia, B.A., Price, R.W. (1986). Neuropathology of acquired immunodeficiency syndrome (AIDS): An autopsy review. *Journal of Neuropathology and Experimental Neurology,* 45: 635–646.

5. So, Y.T. (1990). Neurologic dysfunction: Intracranial disorders. In P.T. Cohen, M.A. Sande, P.A. Volberding (Eds.) *The AIDS Knowledge Base.* Waltham, Mass.: The Medical Publishing Group.

6. Halen, R.E., Yudofsky, S.C. (1987). *The American Psychiatric Press Textbook of Neuropsychiatry.* Washington, D.C.: American Psychiatric Press.

7. Belman, A.L., Diamond, G., Dickson, D., et al. (1988). Pediatric acquired

immunodeficiency syndrome: Neurologic syndromes. *American Journal of Childhood Diseases.* 142: 29–35.

8. (May, 1989). Neurological and Neuropsychological Complications of HIV Disease Conference. Quebec City, Canada.

9. Berger, J.R., Kaszowitz, B., Post, M.J.D., Dickinson, G. (1987). Progressive multifocal leukoencephalopathy associated with human immunodeficiency virus infection: A review of the literature with a report on sixteen cases. *Annals of Internal Medicine.* 107: 78–87.

10. Levy, R.M., Rosenbloom, S., Perrett, L.V. (1986). Neuroradiologic findings in AIDS: A review of 200 cases. *American Journal of Neurologic Radiology.* 7: 833–839.

11. Price, K.W., Brew, B., Sidtis, J., Rosenbloom, M., Scheck, A.C., Cleary, P. (1988). The brain in AIDS: Central nervous system HIV-1 infection and AIDS Dementia Complex. *Science.* 239: 586–592.

12. McArthur, J., Cohen, B., Farzedegan, H., Cornblath, D., Selnes, O., Ostrow, D., Johnson, R., Phair, J., Polk, F. (1988). Cerebrospinal fluid abnormalities in homosexual men and without neuropsychiatric findings. *Annals of Neurology.* 23 (supplement): 534–537.

13. Tourtellotte, W. (1989). Use of cerebrospinal fluid in diagnosing and monitoring AIDS dementia. Basic Science Workshop AIDS Clinical Trial Group (ACTG) Meeting. July, 1989.

14. Post, M.J., Sheldon, J.J., Hensley, G.T., Sorla, K., Tobias, J.A., Chan, J.C., Quencer, R.M., Moskowitz, L.B. (1986). Central nervous system disease in acquired immunodeficiency syndrome: Prospective correlation using CT, MR imaging, and pathologic studies. *Radiology,* 158: 141–148.

15. Kieburtz, K., Ketonen, L., Zettelmaier, A.E., Kido, D.K., Caine, E.D., Simon, J.H. (in press). MRI findings in HIV cognitive impairment. *Neurology.*

16. Tross, S., Price, R.W., Navia, B., Thaler, H.T., Gold, J., Hirsch, D.A., Sidtis, J.J. (1988). Neuropsychological characterization of the AIDS Dementia Complex: A preliminary report. *AIDS,* 2(2): 81–88.

17. Winiarski, M.G. (1991). *AIDS-Related Psychotherapy.* New York: Pergamon Press.

18. Kermani, E., Drob, S., Alpert, M. (1984). Organic brain syndrome in three cases of acquired immunodeficiency syndrome. *Comprehensive Psychiatry,* 25(3): 294–297.

19. Kermani, E., Borod, J.C., Brown, P.H., Tunnell, G. (1985). New psychopathologic findings in AIDS: Case report. *Journal of Clinical Psychiatry,* 46(6): 240–241.

20. Perry, S.W., Markowitz, J. (1986). Psychiatric interventions for AIDS-spectrum disorders. *Hospital and Community Psychiatry,* 37(10): 1001–1006.

21. Kieburtz, K., Zettelmaier, A.E., Ketonen, L., Tuite, M., Caine, E.D. (1991). Manic syndrome in AIDS. *American Journal of Psychiatry,* 148 (8): 1068–1070.

22. Schmitt, F.A., Begley, J.W., McKinnis, R., Logue, P.E., Evans, R.W., Drucker, J.L. (1988). AZT collaborative working group, neuropsychological outcome of zidovudine (AZT) treatment of patients with AIDS and AIDS-related complex. *New England Journal of Medicine,* 319(24): 1573–1578.

23. Jenihe, M.A. (1989). *Geriatric Psychiatry and Psychopharmacology: A Clinical Approach.* Chicago: Yearbook Medical Publishers.

24. Boss, P.G., Caron, W., Horbal, J. (1988). Alzheimer's disease and ambiguous loss. In C. Chilman, F. Cox, E. Nunnally (Eds.) *Families in Trouble*. Newbury Park: Sage.
25. Falloon, I.R.H., Boyd, J.L., McGill, C.W. (1984). *The Family of Schizophrenia: A Problem-Solving Approach to the Treatment of Mental Illness*. New York: Guilford Press.
26. Anderson, C., Reiss, D.J., Hogarty, G.E. (1986). *Schizophrenia and the Family: A Practitioner's Guide to Psychoeducation and Management*. New York: Guilford Press.
27. Goldstein, M.J., Hand, I., Hahlweg, K. (Eds.) (1986). *Treatment of Schizophrenia: Family Assessment and Intervention*. New York: Springer–Verlag.
28. Wegscheider, S. (1981). *Another Chance: Hope and Health for the Alcoholic Family*. Palo Alto: Science and Behavior Books.
29. Bonjean, M. (1988). Helping families cope with Alzheimer's disease. *Family Therapy Today,* 3(6): 1–4.
30. Ware, L.A., Carper, M. (1982). Living with Alzheimer's disease patients: Family stresses and coping mechanisms. *Psychotherapy: Theory, Research and Practice,* 19(4): 472–481.
31. Zarit, S.H., Zarit, J.M. (1982). Families under stress: Interventions for caregivers of senile dementia patients. *Psychotherapy: Theory, Research and Practice,* 19(4): 461–471.

# CHAPTER 8

# Psychotherapeutic Intervention: From Individual Through Group to Extended Network

## *J. Landau-Stanton, C. D. Clements, M. D. Stanton*

### THERAPEUTIC PERSPECTIVE

In Chapter 2, we were introduced to the biological, psychological, and social aspects of Kevin, Helene, and Mary, and we learned the benefit of using a wide angle lens to let us see the total picture of their lives. In the same way, the perspective selected by the psychotherapist influences the therapist's therapeutic direction, as well as the therapy outcome.

In the case of patients with HIV infection, it becomes almost impossible to narrow the lens. They are embedded in their social networks and cannot be viewed from a purely individual perspective. However the issues are presented, the AIDS patient's significant others are inevitably involved. This involvement may be limited to their concerns about their own vulnerability to infection or extend to their feelings about losing someone they love. In addition, this disease involves significant responses from the community. Community agencies, self-help groups, and medical care providers have become intensively involved. Patients may also be connected to the legal system or be a member of a political action group.

Why should the psychotherapist be concerned about these systems at the clinical level? Although Mary's therapist saw her alone, it was impossible to view her without considering her children, her mother, her boyfriend, her socioeconomic background, her hopes and dreams. It was crucial for the therapist to understand these multiple systems levels, regardless of what form of clinical intervention was to be used. In the same way, Kevin's main concern was the care of his mother after he was gone. He hoped his spouse/ lover would continue to be a son to her. Kevin also dreamed about leaving a legacy to the community. He wanted to contribute to AIDS prevention and education—but not at the cost of those he loved.

How can we as therapists understand enough and deal with all the systems levels that concern our patients? In Helene's case, the therapist's sensitivity not only to her nuclear family system but also to her extended family and cultural background became critical. If we apply the model described and diagrammed in Chapter 2, we can more easily identify the systems of which we need to be aware in order to provide her with good clinical care. Following the diagram, and starting with (i) the biopsychosocial level, we expand to (ii) the level of the natural support system: Helene's nuclear family, extended family, boyfriend and intimate friends; her student colleagues and work system; her minister and religious community, and her primary medical care system (family doctor), and her community agency support (AIDS community service, AIDS Hotline). This brings us to (iii), the level of ancillary or artificial support system: the specialty AIDS Clinic, Helene's nurse and psychiatrist, her group therapist, and the group members in the AIDS Women's group within the psychiatric service.

In Helene's case, in order to obtain a truly ecosystemic view,[1] we need to consider the next level. Level (iv) includes cultural, spiritual, and philosophical world views and incorporates world events at economic, political, geographic, and even geological levels. For Helene her cultural tradition was extremely important, and her migration away from her traditional context was motivated by political/economic factors.

In certain cases, issues pertaining to membership of minority groups (either gay, racial, or ethnic), disenfranchisement, and prejudice may need to be addressed. These issues impact at a political and economic level as well as at a personal level; failure to consider them may lead to failure of therapy. Patients might also be discriminated against for their behavior patterns, such as substance abuse, (which, of course, is a very high-risk behavior for transmitting the disease). Substance abusers are engaged in self-destructive behavior and have frequently given up hope at the social levels. Risk of HIV infection, or the disease itself, requires attention to the special characteristics of substance abusers and their families in contrast, for example, to those who are at risk or have acquired the disease through blood transfusion. The issue of vulnerability in self-destructive behavior is best viewed from a larger systems perspective and will be discussed below.

Not only the disenfranchised (although this group is perhaps most vulnerable), but anyone facing the possibility of HIV infection feels guilty, deserving of blame, and shamed. These feelings make it difficult for patients to engage in therapy and particularly difficult for them to bring their significant others into therapy sessions. In the pages to follow, we will present a number of methods and techniques for working with the resistance and for successfully engaging the extended system.

Joining the extended family system, both literally and figuratively, of patients with HIV disease becomes critical for many reasons. These are patients facing chronic illness and death. Despite the frequency of apparent cut-offs, connection to family takes on an urgency. Time is compressed for AIDS patients and their families—development and resolution of relationships that should take many years need to occur in a very short period. The disease also distorts, even to the point of reversal, the natural family life cycle. Children become critically ill before their grandparents and parents, often leaving their children to be cared for by the elders of the family. Even the future of the next generation may be threatened, if an only child is infected with HIV and cannot continue the family line by producing descendants. This signifies far more than the loss of an individual for it may be the loss of an entire family's future. Reconnecting the family's transitional pathway across generations, while looking for meaning in their value systems and contributions, becomes essential; helping them to deal with issues of death, dying and the loss to be suffered by survivors is key.

Therapists are not usually trained to deal with the imminent loss of young patients unless they have specifically worked in the area of oncology or Medical Family Therapy.[2,3] They may also not be attuned to dealing with the family following the loss of their patient or to helping the patient and the family plan for the death of the patient and placement of his or her children. Where does the responsibility of the therapist lie? With whom is the primary relationship? Where are the boundaries? Does the therapist visit the patient in the hospital? At home? Who attends the funeral and who helps the family after the death? When does involvement in these activities become overinvolvement, or excessive countertransference?

The threat of loss colors every aspect of the therapy. It is usually perceived in terms of its negative consequences. However, there may be major positive effects of this time compression and urgency of reconnection. If the therapist is open to engaging the extended system to its full capacity, a great deal of healing across the system becomes possible.

All of these issues can be addressed within a systems approach to therapy. The model detailed below is an adaptation of the Rochester Family Therapy Model which, in line with the seminal work of Speck and Attneave,[4] applies network theory as an effective means of change. Unlike Speck and Attneave, who used family networks as a component of therapy, usually as a "last resort," the Rochester Model considers it the method of first choice.[5-14] Similar to Speck and Attneave's conclusions, we've found that the more extensive the network, the more effective the treatment. Also, the earlier the involvement of the larger network in therapy, the more rapid is the healing process. Various other network therapy approaches have developed over the years, following Speck and Attneave's work.[15-19] However, the following pages reflect the use of the Rochester Model.

## THERAPEUTIC PRINCIPLES AND TECHNIQUES
## PART I. OUTLINE OF THE THERAPY SESSION

### 1. Joining and Determining the Level of Intervention

Therapists need to be particularly sensitive to generational hierarchies, non-traditional family constellations and issues of gender when working with these clients and their families. We find it helpful to encourage all present to greet each other by physical touch, which normalizes the process and helps it resemble everyday social exchange. Joining techniques such as utilizing one's position in the room and the sequence of handshakes and verbal participation are also useful.

The complexity of levels that become evident during the joining process and bear consideration when treating people who are infected with the HIV virus is further illustrated by the case of Amy:*

> Amy was a 39-year-old woman who abused cocaine and was diagnosed as being HIV positive. Amy presented for therapy stating that she was severely depressed and experiencing great difficulty in managing her teenage children. Shortly into the session, Amy revealed another purpose to her visit when she produced a disability form, which required urgent signature as she was out of funds. Her economic crisis had arisen because, being only HIV positive and not diagnosed with AIDS, she had no access to medical care.

As Amy's personal history unfolded, it became apparent that her case could easily have confounded an individual therapist committed to the confidential psychiatric care of his or her patient. It could also have stymied the enthusiastic therapist committed to the immediate resolution of the patient's problems. Amy's situation raised questions of what level to intervene at, which treatment systems to include, what priorities to set, how to identify manageable goals for treatment, and how to design the process to achieve the desired outcome of therapy.

> History revealed that both Amy and her fourth husband, Brian, had been heavily implicated in the cocaine trade. Both of the children hated Brian and blamed him for bringing cocaine into the house.

---

*Therapist, Ann Zettelmaier Griepp, M.D.; supervisor, Susan McDaniel, Ph.D. This case was treated in the Family Therapy Training Program of the University of Rochester.

Violence had become a common occurrence in the home and the children had also witnessed their parents' involvement in outbursts of violence in the streets.

Amy's own family lived in Europe and was not easily accessible to her. Her move was partially an attempt to expand her family support by including the children's own father and his extended family who were from the area. She wanted to ensure that the children would be taken care of in the event of her death. Her contact with her ex-husband had been minimal, however, and when she arrived in upstate New York she found that he was no longer living there.

Mental health status examination was essentially normal, with evidence of some anxiety and depressed mood. There was no sign of major depression or suicidality, nor was Amy psychotic. Her cognitive functioning was normal and there was no sign of neuropsychiatric problems.

From the above, the therapist determined that the issue of psychiatric disability was marginal, particularly since HIV infection was not then seen as qualifying the patient for disability. In order to resolve the therapeutic dilemma, the therapist decided to employ the patient's motivation for disability to aid her in the therapy. The therapist insisted that she was unable to make a clear determination without the assistance of Brian and the children. The therapist was now involved at both the individual/biopsychosocial and nuclear/relational family levels.

## 2. Establishing Strengths and Resources

Amy, Brian and the two children presented for the second session. Shortly after the therapist had developed rapport with Brian and the children, and reconnected with Amy, the session commenced with Brian's statement, "Doc, here I am, HIV positive. It's a bitch to be dying of AIDS in the 80s."

The therapist hastened to look for positive metaphors and reframes to establish what strengths the family had to draw upon to help them deal with the overwhelming events. Families facing infection with HIV are invariably anxious, fearful, and somewhat depressed. They have frequently given up hope and feel responsible and guilty, or blamed, for their predicament. Many AIDS families belong to devalued, disenfranchised, or denigrated groups. These include the gay population, minority groups, inner-city lower socioeconomic families, substance abusers, and people who sell sex. They are already acutely aware of the manner in which they are viewed by society; AIDS only intensifies the self-denigration, guilt, rejection, and inevitable blame. Their cups are always half empty and it is difficult for them to envisage a future. Thus they are less likely to seek external resources that could assist them with their problems. Helping them to view their difficulties from a more positive perspective allows them to uncover options that may not have occurred to them.

A caveat is that positive reframes and metaphors intended to assist families must always be reality-based and the therapist needs to believe in them. An empty Pollyanna promise is of little benefit, since it undercuts the credibility of the therapist and prevents the building of a trusting relationship, an essential for successful therapy. In looking for a positive perspective to share with families, it is useful to explore the relationships prior to the current problems. Helping family members to get in touch with the positive aspects of their earlier relationships helps them to gain motivation, self-confidence, and hope for dealing with current problems.

> Brian was Amy's fourth husband; they had been married for one and a half years. Amy said that this had been her longest relationship since the dissolution of the abusive first marriage to the children's father. Amy had fallen in love with Brian, a likeable, funny disc jockey living a very glamorous fast life, who provided her with constant excitement. They were both facing the loss of this lifestyle and confronting the real possibility of their death. The therapist reframed Brian's earlier statement by suggesting that they all work out a formula not for "dying with AIDS in the 80s'" but for "living with AIDS in the 90s.'"
>
> This created an immediate mood shift in the therapy session by focusing their attention on living one day at a time and gaining as much enjoyment as possible from those days.

In addition to helping the immediate family gain a more positive perspective, it is important to use a multigenerational perspective. The intergenerational models of family therapy have stressed the importance of the family context through time, generally including at least three generations.[20,21,22] With AIDS cases, it is particularly crucial to provide such a perspective, since both patient and support system could be easily demoralized if they looked only at the immediate situation. The rationale for this will be described in more detail later in this chapter in Part Two on the explication of the therapy model.

We have found that the further back one goes the greater the positive information one derives. An effective method for allowing patients and families access to their own competence is encouraging them to look for strengths and resources across the multigenerational extended family and the natural support system. In order to do this, we ask them to list family strengths that have come down to them across time from previous generations and that they would wish to have perpetuated in their children and grandchildren. A list of family strengths developed by Emily's family may be seen in Table 8-B later in the chapter. The list of strengths may be compiled during the initial phase of the session as part of the joining process and then expanded during the mapping process or it may be elicited during the mapping process. In either instance, it may be added to throughout the process of the therapy.

## 3. Mapping the Natural and Artificial Support Systems

*Extended family and natural support system.* Another method for assisting the family in the development of a multigenerational perspective is through the construction of a genogram, which is a graphic display of the extended family over at least three generations.[23] This allows us to explore births, deaths, marriages, separations, and divorces across the extended family system and to gain an impression of multigenerational patterns. Genograms provide ". . . a quick gestalt of complex family patterns and a rich source of hypotheses about how a clinical problem may be connected to the family context and the evolution of both problem and context over time."[23] The method and symbols we use for our genograms are those developed by Bowen[24] and detailed by McGoldrick and Gerson.[23] An example of the genogram may be found in Emily's case, in Figures 8-1 and 8-2, later in the chapter.

We then expand the genogram into a transitional map, further examining and diagramming the many facets of change across time and how they may be connected to present difficulties. In an attempt to determine how the wider context may have interfaced with family life-cycle events depicted on the genogram, we include, for example: culture and country of origin and any changes over time; changes in values, traditions, rituals, religion or spiritual culture; geographic moves; major economic or political changes; natural disasters and any other major events.

Once these have been added to the genogram, we explore with the family whether there have been any family life cycle stages or other transitions that have been difficult for them, and whether these difficulties have been repeated over time across the generations or across sibling and cousin subsystems (i.e. vertically or horizontally on the genogram). If these appear, we mark them with the symbol for transitional conflict. This stage of mapping Emily's family will be found in Figures 8-3 and 8-4.

Since we generally use a color code to simplify the interpretation of complex lines, we have divided the genogram and transitional map of Emily's family into four figures to demonstrate the stages of their development (Figures 8-1 through 8-4). The color code we use in order to consolidate the transitional mapping process into one diagram is: black for all factual information, family members, and members of the natural support system; blue for natural support system relationship lines; red for problem areas or symptoms, as well as for members of the ancillary support system and their relationships to the family; and green for all transitions and transitional conflict lines.

Once the transitional map is drawn, the interpretation is completed by discussion of the strengths, resources, patterns, and themes that appear across generations. This allows the family to realize the inherent assets of their traditions, heritage, and values, seeing how these may have extended across generations and reaching a blame-free understanding of current events. [25-29] The information is then consolidated into a time line, which provides a clear graphic of the coincidence of time-events and how they impact on the current situation. [30] Emily's time line may be found in Figure 8-5.

During the session, we have found that the easiest way to include the family in the mapping process is to use a large sheet of paper attached to an easel. This can then be brought to subsequent sessions for review, addition, or interpretation.

Through mapping, using the methods described above, the therapist was able to discover many strengths and resources in Amy and Brian's family, despite the obvious difficulties they faced. She began by praising them for their move, emphasizing that they had brought the children to a place of safety. The therapist then extended the transitional map to include both Brian and Amy's extended families, as well as that of the children's father. The therapist identified an apparent cut-off between Brian and his family as an area to explore later in the therapy.

In dealing with AIDS families, the process of mapping the family and exploring the strengths and resources of the extended system raises several issues of particular importance. In particular, unresolved grief, loss, and apparent cut-offs are common and deserve the therapist's special attention. The inclusion of members of importance in the support system, beyond the extended family, was also necessary in the case of Amy and Brian.

Amy had two very close friends living in the area, and one of these became her major resource during this time. Amy, Brian, and the children lived in the friend's home and the friend took very good care of them. If one fails to include the friendship network in one's questions, important information and resources may be missed. In addition to friends, inquiries should be made about linkages with other natural support system resources such as family doctors, clergy, neighbors, employers and work colleagues, and community support agencies. Amy had not had time to make these connections, and, in fact, had not even found a primary care physician by the time she presented for psychiatric help. The therapist was able during the mapping process to identify this deficiency and took responsibility for linking her with the local AIDS clinic.

*Ancillary, professional, or artificial support system.* Although Amy had not had time to connect with an ancillary professional support system, her application for disability was steering her in this direction. It had begun to activate the relevant social support services. In dealing with HIV disease, therapists and counselors generally find that multiple services and professional helpers are involved during the course of therapy.

*Healing losses, apparent cut-offs and unresolved grief:* Amy appeared to have very little contact with her family in Britain, with the least contact occurring between Amy and her mother. Amy had left her mother, a prescription addict and alcoholic, in anger 20 years before and had no idea how to bridge the gap. The lack of contact had reached a stage of almost total cut-off between them. She had, however, maintained contact with her brother, thus keeping up with family events. She knew that her mother had cancer and was dying.

Amy's capacity to remain informed about family events despite her apparent cut-offs is not unusual. Research into substance abusers who appeared to be totally out of touch with their families has shown us that cut-offs are often more apparent than real. The substance abusers maintained detail knowledge about important family occurrences through a roundabout route of communication.[31] In our clinical experience, the same applies within the gay population and with others at risk for this terminal illness.

Therapists may be pleasantly surprised if, in exploring this issue, they initially refrain from asking about close contact, instead asking about important family events such as births, deaths, illnesses, graduations, and marriages. Then, the inquiry can pursue the means by which this knowledge was acquired. Once the therapist has allowed the patient to express concern for the family and for to individual members, the patient will find it easier to deal with resolution of the cut-off. This is of particular urgency in HIV disease, since people die unpredictably and time for resolution and healing is limited.

> Amy expressed intense guilt about the cut-off from her dying mother and sadness that she was unable to afford a trip to Britain or even a phone call. While facing her own death, she realized that she would never have contact with her mother again.

## 4. Establishing Treatment Goals and the Therapy Contract

When dealing with people who are overwhelmed and feeling unsure about being able to make any positive changes in their lives, it is useful to establish clear treatment priorities and goals. Instead of identifying problems as such, the family may be encouraged to convert them into specific goals. Drawing upon the strengths and resources identified earlier in the session, the therapist might ask the patient and family, "What would you like to achieve using the multiple strengths that we have discovered?" Patients and families are frequently able to identify particular strengths that would be useful in achieving objectives that earlier in the therapy session seemed out of their reach.

Amy and Brian identified two primary goals as part of this process: their children's safety and ensuring that the children would be taken care of after their death. They were also able to express their wish, with some uncertainty as to how they would achieve it, to reconnect with their families. In addition, they agreed to work on their own issues with death and dying. Another goal was to maintain a sense of living life to the fullest while facing death.

The challenge for Amy and Brian's therapist at this stage was how to help them develop a realistic plan to deal with their request for disability and when (and even whether) to take on the issue of their substance abuse, since the latter was not listed among their goals. The therapist made several decisions about therapeutic choices and directions. She elected not to take on Brian and Amy's drug use at the initial family session, feeling that this would ensure their not returning for further therapy, especially since drug treatment was not their immediate priority. It was necessary to join the family and allow them to achieve some concrete sign of success in their stated goals before the other problems could be tackled. However, even if a family does not deal with an issue of this magnitude fairly early in the therapy, the addiction, and whatever other problems are being denied, will eventually have to be confronted. From the clinician's standpoint, it is primarily a matter of timing.

## 5. Enactment

In order to show the family that they are capable of meeting their goals, and that the strengths and resources that they have identified will enable them to do this, it is useful to employ the technique of *enactment* in the therapy session.[32] Patients are encouraged to identify a primary goal, to state clearly which strengths they will be drawing upon to achieve it, and to start practicing how to do it right there in the session. If this is not done and the first attempt at home fails, they may lose their confidence in themselves and in the therapist. It may be extremely difficult for the therapist to help them regain at a later stage the feeling of competence that they have lost. When one is determining the goal for enactment, it is advisable not to choose the entire goal, but rather to identify a smaller, realistic component of it, so that success may be ensured. A little success is far better than a major failure. In Amy's case, the goal that she and Brian identified as their first priority was reconnecting with their families. They both felt that the most urgent agenda was getting in touch with Amy's dying mother.

The therapist suggested that Amy call her mother immediately from the session. Amy was too frightened and did not feel ready, so the therapist assisted Brian in working with Amy to help her prepare to make the call at the next therapy session. Once she had become more comfortable with the idea and had successfully role-played the phone call, Brian was asked to practice again with Amy at home. Amy felt better as a result of the in-session enactment, supported by the homework, and was able to speak with her mother. The healing had begun.

## 6. Homework

Once the enactment is successfully concluded, homework tasks need to be set, again based on goals, strengths, and successful enactment.[14] In Amy's case, the homework was an extension of the in-session enactment, drawing upon the strength of the marital relationship and the couple's determination to resolve relationships for the sake of their families of origin and their children. Homework needs to be circumscribed, realistic, and highly likely to succeed. For this reason, basing it upon the in-session enactment that the therapist and family have seen succeed is very helpful. Should the family return feeling bad about failure, the therapist needs to take full responsibility for having set unrealistic tasks. In Amy's case the therapy proceeded successfully. Amy had been able to have a meaningful talk with her mother and to resolve their cut-off in a warm and loving way during the in-session enactment. It appeared that she and Brian would be capable of following up the family networking and reconnecting outside of the therapy sessions.

The principles outlined above form a useful outline for both the first and subsequent therapy sessions. Again, it is important to establish strengths and resources early in the session, during the joining phase and while constructing the maps. Doing this makes it far easier for the family to establish realistic goals with hope of a good outcome. It is also useful to ensure that closure of the session is formalized.

## 7. Session Closure and Formalized Greeting

During formal closure, repetition of some of the joining techniques are very useful. For example, shaking hands with AIDS families takes on far more meaning than in other contexts. It is important during both the opening and closing joining to ensure contact between all members of the group present (including patient and therapeutic systems). This formality also assists in normalizing the session by helping families to feel the similarity between this ritual and those of other normal family events (such as financial distress, relocating, career planning, births, weddings, and funerals).

## THERAPEUTIC PRINCIPLES AND TECHNIQUES
## PART II. EXPLICATION OF THE THERAPY MODEL

The previous section provided some specifics for organizing the first therapy session. It gave a feeling for how treatment is initiated and for some of the particular interventions we use with such cases. This section presents the major components of the Rochester Model that apply to the treatment of HIV disease:

1. Cooperation across systems and the engagement and building of a therapeutic team
2. Explicating the transitional pathway.
3. Resolution of unresolved grief, loss and cut-offs.
4. Recognizing scripts, themes and issues of loyalty.
5. Exposing secrets.
6. Resolving transitional conflict and its sequelae.
7. Sensitivity to issues of culture and gender.

### 1. Cooperation Across Systems and the Engagement and Building of a Therapeutic Team

If one is thinking systemically, one has to be aware of all of the levels of the system and their impact upon each other. In HIV disease this is crucial because the biological component will have a major impact at all levels and will cause significant stress across the system.

If therapists remain unaware of the patient's connections with other individuals and systems, they may find that their work is apparently being undercut by others. This may not be intentional, but if communication is incomplete, goals and directions may not be synchronized. As a result, despite the best of intentions all around, people may end up working at cross-purposes. At best, resources that are not pooled may be missed; yet, these cases need all the support they can get.

When one first engages the patient, it may be difficult to persuade him or her to attend the first session with other members of his or her significant network. At the same time, the further the therapy goes, the more difficult it becomes to engage these others. At the least, the therapist should make a careful effort to list all the other members of the extended family, natural support system, and professional system interacting with the patient at a significant level. One may easily achieve this by asking the patient, "Who cares about you and what happens to you? Whom do you see regularly? With whom are you in contact by phone, letter, or visit?" It is often helpful to persuade the patient that we as therapists do not have a history with them, we haven't raised them, and care as we might, we can never love them as their family does. Stressing that we need help in order to provide the best possible therapy assures our patients that we will not blame or scapegoat beloved family members.

Patients may resist involvement of their family members in order to protect them from the horror of the disease. Many of these patients (particularly those with a history of substance abuse, but also those whose families have experienced major losses through time) are scripted to die early,[33] are extremely protective of their families, and are resistant to their coming to therapy. They may be scripted as the saviors of their families, which makes them even more protective.[34] Convincing them that the family will not be harmed, judged, or blamed, but used as a major resource, with acknowledgment of their inherent strengths, lessens the patient's resistance to involving family members in the therapy. Ascribing a noble role to their resistance aids in this process.[31]

While one is engaging key members of the system, however, the other members of the natural and professional support system need to be included in the planning of the therapy. Minimally they should all be contacted; as many as are relevant should be included in the therapy team. Therapists may be surprised by the readiness of the family doctor, the employer, the teacher, the close friends, and others to become involved in helping the patient. This may take considerable effort on the therapist's part, but the result makes the effort worthwhile.

In contacting members of the professional network, one of the basic questions is how the medical team can best work with the mental health providers, the patient, the natural support system, and the rest of the professional support system, including the therapist. In AIDS there are important medical questions, such as the side effects of AZT and DDI, that the entire team needs to take into consideration. There are negotiations with all members of the team about how involved each member should be and how roles should be delineated. Who should be informed about medical complications, or about emotional stress? Where should boundaries be drawn? If consultants are involved, how much should they be included in the intimate family information?

These issues are particularly important for mental health professionals such as psychiatric nurses, social workers, psychiatrists, psychologists, and counselors, all of whom have had some training at various levels in medical science, but who through their identification with behavioral issues may not be regarded by the medical team as legitimate team members. We need to be cooperative team members, without being intrusive or unintentionally undercutting the medical treatment. At the same time, we need to assist the team in being aware of, and sensitive to, the patient's personal, social, and psychiatric situation. A constructive approach is to remind the medical team members of their inherent knowledge of psychiatry and families, thus drawing upon their expertise, rather than lecturing to them.

Stanton, Todd and associates describe many effective techniques for engagement of drug abusers and their families that may easily be applied to this population.[31,35] In addition, Table 8-A provides a listing of frequent resistances to involvement of both natural and professional support systems and some possible responses to them.

### TABLE 8-A
### Engaging AIDS Patients and Their Families

| RESISTANCE | RESPONSE |
|---|---|
| *Logistics & Geography* | |
| "My family lives too far away; I haven't spoken to them in years." | "Well maybe we can just involve them on the telephone." |
| "I don't know where they are." | "It must be very hard not having them know the children. Maybe I can help you trace them." |
| "We live so far away and I'm afraid to drive." | "Well maybe your Dad will make this trip when he knows how important it is." |
| "They're too old to make that trip." | "Wouldn't they be hurt if you didn't give them that choice?" |
| "My husband couldn't possibly take a day off work." | "How about meeting after work next time?" |
| "He's in prison." | "Why don't I speak to the warden and we can all meet there." |
| "They don't even speak English." | "Well, we're fortunate to have an interpreter in the hospital" or "Could you or your wife translate?" |
| "My doctor/minister/therapist is far too busy to come." | "Why don't I give it a try and see if we can coordinate something?" |
| "Don't call my counselor/doctor. I haven't seen him/her for years.' | "It would be really helpful to catch up on some of the details of your earlier history in light of the present." |

### Secrecy, Privacy & Protection

"They don't know about . . . my being gay . . . an addict . . . the rape . . . "

I don't want to hurt them."

"Our family doesn't talk about things."

"My mother is critically ill with heart disease. My father's been sober for so many years this would drive him back to drink and kill my mother."

"This man is my family and he would be hurt if I asked my parents in."

"I don't know who or where my father is."

"How can you make him suffer in his dying days, why can't you let him die in peace?"

"I don't want my children to know. I want their last days with me to be happy."

"My father would never forgive me if he knew. I don't want him to know. I don't want to see him because he'd find out."

"I want them to remember me as I was."

"Well, why don't we just start by asking their advice about the things they do know? You and I can decide together when it's time to share the rest with them."

"Maybe they're not as fragile as you think. When your kids are grown, would you want to be excluded from something this big?"

"Well, maybe this happened to create something so important that it had to be talked about."

"Wouldn't it be more likely to hurt them if they find out only after your death, and you're not there to help them through it?"

"Doesn't he love you enough to want what's best for you? I'm sure you have enough love for them all."

"Let's invite in the others who played a fatherly role in raising you to help me help you. Maybe they also know where we can start looking for him."

"Since we can't guarantee his dying before you, do you really want him to have to deal with this alone?"

"Perhaps it would be kinder to the children to have the mother they've always relied on to help them through tough times be there for them to deal with this? It's the toughest situation they've ever faced. Let's not let them do it alone."

"Maybe he'd rather hear it from you than from others. Are you so sure he'd never find out? I can help you share it with him in a gentle way."

"Didn't your parents change your diapers and clean your vomit when you were small? Don't you think they'd regret missing precious time with you? Would you not visit them if they were frail and smelly?"

"My family would never be able to go back to church."

"Isn't that the best place for them? Is it not a truly Christian/Jewish/Muslim place of forgiveness, community and friendship? Isn't that where they'd receive their best help after your illness? Have no sinners ever been forgiven there?"

"We live in a small town, everyone will know."

"Yes, that is hard. But it can also be a relief when everyone knows and the secret is finally shared. It will also make it easier for the family to have support through this hard time."

"My father/husband/wife will lose his/her job if they find out."

"Isn't it more important to give him/her an opportunity of protecting himself/herself?"

"My kids will have trouble at school."

"There are very few good teachers who wouldn't want to know what the kids were going through so they could help. Why don't you start by sharing with the teacher that you're critically ill, and let's take it step by step from there?"

"They've lost so much, why drag them in to suffer more?"

"Aren't they going to suffer more by being excluded and having to deal with it all of a sudden? Including them now will allow you to help them get used to it all gradually."

"He really wouldn't want to see me after all these years. He wouldn't want me to see him like that."

"Wouldn't he want to make his peace with you?"

"He thinks I don't know that he's gay/IV drug abuser/was in prison . . ."

"Secrets in families are never really secret. The fact that you know shows that. He realizes as you do that people who love each other always get the news somehow."

"I don't want my mother to know my baby has AIDS."

"Don't you want your mother to be able to protect herself from infection? How can she do that if you don't tell her? Is there anyone to help you tell her?"

"Well maybe that's a start."

"We'll tell them he has cancer, they're too young to understand."

"They'll just talk about their problems and not listen to his . . . it'll be more painful for him."

"I have a lot of experience with family sessions like that, and you'll be pleasantly surprised at how they'll tune in when they realize how important it is to him."

### Apparent Cut-offs & Scapegoating

"You're not going to be able to get them in. I won't bother to give you their address because they've never come when I've asked."

"I'm the black sheep. They really don't want anything to do with me."

"They'll come in but they're not very . . ."

"She's always been the one who causes trouble."

"We're not going to bring our brother and sisters in; they haven't been drinking; they don't have AIDS."

"You'll never know if we don't try. How much worse can it get? If you were in their shoes, wouldn't you want to be given a chance?"

"Are you going to write off the possibility of a change? Maybe when they know how serious it is, they'll respond differently."

"Never mind, I'm used to dealing with that."

"Well, maybe this is her chance to turn it around. Let's give it a go."

"Maybe they've always felt helpless around you, and now there's something that they can do."

### Threats

"If you bring them into the same room, they'll kill each other."

"They're all addicts, and they'll make me relapse."

"He's responsible for all this and I might kill him."

"I don't want my parents to have the children. If they come in, they'll fight my husband for custody."

"You don't really want my ex-husband here? He's never been a father to them and will just make them miserable."

"This isn't how I want to handle it. If you bring them in, I won't come back."

"We haven't had a murder in this room yet, and we've seen a lot of people who felt this way. We'll stay with the topics they agree on and avoid the rest for now."

"I don't believe that your sobriety is that fragile. Maybe you can also help them now."

"Who else needs to be here to make sure that doesn't happen?"

"And if they don't come in, they won't? Surely the only hope of negotiation is while you're still around to help them, and I've done this a lot."

"He's still their father, and maybe you can help them see the man you married while you're still alive. Otherwise, they have no hope of ever thinking enough of themselves with a father like that."

"What are you afraid might happen? I know from getting to know you that your parents must be really special people who could help us both a great deal."

### Denial

"He's not that sick, if we come he'll think he's dying."

"Well, maybe you need to explain to him that it hurts you to think of missing lots of time to be together before he becomes really ill."

| "I'm not ready to deal with their grief, I'm not really sick. This could take years, why bother them now?" | "Maybe you can plan a fun visit so they'll have lots to remember when you do get sick." |
| "Why bring in my doctor, this is just a cold." | "Isn't he the best judge of that?" |

Engaging Kevin Frost's family provided an interesting challenge to the therapist. The initial phase of engagement and joining had been easy. Both Kevin and Bill were forthright about their issues, open to the therapist's discussing the case with Dr. Brown, their family doctor, and even to inviting him to a session if necessary. They assured the therapist that there were no secrets that they had to keep from each other and each declined the opportunity to spend a portion of the session alone with the therapist.

When it came to including Kevin's mother, however, resistance was apparent. As Kevin and Bill mentioned her, they were very quick to explain why it would be inappropriate to include her at the next session:"She's old; she can't make it in because she's bedridden and in a wheelchair; and anyway, we're going to New York for a few days." The therapist went with the resistance, quietly insisting that she would work with them to resolve the physical difficulties of getting mother in. The therapist promised maximum flexibility. She offered to arrange for special transportation and to have the session at any time that suited them all; if the mother could still not be at the next session, she made it clear that the session would be devoted to planning how to get mother in.

The next session was held in the hospital. Kevin required emergency admission shortly after his return from New York. The therapist realized that time was running out and decided to invoke the assistance of other members of Kevin's network. Once the social worker was in contact with Kevin's mother, the rest was easy, as it generally is. Most mothers do choose to visit their sons in hospital and the social worker was able to organize the visit.

In cases like Kevin's where the patient is so reluctant to involve people who love him, it is often helpful to find a way to give the choice of contact to those people in order to get around the issues of protection. The therapeutic team at this stage consisted of Kevin, his spouse, his mother, his family doctor, his therapist, the case manager and members of his support group from the community service AIDS agency, the hospital social worker, and other hospital staff. The therapy could proceed.

## 2. Explicating the Transitional Pathway

Treatment interventions are best designed to create continuity between past, present, and future. The therapist needs to ask "Why now" when therapy is requested.[30] This question, asked in a gentle nonjudgmental way, allows the patient and family to explore the interface of what is happening with regards to their HIV infection in conjunction with what is happening across the nuclear and extended families. This is done by exploring family life-cycle stage, developmental stage, ethnic and cultural background, and the resolution of transitions or presence of transitional conflict. We have found that this interface allows the therapist and family to understand the context of the presenting problems. Emily's story, and her genogram, transitional map, and time line (Figures 8-3, 8-4, and 8-5) will illustrate this.

Once this is done, the information can be normalized by the therapist rephrasing it in terms of the events and changes that the patient and family have experienced. The family is able to see that earlier patterns that have become entrenched, and often problematic, were originally adaptive solutions to unavoidable events. This enables them to recognize the relationship between events over which they had no control and the emergence of their current difficulties. The transitional perspective allows them to hope for change, often for the first time, and to realize that they have a choice of whether or not to perpetuate the patterns. It also alleviates blame and guilt, since the origin of problems is understood in a logical, sequential, and broader way. They are freed to view their current problems or dilemmas in terms of past experiences across a multigenerational history, hence allowing them to make logical choices for their future.[13] This is accomplished by assisting the family and natural support system to produce an extended genogram or transitional map upon which details of changes such as geographic moves, losses, spiritual philosophies, ethnic and cultural traditions, and value systems can be mapped (as illustrated below).

The confluence of events, both vertically down through generations and laterally across sibling systems, allows both therapist and family to understand themes, scripts[25,28,29,36] and current events in terms of where the family came from.[13] When the transitional pathway has been explicated—that is, once they understand where they come from—they are able to envisage where they are and to take control of where they wish to go.[13] The transitional pathway is thus connected from past through present to future. This is explored further in the section describing the importance of family themes and scripts. A graphic method for drawing these confluences that is particularly easy for families to follow is the time line.[30]

Where families have major difficulties in negotiating a particularly problematic phase of their lives, normalizing this difficulty is therapeutically very helpful. By explaining to families that it is normal to experience difficulty when under siege, one frees them up to be able to start the resolution process.[37,38,39,40,41] Landau also determined that more than three stress events happening concurrently or within a short time period precipitated symptoms in the family.[13] Many families, surprisingly, do not realize how many stressful events are involved in the current problem. When they do, they can appreciate that their difficulties may serve a purpose and may, in fact, be a means for adapting to the stress.

Kevin's therapist, with the assistance of his natural support system, was able to construct a transitional map that formed a key component of the therapy. Kevin's older brother had committed suicide at a young age and his only other brother had been taken from the family through a court order while in his teens.

Clara, Kevin's mother, was extremely attached to Kevin and constantly reminded him of his importance to her since the loss of her other two sons. As is common in families who have lost children, the remaining child has an enormous responsibility to fulfill the roles of those who are lost. As a result, he never wandered very far from home and he and his mother had not managed to negotiate the "leaving home" family life-cycle stage.[42] Losing children is a reversal of the natural family life cycle and frequently results in unresolved grief and difficulty in negotiating subsequent life-cycle stages.[43,44,45]

When a confluence of life cycle or externally induced events results in a member, or members, of a subsystem moving at a pace or direction different from the rest of the system, a transitional conflict results.[8] This delays the resolution of the next stage. Families may appear to be stuck at that transitional or life-cycle stage. However, in reality, family members are oscillating rapidly between the extremes of the transitional poles, but not moving forward to resolution, thus appearing stuck. For example, in Kevin's case, he tried very hard to leave home, moving halfway across the country, but failed abysmally, and returned to his hometown, where, inevitably he ended up living with his mother.

The therapist subsequently learned that Kevin's father had died a long, lingering death from cancer five years before and that Kevin felt that his father had died in an extremely brave and honorable way. Kevin had been able to deal with the probability of his own impending death, but struggled with his mother's pain. His strength was a script handed down by his father. Kevin was determined to follow his father's example and die with as much dignity as he felt his father had. In fact, he believed that this way of dying would serve as a memorial to his father and leave a very meaningful legacy to the family left behind.

In addition to all these losses, Kevin's mother had experienced a recent illness that made it impossible for her to live independently, necessitating the move to Kevin and Bill's apartment. Kevin's mother had not really dealt successfully with all her grief and, with Kevin being her only remaining child, it was not surprising how reluctant he was to put her through more pain or to have her know that he, too, was going to leave her. Once the therapist understood this, she also understood his resistance to involving his mother in the therapy and realized the critical significance of doing so.

## 3. Resolution of Unresolved Grief, Loss and Cut-Offs

Kevin's mother more than met the criteria of three or more major transitions occurring around the same time in her life. Two of the losses were both unpredictable and out of synchrony with the expected family life cycle. Loss of children in itself constitutes a reversal of the family life cycle, and parents have enormous difficulty resolving this type of event.[46]

In most AIDS cases, the reversal is a probability; however, in this family's case these losses represent not only a *reversal of the life cycle*, but losses of an atypical and overwhelming magnitude.[38] Patients dying with AIDS who are able, like Kevin, to find a spiritual strength and come to terms with dying, often unintentionally aggravate the reversal of roles by becoming parental caretakers for their elders' grief.

The three central principles in dealing with loss (as with other transitional conflicts) are *reconnection, continuity, and recalibration*. These need to be achieved in order for the family to perceive the complete transitional pathway so that they are free to hope and to plan for a meaningful future. The therapist's first task, after identifying cut-offs and losses through the mapping process, is to help the family assess the possibility of physical reconnection. By drawing upon the family strengths and with the assistance of any or all members of the natural support network (and where necessary, the professional support system), connections that have not been dreamed of become possible. Unfortunately, in this case, reconnection with Kevin's brother proved an impossibility since the social service agency was unwilling to facilitate its happening and would not disclose his new identity or place of residence.

When Kevin's family realized that reparation of the cut-off was impossible, they nonetheless felt a great deal better for having tried. The guilt associated with the cut-off had been very destructive and some of this was relieved by the effort. In this instance, as in most cut-offs, the disconnection was associated with considerable ambivalence, which is an invariable component of the loss and guilt. In Kevin's case, he had taken responsibility for being the "good son" replacement for two brothers and the energy and discussion around the reconnection attempt relieved him considerably. This allowed the therapist to question his need to remain the "good son" around his process of dying and around the "secret" of his homosexuality.

Once contact or the possibility of contact across a cut-off has been initiated and the family is feeling more competent and hopeful, issues of loss through chronic illness and death may be dealt with. With AIDS cases, one is dealing not only with resolution of past losses but also with the probable or real loss of the patient.

AIDS, unlike many chronic illnesses, may resemble the *intermittent course* of cancer, or even of malaria, in some ways. This potential rapid recycling of the illness makes it very difficult for both the patient and the people who love him or her to continuously readjust. At one moment they are in deep grief, saying their farewells and planning the reorganization of their lives (for example, who will take care of the children, where the patient will be buried, who will carry on his or her role in the family). Then, at another moment, a sudden remission occurs, and he or she is back at work, taking care of the children, and needing to be taken back immediately into his or her original family role.

Therapists need to help families prepare not just for the eventuality of death, saying farewell, and planning the ongoing life of the remaining family members, but also for helping the patient and family plan how to deal with dying—and living—dying—and living—possibly numerous times. This is particularly difficult for the parents of the patient and for any children he or she may have. This cycling may happen with remarkable rapidity. Family members may eventually get to the point where, having said their goodbyes several times and gone through as much anguish and grief as they can handle, they wish the patient dead. This causes unutterable guilt and remorse. Unless the therapist is particularly sensitive to this issue, it will never be mentioned and may leave long-term emotional scars.

Therapists need to normalize the reaction of family members to this intermittent cycle, explaining that when people love deeply, the pain of constant leave-taking and the peaks and valleys of hope and despair become intolerable to anyone. When something becomes unbearable, we all wish it away. Helping family members share their feelings with the patient allows the patient to forgive them feelings that he or she is bound to understand, if not share. This also allows the patient to expose his or her wish to be out of this impossible situation, without feeling the guilt of the suicidal person (who chooses to leave beloved family members behind to suffer). In fact, this level of sharing can increase the closeness between patient and family, making the rest of the time they do have together much more meaningful. It also allows families additional time, for which, once the guilt is alleviated, they may be grateful. They have more time than expected to redefine the mission of the family, reallocate family roles and expectations, plan the funeral together with the patient, and decide which family strengths and values precious to the patient will be continued to future generations, and by whom. In this way, patients and families may consciously take charge of recalibration, so the family is not disorganized by the death.

HIV disease is both chronic and debilitating, resulting in many significant physical losses for both patient and family. Patients frequently fade away, losing their physical attractiveness and sex drive. Their faces change, they lose their hair, and they may be covered with unsightly lesions. They generally lose their energy and as a result lose their jobs and their capacity to support themselves. Their social life is inevitably curtailed, and they frequently feel like pariahs of society. Their self-confidence and self-image are badly impaired. They may become significantly depressed and, in addition, may develop neurological symptoms and signs, including dementia—a loss, at best, of intelligence, and, at worst, of self as has been described in Chapter 7.

In Kevin's case, he developed mild cognitive impairment, leading to episodes of confusion. He needed to learn several techniques to organize his memory, such as the use of a daily pillbox for his medication so that he could check at any time and know what he had taken. He also kept a notebook and diary, so that he would be able to reacquaint himself with periods of time that might otherwise have been lost to him. The therapist worked very closely with Kevin's spouse, Bill, and other family members to assist them in both developing and maintaining these tasks.

How can a therapist help a family deal with unresolved loss and grief from the past, while not losing sight of the enormity of present issues? Because of *compression of the time-clock* with these cases, therapy needs to be particularly goal-oriented and brief, as discussed earlier. Tasks that are past-related need to be very clearly defined in terms of present gains. They need to be both practical and concrete, with clear reward to patient and family. Kevin's mother was about to lose her last son, and Kevin was about to end the family line. Connection with the extended family was clearly of critical significance in this case (as in all AIDS cases) since *continuity of the family values and heritage* would have to occur through extended family. Guaranteeing this continuity allows hope to emerge and energy for dealing with emotional pain. The therapist was able to help Kevin identify members of the family who he felt would remain connected with his mother, in addition to ensuring that she and Bill would remain in touch. In order to take care of Bill, and his mother, Kevin also made close ties with the local AIDS community service agency.

In terms of Kevin's passing on the baton of his mission and value system, he decided that he wanted to leave a legacy of education about HIV disease that would be a constant reminder to his family that he was still with them in spirit. Many AIDS patients have chosen this means of contribution and connecting.

In addition, Kevin helped his family to design a quilt piece that they would always know contained his thoughts and emotions as well as theirs. The Names (Quilt) Project,[47] similarly to the Vietnam war memorial, serves the function of a communal graveside marker that can be shared in the abstract by many and at a personal level by those who are directly involved. This Project is a collection of quilt pieces handmade by families, friends, and loved ones as mementos of persons who have died of AIDS. It is now 10 football fields in length and too large to be transported intact. Sections of the Quilt are exhibited throughout the U.S. and memorial rituals are held. In this way, families, health care providers, and communities may share their losses and their hopes for the future.

In order to allow patients and families to deal with impending death, therapists need to pay specific attention to resolving prior losses. In Kevin's case, the grief that was in some part unresolved was recent in the family's history. Frequently, unresolved loss may go back generations. It may include loss of a country in the cases of immigrants; it may result from divorce and subsequent cut-off; it may have been initiated by the loss of many babies through spontaneous abortion or during an epidemic (the 1918 Influenza Pandemic, the Ethiopian Famine of the 1980s) or through genocide (the Armenian and Jewish holocausts). Even where several losses are apparent in the present or recent generations, therapists need to inquire carefully about past losses, geographic moves, divorces, and migrations, since prior losses might well be aggravating the lack of resolution of present losses.[44,45,46,48] Unresolved mourning and loss within the nuclear or extended family are commonly associated with suicidality, as is illustrated by the following case.

Families may not deliberately conceal such losses, but instead may actually be unaware of how these losses could relate to the suicidal family member.[14] Therapists can take the family directly into the mourning process, compressing them to the original and unresolved point of transitional conflict and then moving them through this point in a new way so "they can complete the transitional pathway from the past, through the present and into the future. Because the different family subsystems may, perhaps, have been 'out of synch' ever since the point(s) of loss, this approach takes them phenomenologically, experientially, and structurally to an earlier point, holds them there briefly, and guides them forward."[7,14]

Julian Levine's losses covered many generations, including the loss of three of his nephews and nieces (i.e. the next generation). Julian, a 30-year-old homosexual Jewish son of divorced parents, was admitted to the psychiatric inpatient ward with AIDS and suicidality.* He had

---

*The therapy team consisted of A. Griepp, M.D., the referring psychiatrist; S. Scheibel, M.D., the infectious disease specialist; S. Baldwin, A.C.S.W., C.S.W., the family therapist (originally functioning as the supervisor to B. Grimstead, C.S.W.); J. Landau-Stanton, M.B., Ch.B., D.P.M., supervisor of S. Baldwin; the inpatient activities therapist, Laura Napolitano; the inpatient social worker, Yvonne Dohr; the outpatient social worker, K. Deuter, C.W.W.; and a chemical dependence counselor, R. Tocco, M.S., C.A.C.

been depressed for about 10 months with increasing vegetative symptoms (sleeping much of the time, and eating little) and had become progressively more isolated. He was not complying with his medical treatment, nor was he reliable in taking his medication.

Julian lived with a female maternal second cousin, Cathy. Cathy was the same generation as his mother, the daughter of his grandmother's brother. Prior to this he had resided consecutively with his mother and father throughout and after their divorce, which occurred when he was eighteen, until their subsequent remarriages. He had made a brief excursion to California during the stress of the divorce.

Julian was the youngest of three siblings, from an upper middle class family. John, the oldest, was married to Pamela and had one surviving child, a little boy aged nine months. John and Pamela had lost two babies through miscarriage, and their little boy was a surviving twin. John's and Julian's sister, Willa, the middle child, had a two-year-old son and was pregnant. Julian and John were not at all close, but Julian was extremely close to both Willa and Pamela, and shared time with them equally. However, after the death of Pamela's twin baby, Julian spent more and more time with her. Pamela's sister had died from suicide following a severe depression, and she really understood Julian's suicidality. Without AIDS, suicidality is extremely common in families that have experienced catastrophic losses. In Julian's case, his physical malaise and the knowledge that he was going to die, along with the family grief, created in him the wish to die quickly. In fact, the metaphor used by the therapy team was, "the horizontal man." It was as though he were already dead.

Apart from family, Julian had no close relationships. He had never been involved in a long-term relationship and had come to terms with his homosexuality. The family therapy team encouraged Julian and his parents to bring in all the members of the family and friendship circle who cared about Julian, and would want to help the therapists. The members of the extended family who attended various therapy sessions, sometimes together and sometimes in subgroups, were Julian, his mother and stepfather, his mother's sister, his father, his brother John and wife Pamela, his sister Willa, and Cathy, the cousin with whom he lived. The natural support system was further augmented by a close grandmotherly friend of the family and the case worker from the local AIDS community agency.

In addition, the professional network was mobilized and participated actively, in varying combinations, throughout the therapy process. This professional group included the referring psychiatrist and infectious disease specialist, the in-patient team comprising the primary nurse, the social worker and the activities therapist, and an out-patient team of family therapists, social worker, and substance abuse counselor.

In the case of severe depression or suicidality, it is extremely helpful to mobilize as extensive a support network as possible to amplify the immediate family's efforts to save the life, or improve the quality of life, of someone they love.[14] Where immediate family members are intimately involved in the depression or suicidality, they may be rendered incompetent since the stressors impacting on the patient are also affecting them. In order to look for resources whose competence is not undermined by the acute stress, the therapist needs to expand the system by involving extended family and natural support systems. This invariably results in the inclusion of network members with a different perspective and without the same loyalty and other binds. A positive shift occurs and the patient and immediate family are influenced by the larger system, becoming more hopeful, and working together towards healing.

After the joining process, a family transitional map was constructed and an extensive list of family strengths established, as were goals for Julian. These focused on his quality of life and survival. The metaphor used by the team was Julian's converting from "horizontal man" to "vertical man."

An enactment based on these goals and utilizing the family strengths followed. The family had listed supportiveness and loyalty as key strengths, and their wish to take care of Julian as a primary goal. They identified his taking his pills as the most urgent priority. The enactment incorporating all of this was for mother to take Julian around the room to ask each member of the network in turn whether he or she would be there for him if he took his pills. They responded by surrounding him physically and all wept quietly while reassuring him of their love. He was able to tolerate this, at least briefly.

The task of Julian's taking his pills was reinforced by subsequent homework. This was designed while his parents sat on either side of him, ensuring him of their support. They promised to purchase a special daily pillbox, so that he would always know which pills were needed. They also promised to assist him by supervising his pill-taking. The family agreed to be there as backup.

The therapy team realized that Julian's suicidality could not be resolved until he understood the larger issues of loss in the family and how it was that he felt the only way he could serve the family was by dying. Pamela was able to describe how she had experienced the loss of her babies. She wept copiously and begged Julian to enjoy each day of his life. The older members of the family were also able to share their grief at the loss of their elders, as well as the loss of the family future. They added their pleas to Pamela's.

Rather than oppose the natural direction of the family, which at this stage was rather morbid and leaning towards an intense concentration on the impending death of Julian, the therapy team commenced *an intense compression move*[10] *by going with the natural direction of the system.*[8]

The therapists encouraged Julian to "explore death with clarity." They encouraged him to go with his father to view the burial plot that his father had selected for himself to see whether he would like one there, too. The therapists advised him to go with his father to choose a coffin, but discovered that since he was an observing Jew the box had to be simple pine. In addition, they advised Julian to write a living will with the assistance of those who loved him.

While dealing with intensity in this manner, it is very helpful to employ the polarization technique of the "Pick-a-Dali Circus" approach, maintaining intensity at both poles equally and simultaneously.[11,12] In Julian's case, the poles being dealt with at this time were "to live" or "to die." It is important to maintain intensity at both extremes so as to avoid pushing the patient and family to either extreme. By the therapists going further at each end than the family would dare, the exaggeration allows the family members to moderate their positions and move towards a less extreme stand.

At the other pole, the therapists suggested that Julian affirm his status as a member of the living by joining his father and stepmother for dinner at his brother's house.

In this manner, planning for his death and experiencing the intensity of what dying would mean were balanced by the proposal that he really enjoy each day of his life by reconnecting closely with the family who wished to enjoy it with him. Another important component of the compression move was to advise the family that Julian should go home to live with one of his parents, since in many ways he was living like a three-year old who could not make life-preserving decisions for himself (refusing to eat, take his medication, and sleeping all the time). Sending him back home again (even hypothetically) would allow him to grow to the leaving home stage sufficiently to take care of himself and leave home properly later.[14,22]

The outcome of the therapy was that, shortly after moving home and being taken care of, Julian decided to take responsibility for himself and become a "vertical man."

In Julian's case, the unresolved grief was dealt with by exposure, compression, and helping Julian and his family to understand the role of previous losses in Julian's current suicidality and to bless his living. In some instances, it is useful to go further with the unresolved bereavement, to the extent of a memorial service or graveside visit.[14,49] As in Julian's case, however, families first need, through a process of mapping and gentle revelation, to get in touch with the impact of the losses they have suffered. The therapist also needs to help both patient and family understand the role of the patient vis á vis those lost. Once this has been achieved, a ritual memorial ceremony may be extremely helpful in order to give the patient the motivation to go on living and to successfully stop the scripting with those dead.

The memorial ceremony, or graveside visit needs to be designed in a culturally and spiritually appropriate way for each family. Careful consideration also needs to be given to the member(s) lost in terms of what would be most fitting. In some instances, a key ancestor may be identified, frequently someone whom the current index patient has been selected to follow and represent within the family. Additionally, there may be other losses, such as the children of the next generation, as in Julian's case. Where the loss covers both past and present in this way, it is important to ensure that both are honored. It is usually better, and of more impact, to select the most powerful deceased member's grave as the symbolic center of the grieving. Surprisingly, many family members in a family dealing with unresolved grief may not even have attended the original funeral or visited the grave in the past.

These ceremonies need to be planned by as many members of the natural support network as are accessible. Those who are unable to be included in the therapy sessions may be contacted by telephone from the session, or receive letters from the natural and professional networks present at the session, or be given audio or videotaped recordings of the session in which the planning occurs. In addition to the members included in this way, special effort should be made to ensure that any religious traditions appropriate to the family be considered and that ministers should be included in the planning where appropriate. If the grave identified is too far away for the ceremony to be held there, a spiritually appropriate alternative should be selected by the family, with the therapist's assistance.

In the case of Sal Bertoli, an 18-year-old adolescent with AIDS, the family had never resolved the immense grief resulting from the loss of the patriarch, Sal's maternal grandfather, Vince. Sal, like many AIDS patients, had lost the will to live. The family felt that a memorial graveside visit at Vince's gravestone would mean a great deal to them all. Sal's grandmother had not been to the grave since the funeral and was very reluctant to face the emotional pain of this ceremony. However, as she said to the therapist* at the graveside during the cer-

---

*Therapist, R. Epstein, M.D.; Supervisor, S. Baldwin, A.C.S.W., C.S.W.; Supervisor of Supervision, J. Landau-Stanton, M.B.,Ch.B.;D.P.M. This case was treated in the Family Therapy Training Program of the University of Rochester.

emony, "I didn't want this thing tonight, but I did it to help my grandson."

Close family members are often reluctant to face this kind of ceremony, but, as with Sal's grandmother, can usually be motivated to participate for the love of the living. Generally, the reluctant member(s) are the ones who most need to resolve their own grief in order to free both themselves and other members of the family—most especially, the index patient who is frequently scripted to represent or replace the lost member. Grandparents are extremely important members of the family. Their distress can reverberate across the system, and their assistance as resources in therapy can be crucial.[50,51,52]

The underlying principle of this intervention is to join the contributions made by deceased members (rather than the grief and loss of the past) with the potential of the future. "The ceremony (should) include a joyful recognition both of the valuable attributes and unique gifts of those who have died, and of the ways in which these have been, and would continue to be, carried into the future by succeeding generations."[14] In this manner the transitional pathway is reconnected with hope.

In order to achieve this, members are asked to prepare statements recalling beloved, joyful, or special moments and shared experiences, to bring photographs and other memorabilia, poems, stories, musical recordings, and so forth. In some instances, families have asked ministers to give the same sermon that was given at the original funeral, so that younger members of the family might share it. This can be a very powerful experience for all involved. Older members of the group are asked to share with younger members of the group particular ways in which they may represent the best of their forebears in their own future lives. This allows them "to ascertain where they had come from and where they are going, (so that) they (can) see a pathway along which they could proceed."[14] Family members are encouraged to design the ceremony in the most natural way for their particular family. They may bring food and drink, arrange to get together socially afterwards, or find some other means of being together to continue the process.

The whole Bertoli family met at the gravesite in the pouring rain. The therapist welcomed the family by saying, "We are here together to grieve the death and also to choose life. Now is the time to remember the lessons, the values, and also the caring that grandpa Vince gave to you as a family. This is a time for each to take from back generations what he would want for the generations to come." The therapist then asked the family to bring out the objects they had brought to share with each other and to describe why they were of significance. Family members had brought a variety of things, including photographs, poems, flowers, and music, in addition to items of personal significance.

Vince's niece, Marianne, shared first: "I brought coleus seeds. Your grandfather had real beautiful coleus plants in his yard. I figure that you could put them in the ground yourself and watch them grow."

Vince's wife, Millie, closed with a moving, tearful statement to her husband: "We miss you and we'll always love you." The atmosphere at the graveside changed as Millie said goodbye to her husband for the first time. Others wept quietly and felt free to share their feelings.

In this way, during a memorial ceremony, the family inevitably finds a positive way to say farewell to the lost ones, and to give blessing for the living to continue without grief, but rather in celebration of the good contributed by those deceased. In addition, the intense emotional atmosphere generated at the graveside and the feeling of forgiveness that goes with it frequently allow the freeing of former binds, such as those of loyalty and scripting, and allow the family to voice their appreciation of the deceased, along with separateness. They are then ready to resolve past problems and employ the transitional perspective to give them and the next generation hope and direction for the future, based on the wisdom and strength of the past. This ceremony frees the family to share both information and "secrets" openly in a warm and trusting environment, permitting the effective use of the family's combined resources to cope with the future.

Frequently, the ritual expands to include memories and experiences of the people who were not directly involved with the deceased, but have their own grief to share about other situations. When appropriate, the professional network may become involved in this process as a way of sharing the intensity, and showing the family the universality of grief and loss.

### 4. Recognizing Scripts, Themes and Issues of Loyalty

In Sal's case, he was scripted by the family to represent his grandfather in the grandchild generation. Families operate under three basic sets of rules: (i) the interactions within the immediate family, (ii) the interface with external systems, and (iii) the extended family system's heritage. As a number of investigators have noted, this third area is passed down from previous generations to the present: the family responds intrinsically to guidelines from the past.[25] Such guidelines affect the extended family's decision-making both as a family and in terms of "how its various members are regarded and differentially treated or reinforced." Although these rules are often preconscious, everyone in the family knows them.

As families develop concepts of themselves that are passed on, *ideas or themes* make each family distinctive and give it a sense of shared identity. Such themes provide a sense of continuity and are sometimes called historical themes[53] or legacies[54,55,56] or scripts and legends.[57] Themes can include ethnicity/culture, vocations, recreation, values, stories and legends, health, personality descriptions, or death and dying. Themes may also exhibit *generation-skipping*, in which themes disappear in one generation only to reappear in the next. The disappearing theme is retained in the family's memory and is expressed later down in the line. Even if there is no generation-skipping, some mechanism of balance appears to be operating in a family.

The vehicle by which a family's identity (theme) is specifically conveyed to its members is the concept of the family script.[29] Certain individuals are encouraged or reinforced to carry out specific scripts. These scripts (i) maintain a family's theme and (ii) ensure that themes are balanced across a generation. "Family scripts, themes, and balance are the cornerstone of this theoretical paradigm of multigenerational family functioning."[13] Scripts are conveyed and reinforced by many people in a family and generally predate the birth of the scripted person, unlike roles, which are present-oriented, more flexibly assigned, and may circulate within a family. Scripts may also be crossgenerational, as was the case with Sal, who was scripted to represent and replace his grandfather, Vince.

As with Sal, scripts may extend from the death of a family member. Young or even unborn children can be identified with recently deceased loved ones, keeping the memory of the deceased alive and alleviating the sense of loss. The child becomes a *"revenant,"* a revered replacement of the one lost, and represents that person to the entire family.[13,48] In Sal's case, as with other AIDS cases, the family was being threatened with the loss of the "revenant" and their reaction to his illness was thus greatly intensified. If measures are not taken to resolve the prior loss of the key family member and to deal openly with issues of continuity of themes, the stress to the revenant is extreme and the family as a whole may be threatened. In fact, there appears to be a dynamic process involving three general stages:[25]

*"Onslaught:* If an extended family's system of themes, scripts and balance is assaulted by a combination of (a) societal pressures that challenge it . . . ; (b) a series of both normal and stressful life cycle events . . . especially involving the unexpected loss or incapacitation of central family figures . . . ; and (c) these events impinge concomitantly or in close succession, an onslaught has occurred.

*"Rigidification:* To protect itself in the face of onslaught, a family will tend to 'dig in,' clinging to its traditions and its identity in almost ter-

rified desperation. Commonly it will resort to stereotyped, tried-and-true coping methods and strategies—whether they work or not—across a wide range of problem situations and contexts.

"*Isolation:* . . . The family closes itself off from outside influences . . . and the extended family's cohesion . . . is sacrificed as it attempts to ignore the world as best it can. In addition, its ties to the kinship network may begin to erode. . . .

In the case of Sal and his family, the therapy culminating in the graveside memorial ceremony dealt specifically with the issues of celebrating the lives of those deceased and renewing the family's pledge to perpetuate the strengths and gifts of the family. These actions ensure the continuation of healthy family themes across the entire family system, as opposed to their remaining the responsibility of one "revenant." In addition, preventive work was done during the ceremony to prepare the family for their farewell to Sal, the "revenant," thereby freeing him up to enjoy the rest of his life rather than hastening to join his grandfather.

## 5. Exposing Secrets

Secrecy is invariably an issue when one is treating HIV disease. The question always arises about, "Who should know? Whom should I tell? Whom do I dare not tell? What will happen if so-and-so finds out?" There are real concerns with these issues that might apply to any illness. Where HIV is involved, they become particularly critical in light of the political, economic, and ethical considerations associated with this diagnosis. How does this impact on psychotherapy?

In the case of Emily, a 25-year old student and mother, the issue of secrecy became important. Emily and her two-year old son, Mike, were both HIV positive. Emily, unlike many other HIV positive patients, was willing to share the news with her family soon after the diagnosis, but was hesitant to tell her friends and other members of her community. She wanted desperately to protect her little boy from the potential dangers of ostracism and cruelty.

As in the case of Emily, parents struggle far more with the secret of HIV disease in their children than with their own diagnosis. Gillian Walker, in describing one of her cases involving the secret of a child who had contracted AIDS from a blood transfusion, discusses both the good and bad consequences of secrecy:[58]

"Secrecy permits the child to have as normal a life as possible. But secrecy also torments the wife, who worries about the inevitable ostracism if the child's illness were revealed; who worries that someone could become infected because he or she was not informed. Secrecy also binds the couple together, strengthening a fragile alliance, placing boundaries between them and their families of origin, to whom they are both deeply attached."(page 131)

Emily's openness about sharing her HIV status early with her family was unusual. Her wishing to keep it secret from others, outside of the family, was not. Most HIV positive people are embarrassed, ashamed, and concerned about prejudice. More importantly, they do not trust the response of their family and friends, expecting rejection and punishment. Even if people are comfortable sharing their HIV status with family and friends, informing the community at large may be seen as highly dangerous. In Central Africa, HIV status remains a highly guarded secret because of the community's typical reaction to the information. The individual and family can be ostracized, and people with AIDS are expected to die quietly and out of sight. It took a great deal of effort for the media in those countries to even mention AIDS. In one African country, it was only by the President's meeting a popular singer who was known to be HIV positive that AIDS education and prevention could be initiated.

> During a family therapy session that included Emily's natural support system, Sandra, her best friend, expressed her admiration for Emily's mother who, "Had such courage with the HIV (diagnosis). To her there was no choice but to accept Emily and to love Emily." Sandra also shared her sorrow that, "You know a lot of parents don't know that."

Many HIV positive patients feel certain of rejection by their parents and families. It is difficult for them not to interpret as rejection and blame what is frequently a desperate response.

> During a session, Emily's mother shared how she had felt when Emily told her of the diagnosis. She described her intense feelings of identification with the mother in the movie "Steel Magnolias" as follows: "The daughter had been told not to have a baby (because it could kill her). She was standing at the grave saying, 'I'm mad, and I hate the world, and I don't know why it happened to me.' . . . She's standing there stamping on the grave, and I'm sitting there crying. But I have the feeling that I can't face the world that way every day."
> The therapist's* response to this intense emotional statement was, "What would life be worth if you did? . . . What you're doing is living

---

*Therapist J. Landau-Stanton, M.B., Ch.B., D.P.M. accompanied by faculty of the AIDS Training Project: Colleen Clements, Ph.D., Ann Z. Griepp, M.D., Jackie Nudd, Alexander Tartaglia, D.Min., Robert Tocco, M.S., C.S.A.C.

and enjoying these kids. Angry? Yes, like 'Steel Magnolias,' angry at her; furious at times, or for periods of time, because she's killing herself. But loving doesn't stop, because the anger comes from the intensity of loving. Youngsters with HIV run and hide from their parents because they think their parents will judge them. Every set of parents that we've grown to know loves their children."

Therapists can rest assured that most parents, when dealt with in this straightforward manner and when given an opportunity to share with their children, will do so without rejecting them. Since they may also express anger, or even fury, which chases the children away by confirming their worst fears of rejection, therapists need to predict this response in advance so it can be expected and dealt with appropriately. Therapists should explain that such a reaction is caused by the pain of loving and the fear of loss as in parents tempted to beat little children who have exposed themselves to danger or returned from a brief period of hiding away. By sharing these dynamics with families, the therapist frees them up to express their feelings and to become closer.

While Emily was able to share her news with her family, dealing with the community posed a more serious problem for them all. Her older brother, Adam, was really concerned that anybody outside the family might find out that his sister was HIV positive. "We didn't want to tell anyone. We thought we'd say she was sick—say it was cancer or something."

As Adam stated, a level of knowledge about HIV disease makes it far easier for people to share the diagnosis. Therapists can assist in this process by offering to educate family, friends, and other members of the natural support system concurrently with the patient. This makes it far easier for everyone to deal with the issue. People are automatically far more frightened of something they don't understand. They feel vulnerable to infection and are frequently unaware of how to protect themselves. This colors their reaction, often leading to apparent rejection of the patient.

In counseling these families, therapists need to exercise caution while advising patients of the costs of secrecy. There are many instances, such as Adam's work situation, where people are not ready to hear the diagnosis of AIDS. Where there is no direct danger of transmission, as in this case, we generally leave the decision to the patient and family. In the case of the natural support system of the patient, however, we feel that the cost of secrecy outweighs the benefit of exposing the secret. We therefore encourage the patient to share the diagnosis, additionally offering either direct education for friends or a list of available resources where they can acquire the information needed to deal positively with the news. A model of how to access this information in your community is given in Chapter 5.

Many patients faced with a positive diagnosis of HIV disease are not just dealing with the stigma of AIDS, but have many other secrets embedded within their family systems. Such secrets may be guarded from the outside world by the family. Secrets may not be known by the entire family, but only by a few members. The populations at risk for HIV are frequently driven to secrecy because of prejudice and the fear of rejection by both family and community. These secrets include such issues as grief and loss, homosexuality, alcoholism and drug addiction, forms of family violence, physical and sexual abuse, and incest. Legal and law enforcement problems may also be secret from all or part of the nuclear or extended families.

Family secrets develop as protective mechanisms, but do not adequately function in that role over time. As was described in the section and table on resistance, secrets invariably end up creating coalitions within the family and dividing family members or subsystems from each other. The burden of secrecy is usually carried lovingly by certain family members and unknowingly by others. In an attempt to protect each other, families may end up being disrupted and pulled apart by secrets. The burden of the secret(s) may also make it difficult for individual family members to function well both within the family and in other parts of their lives, for example with their friends and in their work settings. Secrecy also may divide the patient and his or her surrogate family from their families of origin, creating rifts when they most need to be close to the people they love.

In the case of gay people, where the family is being protected from knowledge of their sexual orientation, this form of rift is extremely common. In the case of Kevin, discussed earlier in the chapter, events had made it difficult to maintain such secrets. His ailing widowed mother had to come to live with him and his spouse, Bill; she had to know about his homosexuality and his illness. However, even in this case, the therapy team had to take responsibility for helping the family overcome the barrier of secrecy and protection before Kevin was comfortable revealing either his sexual orientation or his illness.

> In the case of Peter, a young man who had been separated from his parents and all but one sibling for many years, his homosexuality was still a secret when he was diagnosed with AIDS. The therapist was eventually able, using Peter's older brother's assistance along with many of the techniques listed in table 8-A for overcoming resistance, to gain Peter's permission to call the parents. The session in which Peter shared his history and current problems with them was extremely moving. They all wept and his parents were able to hug him and tell him how much they had missed him. They were able

to forgive him both for their pain and for his choice of an alternative life style, expressing their wish that he had trusted them enough not to exclude them.

Even though these cases may take a great deal of gentle persuasion, the reward for the therapist is well worth his efforts. Secrecy, despite having its origin in loving protection and privacy, is always painful, nor is it ever rewarding to the individual, family, or therapist, in the long term.

### 6. Resolving Transitional Conflict and Its Sequelae

In the case of Emily's family, a family secret around both alcoholism and loss emerged during the drawing of the transitional map. It became a central issue for resolving the transitional conflict that was at the nexus of Emily's problems. Emily had started drinking at the age of nine and had commenced the use of cocaine by the time she was in her early teens. As the therapist drew the genogram (see Figure 8-1), depicting relationships (Figure 8-2), expanded it into a transitional map (see Figures 8-3 and 8-4), and added a timeline (see Figure 8-5), the chronology around the origins of Emily's addiction and the transitional conflicts became apparent.

From the genogram it became clear that Emily's paternal family of origin had experienced multiple, catastrophic losses. Her paternal grandparents had married in Ireland and left their families there to immigrate to the United States. They never saw any of them again. They had lost their first three children; Emily's father, the last-born, was their sole surviving child. Emily's paternal grandfather had died in 1967, her paternal grandmother in 1975, and her maternal grandfather in 1961 According to the genogram, both Emily and her brother, Adam, were adopted since their parents were unable to have babies of their own.

The transitional map further revealed that Emily's paternal grandfather had been senile with Alzheimer's disease around 1961, the year that Emily's maternal grandfather died. Her paternal grandmother had to be hospitalized at one point.

Emily's brother was adopted at birth in 1963, and Emily in 1966. Emily's paternal grandfather died in 1967 while she was still a baby. Both children grew up knowing that after his death the paternal grandmother became a secret drinker and that she was always sad. Emily and Adam were clearly very important to their grandmother, who had lost everyone in her family except her son, daughter-in-law, and two grandchildren. In fact, one might suppose that the grandchildren were, in some way, a replacement for her lost family, particularly Emily, who was born shortly before the death of her husband. Her son and she were extremely

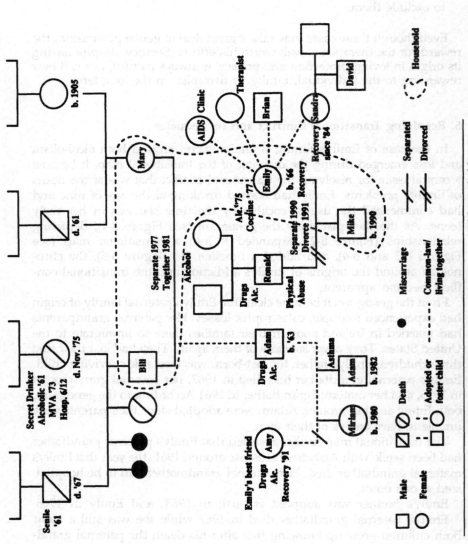

**Figure 8-1.** Emily's family genogram with problem areas and household

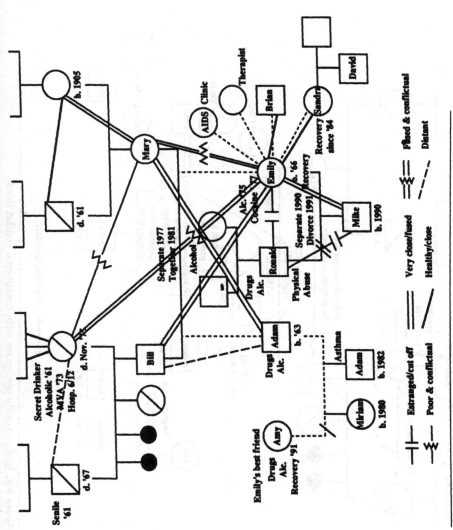

**Figure 8-2.** Emily's family genogram with relationship lines

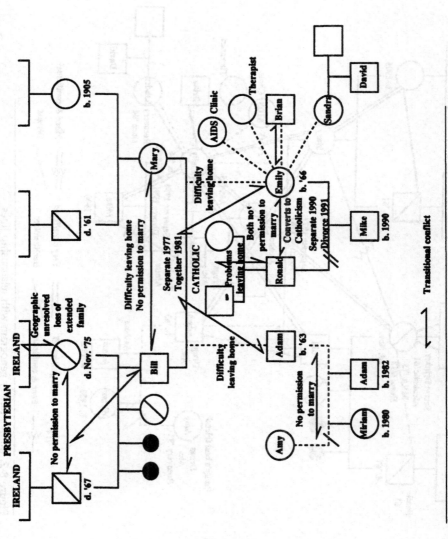

**Figure 8-3.** Emily's family genogram with transitional conflict lines

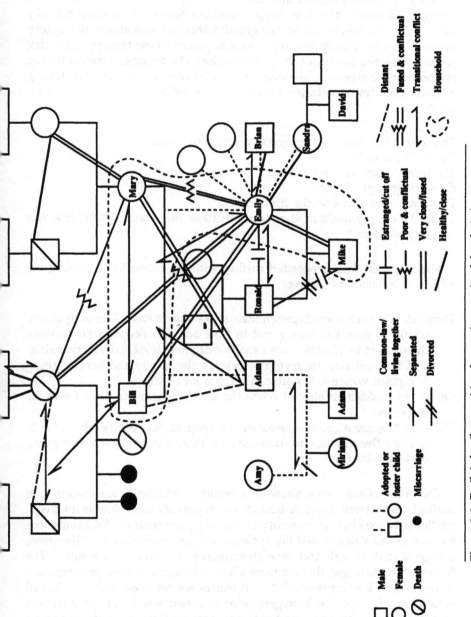

**Figure 8-4.** Emily's family transitional map (text omitted for clarity)

| Symbol | Meaning |
|--------|---------|
| □ | Male |
| ○ | Female |
| ⬚Ø | Death |

| Symbol | Meaning |
|--------|---------|
| - - ○ | Adopted or foster child |
| - - □ | |
| ● | Miscarriage |

| Symbol | Meaning |
|--------|---------|
| - - - | Common-law/living together |
| | Separated |
| | Divorced |

| Symbol | Meaning |
|--------|---------|
| ++ | Estranged/cut off |
| ww | Poor & conflictual |
| ||| | Very close/fused |
| / | Healthy/close |

| Symbol | Meaning |
|--------|---------|
| / = | Distant |
| ⇶ | Fused & conflictual |
| | Transitional conflict |
| ⌒ | Household |

close, since he was the sole survivor, and hence the replacement for her other three lost children.

Emily's paternal grandmother died in 1975, and that was the year when Emily, aged nine at the time, began drinking herself. Even though Emily did not express closeness with her grandmother and was almost derogatory about her in the family session, it was apparent to the therapy team that she was scripted to replace the grandmother. The therapist, concentrating on the positive aspects of the transitional pathway in order to start sharing a transitional frame with the family, had the following conversation with Emily:

*Therapist:* "Are you the first recoverer in your family?"
*Emily:* "I guess."
*Therapist:* "Then you're a pioneer."
*Emily (laughing):* "I guess."
*Therapist:* "Are you also the first addict?"
*Emily:* "Well, my dad's mother was a drinker. She was a drunk. She was independent."

The therapist then proceeded further with the frame by reframing the addicted behavior as follows:

*Therapist:* "Go back enough generations to see how it starts—as adaptation, trying to save the family, not to hurt anyone. People who sacrifice themselves to addiction are usually extremely loyal, extremely loving, and in some way are trying to balance the family and keep it going at a point where it is going through a lot of stress."
*Emily:* "My addiction started when the family was in turmoil, I was the scapegoat."
*Therapist:* "We see it more as savior than scapegoat. Somebody who is ready to draw the attention to themselves to detour from what else is going on in the family."

The onset of substance abuse in a family is frequently associated with multiple concurrent life cycle transitions, especially when loss is involved, particularly the chronic disability or loss of a grandparent.[59] A family that has successfully negotiated life cycle stages previously may find the stress too great to deal with and develop transitional conflict as a result.[13] The family life cycle stages that are most likely to be impacted are puberty, adolescence, and leaving home.[31,42,60] If this is not resolved, the transitional conflict may be repeated from generation to generation, becoming a chronic problem and resulting in repeated transitional conflicts. Also, if a particular life cycle stage is not adequately negotiated, subsequent stages will also not be successful. [42,59]

> "In some cases, generation after generation has repeated the same problematic patterns; conflicts have been perpetuated around similar points of transition. [7,31] One may see cross-generational coalitions, with grandparents parenting grandchildren, and parents failing to become competent. Frequently, the stages of growing up, leaving home, [42] getting permission to marry, [61] and becoming competent parents to an adolescent are not adequately achieved in these families. The therapeutic task is one of helping the family through the transition period." (p. 330) [59]

During this same period, Emily's parents, Bill and Mary, developed serious marital difficulties, perhaps as a result of the change in family structure with the death of Bill's mother. The therapy team postulated that Emily's drinking problem was also a way of keeping her parents focused on her as a detour from their marital difficulties. [60] Emily's brother, Adam, also began to drink and act out around the same time. Bill and Mary separated in 1977, leaving Mary alone in the home with Emily and Adam. Adam took over as the man of the house, holding wild parties and not attending school with any regularity. Emily added cocaine to her drinking.

The situation deteriorated progressively. Adam became sexually involved with Emily's best friend, Amy, also a substance abuser. Amy became pregnant, Adam dropped out of school and left home—only to return in 1980 with Amy and her baby, plus a new pregnancy. He had pulled himself together, taken the high school General Equivalency Diploma examination (G.E.D.), and found a job. Shortly after the birth of the second child, Adam moved out once more. For a brief time Emily and Mary were alone. Father Bill returned to take up his position as head of the household shortly after and Adam gained custody of his two children. Adam brought both babies to live with his parents and found a home of his own. The crossgenerational coalitions were complete.

Upon further examination of the transitional map, it became apparent that once Emily's parents were safely together again, she began to flirt with recovery. Her entry into recovery was assisted by her mother, a close friend, and her boyfriend. Emily started attending a 12-step fellowship program and building relationships within the group.

Emily's mother attended Al-Anon meetings and described the hopelessness of trying to be a successful parent: " When she (Emily) was first dry, she got a job in her favorite watering hole. She had it all planned. No matter what I said, I was always in the wrong. I never wanted to kick her out, but

I didn't give her money, so she'd go to Dad and say she'd pay him back. Dad gave it to her."

Thus the tension between the parents would be enacted, through their daughter, who not only struggled with her sobriety, but also failed repeatedly, maintaining her parents' concentration on her problems and keeping them together. Emily also made repeated efforts to leave home. Madanes stresses that the way in which a therapist views the situation will determine the strategy to be used.[62] In Madanes' framework, Emily could be viewed as having been disobedient and out of parental control, misunderstood, and mistreated, or as a pawn in a parental power struggle. The perspective of Madanes that we feel to be the most accurate and helpful is that Emily was concerned and protective of her parents. Each failure of Emily's to leave home resulted in a renewal of joint parental activity, thus also serving to maintain the marriage.[42] As Emily described in the therapy session, "I'd get an apartment and not even move my furniture—live out of boxes and a sleeping bag, since I knew I'd run out of money and go home again."

Unfortunately, as is common during the recovery from substance abuse, Emily substituted sexual addiction for her free-basing cocaine habit. She embarked on a clearly self-destructive relationship with an intravenous drug abuser, who was openly bisexual. Therapists and substance abuse counselors need to be aware of the importance of sexual counseling during the initial phase of abstinence, since sexual substitution is as common as nicotine, gambling, and eating addictions at this time. In fact, Emily's behavior might be viewed as a combination of sexual addiction and gambling—with her life. Abstinence alone does not resolve the transitional conflicts that lead to self-destructive behavior. Attention to the family factors is a critical component of therapy.

Self-destructive individuals are frequently in denial, not only about the magnitude of their substance abuse, but also about other risk behaviors and the importance of safer sex. Emily later told her therapist that she had assumed that the 12-step fellowship group was a safe haven from the risks of the outside world. She also, like most heavy users, was out of contact with the media and able to maintain a heavy denial about the risk of HIV disease and its connection with substance abuse.

Emily did finally recover from both her addictions, but by then she was already HIV positive, although she did not discover this until 10 months after her son was born. She had married a verbally abusive, drug-addicted man. Her worst fears came true when the marriage ended very stormily once her diagnosis was made. Her husband blamed her not only for her own disease, but for "killing our son." Emily and her baby, Mike, moved home with Bill and Mary. She had selected a marriage unlikely to last; once it failed, she was moved back in the life cycle to the adolescent stage.

The therapist was able to reframe Emily's moving back home as a highly successful choice on the part of Emily and her family. It would give them the opportunity to let her relive her adolescence in a controlled, loving, and appropriate environment. Had she not moved home herself, the therapist would have prescribed this move as a "compression"[10] backwards on the transitional pathway, going in the natural direction of the flow of the family system in order to effect the successful completion of a transitional stage.[13]

Thus, the transitional map was completed. The therapist proceeded with the help of the family to translate it into a structural time line[30] (Figure 8-5).

Emily's family had also come up with a lengthy list of strengths that could be perpetuated in future generations. The combination of transitional map, family strengths, and time line showed clearly how events had clustered and how themes and scripts were being handed down across generations.

**TABLE 8-B**
**List of Family Strengths**

| | |
|---|---|
| Humor | Parents never left |
| Togetherness | Close grandparenting |
| Helpfulness | Tolerance |
| Teamwork | Intelligence |
| We were chosen by people who really wanted us | Capacity to use resources |
| Loving | Socially active |
| No negatives | Sense of mission |
| Honesty | Sounding board |
| Patience | Share freely and know others can be objective |
| Wanting to be understood | |
| Open-mindedness | |
| Never prejudge | Parents validate children's feelings |
| Trust/Acceptance | |
| Freedom to children | Independence |
| Guts | |

These techniques allowed the therapist to construct a transitional perspective for the family that would help them to understand and forgive themselves for their current difficulties in terms of their past history and facilitate their taking charge of designing their future path.

The transitional perspective is given in stages throughout therapy sessions, as relevant information is shared with the therapist by the family. A final summary is given at the end of the total mapping process. In Emily's case, the family was praised for its intense loyalty and togetherness, as well as for not allowing family members to go off alone until they were really ready, even though they were to be praised as a family for their pioneering

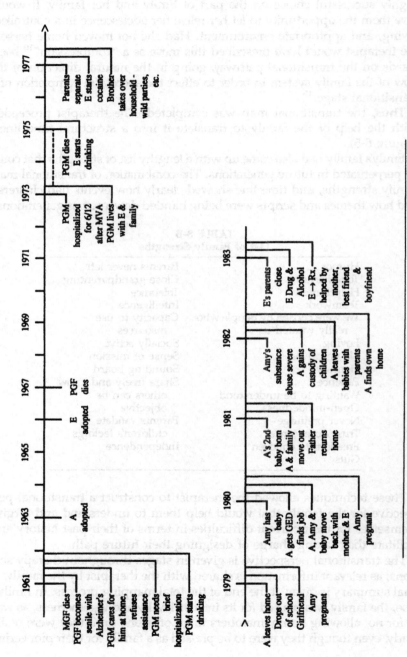

Figure 8-5. Emily's family timeline

spirit. In this way, both the closeness and distance poles were simultaneously validated.[11,12] The family had needed to stay close together since they had suffered such extreme losses and concomitant life cycle changes. The therapist described these as starting back in Emily's grandparents' generation, when her paternal grandparents had left Ireland and their families to come to the United States as pioneers. The family was absolved of all blame, understood the events in terms of loyalty[21] and family ties, and was congratulated upon finding their own solution—bringing Emily back home again.[22]

The transitional pathway was now complete, with past explaining present, and the family feeling that the future was in their hands. The therapist underscored the family's sense of mission. Emily's paternal grandfather, a Presbyterian minister, had come to the United States on a mission; now Emily was determined to fulfill a mission of her own. She planned to embark on a series of talks and educational activities centered around AIDS prevention. She was determined to ensure that she would leave a legacy of pride and meaning for her family. Her father planned to join her in her mission once he had retired from his full-time job. The family was ready to plan for the inevitable deaths of Emily and Mike, knowing that they would leave behind them significant markers of their impact on the world.

## 7. Sensitivity to Issues of Culture and Gender

The cultural and gender context of HIV disease is extremely rich. Members of any ethnic group may contract AIDS, as may individuals with alternative life styles and variations of gender identity. A quick review of the cases discussed shows rich variability of language, religion, education, and lifestyle.[7] Helene came from Haitian descent and her cultural norms were an integral part both of her contracting the disease and of her clinical management. Kevin and Julian were both members of the gay community, living an alternative lifestyle with surrogate families, but of different religious faiths. Julian's family were practicing orthodox Jews, while Kevin's were Catholic. Their religions made a real difference in the planning of the rituals and ceremonies not only around their deaths and reorganization of the family, but also around their living with HIV disease.

In terms of ethnicity and heritage, Mary Porter was an American of many generations, from a rural background and living in a healthy nuclear family. Amy, married to Brian, was British and an American immigrant, while Brian was a nonpracticing Jew. Sal, on the other hand, was of mixed Irish-Italian descent. Emily came from a typical American background, with first generation parents of Irish-Presbyterian descent. She had converted to Catholicism when she married into an Italian Catholic family. Peter came from an old mainline American family, basically atheists who rediscovered their religious roots at Peter's deathbed.

How does the therapist take all of these factors into account in the therapy process? Why are they important? In Sal's case, the therapist was greatly aided by her knowledge of Irish culture and her understanding of the difficulty that Sal's maternal (Irish) family members had in expressing their emotions. The therapist was able to draw upon Sal's father's Italian expressiveness to help the Irish side of the family through their pain. Therapists should attempt to learn, both from the literature and from their patients, as much as they can about the impact of different cultures on the patients and families they treat.[63] However, it is not possible for therapists to learn all about the myriad of cultures with which they may work. Families, as the experts on their own family system and culture, can be excellent teachers; therapists may benefit from allowing families to share their cultural norms and customs with them:[7]

> It is assumed that the family knows more about itself and its culture than the therapist ever could. The therapeutic system is, therefore, composed of two subsystems of "experts"—the family (and extended family), and the therapist aided by the community network (natural support system) where appropriate (experts on the theory and means for bringing about change). (p. 260)

In addition, the therapist may draw upon therapy models that are relatively culture-neutral and employ a methodology that utilizes what knowledge of the family culture the therapist has or is able to acquire. The transitional theory and therapy described in this chapter form such a model. All families are involved in the transitional pathway, so that the transitional frame may be used regardless of culture.[13] In instances where the family is unavailable, for cultural or geographic reasons, a link therapist (a family member who functions as therapist for the family) may be selected, to be supervised by the professional therapist.[13,64] Another transitional method that may be useful in dealing with families where language is a problem is that of *transitional sculpting*. This is a nonverbal, experiential technique for physically explicating the transitional pathway.[13]

> The Roman Catholic religious culture of Emily's in-laws became an important part of Emily's experience with HIV disease. When Emily and Mike were first diagnosed, the family took the two of them to healing masses, blessed them with holy oil, and said many rosaries over them. An intolerant physician or therapist might have opposed these measures and alienated the family. In fact, Emily was touched by their tangible concern.
> A more problematic experience with religion arose in the case of the

Piccolo family, a very religious Catholic Italian family. Their son's wife, Maria, had been diagnosed as HIV positive. The family believed that wearing garlic around the neck was healing and that novenas were more powerful than modern medicine. They also wanted Maria to have a baby, saying, "We want you to live. We want you to produce an offspring. Even though everybody here is positive, we want you to take a chance."

Gino loved his wife dearly, but was also the first son of parents to whom he was very loyal and devoted. He was able to resolve some of his ethical dilemma by refusing to be tested for the virus, despite knowing that his beliefs had put him at risk.

As the editor of *The Family Therapy Networker,* Richard Simon, points out, the power of traditional alliances such as race, class, ethnicity, or culture is very powerful; in addition, gender alliances are also very powerful and the health care professional needs to be sensitive to that power.[65] Homophobia, or fear of homosexuality, is one of the effects of "these primitive tribal forces," creating a "them/us" feeling that therapists need to recognize in themselves and their colleagues. Failure to recognize and deal with gender issue countertransference can seriously impact quality of care and the outcome of treatment, particularly in clients and patients who are already vulnerable. In Kevin's case, his homosexual orientation had the potential of interfering with the therapy if his therapist had not dealt with her own feelings. The special issue of *The Networker* underlines the need to know more about the homosexual and lesbian community, and their family constellations.[65]

Markowitz describes faulty assumptions that therapists still make about homosexuality.[66] She sees these as tending to fall between two extremes. One is that whatever the patient's presenting complaint, homosexuality is seen as the fundamental problem. The other extreme is the therapist's belief that homosexuality makes absolutely no difference at all, downplaying its relevance to the therapy.

Another central problem in providing gender-sensitive therapy to the gay population is the therapist's conception of family.[67] Kevin's therapist's acceptance of the role of Bill as Kevin's spouse was integral to the success of the therapy. Dahlheimer and Feigal describe the varieties of nontraditional families that have previously not been recognized or considered in the context of therapy and how best to approach their treatment. One of their suggestions for therapists who are not experienced in dealing with gay clients and their families is to use gay co-therapists. A second suggestion is to have a gay or lesbian colleague supervise the first few cases involving homosexual clients. Finally, they recommend reading a broad spectrum of gay/lesbian novels and autobiographies for insight into the specific gender issues that arise. There is a wealth of literature of this type written by the homosexual and lesbian community, dealing specifically with the issues of HIV infection and its impact on this community.

Gender issues in therapy can also originate because of male-female differences in the heterosexual community. The different ways in which men and women experience reality, as well as the change in attitudes across generations, also need to be considered by health care professionals, who are not themselves immune to the same attitudes. Walters et al. suggest a list of guidelines which incorporate sensitivity to feminist issues:[68]

1. Identification of the gender message that conditions behavior and sex roles;
2. Recognition of women's limited access to social and economic resources;
3. Awareness of sexist thinking that limits women's options to direct their lives;
4. Acknowledgment that women are socialized to assume primary responsibility for family relationships;
5. Recognition of the problems of child-bearing and child-rearing in our society;
6. Awareness of family patterns that can result in women competing with each other for power, splitting them from each other;
7. Affirmation of female values such as connectedness, nurturing, and emotionality;
8. Recognition and support for lifestyles outside of marriage and family; and
9. Recognition that no intervention is gender free.

They conclude that good clinical work needs to recognize the client's gender socialization. This is clearly of prime importance when one is dealing with HIV disease, since even those clients who are not homosexual or lesbian are still facing a disease with major sexual and gender implications. For example, the primary partner of an intravenous drug abuser, because of her gender socialization and lack of personal authority,[69] may be reluctant to ask that her partner use a condom.

Sensitivity to culture and gender is clearly of paramount importance in dealing with HIV disease, not only since cultural traditions and values impact on human decision-making (see Chapters 9 and 10), but also because of the vulnerability of inner-city populations in which cultural minority groups are over-represented (see Chapter 3).

## CONCLUSION

We have presented a model for the psychotherapeutic treatment of HIV positive and AIDS cases that attempts to be both integrative and comprehensive. It is based on a theory of human and family development which attends to intergenerational structure, support systems and the dynamics surrounding grief and loss. While space prohibits full explication of this "Rochester Model" (for instance, a number of its dimensions are not described here), we hope the reader has gained enough of a sense of it to begin applying it with cases of this type. Those interested in a more complete exposition are referred to the various publications cited.

## REFERENCES

1. Auerswald, E.H. (1974). Thinking about thinking about health and mental health. In S. Arieti (Ed.) *American Handbook of Psychiatry. 2nd Edition.* New York: Basic Books.
2. McDaniel, S.H., Hepworth, J., Doherty, W. (1992). *Medical Family Therapy.* New York: Basic Books.
3. Rando, T. (1985). Bereaved parents: Particular difficulties, unique factors, and treatment issues. *Social Work. 30:* 20.
4. Speck, R., Attneave, C. (1973). *Family Networks.* New York: Pantheon.
5. Stanton, M.D., Landau-Stanton, J. *Transitional Therapy: Theory and Approach.* In Preparation.
6. Landau-Stanton, J., Stanton, M.D. *Transitional Therapy: Special Techniques.* In Preparation.
7. Landau-Stanton, J. (1990). Issues and methods of treatment for families in cultural transition. In M.P. Mirkin (Ed.) *The Social and Political Contexts of Family Therapy.* Needham Heights, Mass.: Allyn & Bacon.
8. Landau, J., Griffiths, J., Mason, J. (1982). The extended family in transition: Clinical implications. In F. Kaslow (Ed.) *The International Book of Family Therapy.* New York: Brunner/Mazel.
9. Landau-Stanton, J. (1985). Competence, impermanence and transitional mapping: A model for systems consultation. In L. Wynne, T. Weber, S. McDaniel (Eds.). *Systems Consultation: A New Perspective for Family Therapy.* New York: Guilford Press.
10. Stanton, M.D. (1984). Fusion, compression, diversion and the workings of paradox: A theory of therapeutic/systemic change. *Family Process, 23:* 135–167.
11. Landau-Stanton, J., Stanton, M.D. (1983) Aspects of supervision with the "Pick-a-Dali Circus" model. *Journal of Strategic and Systemic Therapies, 2* (2): 31–39.
12. Landau-Stanton, J., Stanton, M.D. (1986). Family therapy and systems super-

vision with the "Pick-a-Dali Circus" model. In F.W. Kaslow (Ed.). *Supervision and Training: Models, Dilemmas and Challenges*. New York: Haworth Press.

13. Landau, J. (1982). Therapy with families in cultural transition. In M. McGoldrick, J.K. Pearce, J. Giordano (Eds.) *Ethnicity and Family Therapy*. New York: Guilford Press.

14. Landau-Stanton, J., Stanton, M.D. (1985). Treating suicidal adolescents and their families. In M.P. Mirkin and S.L. Korman (Eds.), *Handbook of Adolescents and Family Therapy*. New York: Gardner Press.

15. Imber-Black, E. (1988). *Families and Larger Systems: A Family Therapist's Guide Through the Labyrinth*. New York: Guilford Press.

16. Callan, D., Garrison, J., Zerger, F. (1975). Working with the families and social networks of drug abusers. *Journal of Psychedelic Drugs, 7:* 19–25.

17. Kliman, J., Trimble, D.W. (1983). Network therapy. In B.B. Wolman, G. Stricker (Eds.). *Handbook of Family and Marital Therapy* (277–314). New York: Plenum Press.

18. Rueveni, U. (1979). *Networking Families in Crisis*. New York: Human Sciences.

19. Schwartzman, J. (Ed.). (1985) *Families and Other Systems: The Macrosystemic Context of Family Therapy*. New York: Guilford Press.

20. Bowen, M. (1978). *Family Therapy in Clinical Practice*. Northvale, NJ.: Jason Aronson.

21. Boszormenyi-Nagy, I., Spark, G. (1973). *Invisible Loyalties*. New York: Harper & Row.

22. Framo, J.L. (1976). Family of origin as a therapeutic resource for adults in marital and family therapy: You can and should go home again. *Family Process, 15:* 193–210.

23. McGoldrick, M., Gerson, R. (1985). *Genograms in Family Assessment*. New York: Norton (page 1).

24. Bowen, M. (1980). Key to the use of the genogram. In E. A. Carter, M. McGoldrick (Eds.). *The Family Life Cycle: A Framework for Family Therapy*. New York: Gardner Press.

25. Stanton, M.D., Landau-Stanton, J. Ancestry: Its role in normality, nonshared environments and dysfunction. In Preparation.

26. Sussman, M. B. (1965). Relationships of adult children with their parents in the United States. In E. Shana, G. F. Streib (Eds.). *Social Structure and Family Generational Relations*. Englewood Cliffs, NJ: Prentice Hall.

27. Denham, T. E., Smith, C.W. (1989). The influence of grandparents on grandchildren: A review of the literature and resources. *Family Relations. 38:*345–350.

28. Stanton, M.D., Landau-Stanton, J. The role of ancestors in family life and nonshared environments: I. Family themes, balance, and generation skipping. In Preparation.

29. Stanton, M.D., Landau-Stanton, J. The role of ancestors in family life and nonshared environments: II Family scripts and replacement. In Preparation.

30. Stanton, M.D. The time line and the "Why now?" question: A technique and rationale for therapy, training, organizational consultation and research. *Journal of Marital and Family Therapy*. In Press.

31. Stanton, M.D., Todd, T. and Associates (1982). *The Family Therapy of Drug Abuse and Addiction.* New York: Guilford Press.
32. Minuchin, S., Fishman, H. C. (1981). *Family Therapy Techniques.* Cambridge, Mass.: Harvard University Press.
33. Landau-Stanton, J., Stanton, M.D. How did it start?: The family process of addiction and other serious disorders. In preparation.
34. Stanton, M.D. (1977). The addict as savior: Heroin, death and the family. *Family Process, 16(2):* 191–197.
35. Stanton, M.D., Todd, T. (1981). Engaging "resistant" families in treatment: Principles and techniques in recruitment; III Factors in success and cost effectiveness. *Family Process, 20:* 261–293.
36. Byng-Hall, J. (1991). Family scripts and loss. In F. Walsh, M. McGoldrick (Eds.). *Living Beyond Loss.* New York: Norton.
37. Hill, R. (1971). *Families Under Stress.* Westport, CT: Greenwood Press. (Original work published in 1949).
38. Holmes, T.H., Rahy, R.H. (1967). The social readjustment rating scale. *Journal of Psychosomatic Research, 11:* 213–218.
39. McCubbin, H. (1979). Integrating coping behavior in family stress theory. *Journal of Marriage and the Family, 41:* 237– 244.
40. McCubbin, H.I., Boss, P.G. (Eds.) (1980). Family stress, coping and adaptation. *Family Relations. 29(4).*
41. McCubbin, H.I., Figley, C.R. (1983). *Stress and the Family: Vol. 1: Coping with Normative Transitions.* New York: Brunner/Mazel.
42. Haley, J. (1980). *Leaving Home.* New York: Jossey-Bass.
43. McGoldrick, M., Walsh, F. (1991). A time to mourn: Death and the family life cycle. In F. Walsh, M. McGoldrick (Eds.). *Living with Loss.* New York: Norton.
44. Paul, N., Grosser, G. (1965). Operational mourning and its role in conjoint family therapy. *Community Mental Health Journal, 1:* 339–345.
45. Hare-Mustin, R. (1979). Family therapy following the death of a child. *Journal of Marital and Family Therapy, 5:* 51–60.
46. Parkes, C., Weiss, R. (1983). *Recovery From Bereavement.* New York: Basic Books.
47. The Names Project, 2362 Market Street, San Francisco, CA 94114
48. Reilly, D.M. (1975). Family factors in the etiology and treatment of youthful drug abuse. *Family Therapy, 2:* 149–171.
49. Williamson, D.S. (1978). New life at the graveyard. *Journal of Marriage and Family Counseling, 4:*93–101.
50. Landau-Stanton, J., Le Roux, P., Horwitz, S., Baldwin, S., McDaniel, S. (1990). Grandma, come help. In T.S. Nelson, T.S. Trepper (Eds.). *101 Favorite Family Therapy Interventions.* Binghamton, N.Y.: Haworth.
51. Williamson, D.S. (1981). Personal authority via termination of the intergenerational hierarchical boundary: A "new" stage in the family life cycle. *Journal of Marital and Family Therapy, 7:* 441–452.
52. Sagan, L. (1987). *The Health of Nations.* New York: Basic Books.
53. Kantor, D., Lehr, W. (1976). *Inside the Family: Toward a Theory of Family Process.* New York: Harper Colophon.

54. Boszormenyi-Nagy, I. (1976). Behavior change through family change. In A. Burton (Ed.). *What Makes Behavior Change Possible*. New York: Brunner/Mazel.

55. Boszormenyi-Nagy, I., Ulrich, D.N. (1981). Contextual therapy. In A.S. Gurman, D.P. Kniskern (Eds.) *Handbook of Family Therapy*. New York: Brunner/Mazel.

56. Boszormenyi-Nagy, I., Krasner, B.R. (1986). *Between Give and Take*. New York: Brunner/Mazel.

57. Byng-Hall, J. (1988). Scripts and legends in families and family therapy. *Family Process*, 27: 167–179.

58. Walker, G. (1991). *In the Midst of Winter: Systemic Therapy with Families, Couples, and Individuals with AIDS Infection*. New York: W.W. Norton.

59. Stanton, M.D., Landau-Stanton, J. (1990). Therapy with families of adolescent substance abusers. In H.B. Milkman and L.I. Seder (Eds.). *Treatment Choices for Alcoholism and Substance Abuse*. Lexington, Mass.: Lexington Books. (p.330).

60. Haley, J. (1976). *Problem Solving Therapy*. San Francisco: Jossey-Bass.

61. Stanton, M.D. (1981). Marital therapy from a structural/strategic viewpoint. In G.P. Sholevar (Ed.). *The Handbook of Marriage and Marital Therapy*. Jamaica, New York: S.P. Medical and Scientific Books.

62. Madanes, C. (1986). *Behind the One Way Mirror: Advances in the Practice of Strategic Therapy*. San Francisco: Jossey-Bass.

63. McGoldrick, M., Pearce, J.K., Giordano, J. (Eds.). (1982). *Ethnicity and Family Therapy*. New York: Guilford Press.

64. Landau-Stanton, J. *Link Therapy: Technique and Theory*. In preparation.

65. Simon, R. (1991). From the editor. *The Family Therapy Networker*, 15 (1):

66. Markowitz, L.M. (1991). Homosexuality: Are we still in the dark? *The Family Therapy Networker*, 15 (1): 27–44.

67. Dahlheimer, D., Feigal, J. (1991). Bridging the Gap. *The Family Therapy Networker*, 15 (1): 44–53.

68. Walters, M., Carter, B., Papp, P., Silverstein, O. (1988). *The Invisible Web: Gender Patterns in Family Relationships*. New York: Guilford Press.

69. Rampage, C. (1991). Personal authority and women's self stories. *Journal of Feminist Family Therapy*, 3 (1/2): 85–98.

# CHAPTER 9

# Spiritual, Cultural, and Community Systems

## *J. Landau-Stanton, C.D. Clements,*
## *A. F. Tartaglia, with J. Nudd,*
## *E. Espaillat–Piña*

Family systems, as they extend and push out, inevitably intersect with cultural, communal, religious, and philosophic traditions and institutions as well as with the ethos or world view carried by those subsystems. A systems approach to HIV disease suggests that no single subsystem can address the multifaceted nature of working with persons at risk. The burden of care is most adequately and responsibly addressed when shared fluidly across subsystems.

Our primary goal in this chapter is to familiarize the health care professional with (1) an awareness of spiritual issues and the tools for spiritual assessment; (2) an awareness of the particular dynamics and needs of different racial and ethnic minorities; and (3) the methods for mobilization of community resources. Underscoring each of these is the message that therapists need not feel alone when counseling individuals and families impacted by HIV disease. Even though the majority of persons presenting for therapy share the same issues—separation, loss, life adjustment, relational conflict, or search for meaning—HIV + persons experience these issues with a higher level of intensity and a greater sense of urgency. Natural support systems and community resources are among the therapist's best allies.

## SPIRITUAL ISSUES AND HIV DISEASE

### Peter's Case

"I have become spiritual, not in the traditional religious sense, but in a very personal way." These are the words Peter, diagnosed with AIDS, spoke when the chaplain* first met him. Raised in a family of self-proclaimed agnostics, Peter had described himself as at best neutral, at worst antagonistic, toward institutional religion. The "church" was, after all, one of those institutions that "condemned me and my (gay) lifestyle."

### Larry's Case

Such also was the case with Larry, an HIV-positive gay white man, admitted to the psychiatry unit for a major depressive episode. He requested a chaplain's visit, then began with the question, "Do you believe in heaven and hell?" As the conversation unfolded, it became clear that the only option Larry saw for himself was hell. He was angry at the Free Methodist tradition in which he was raised, railed at Jerry Falwell, and yet could not see himself moving beyond the internalized moral judgment. The connection between his depression and internalized guilt became clearer. He had brought shame to his family and the only adequate penance was suicide.

Despite Larry's lack of contact with his religious community, the therapist realized that it was important to reconnect him not only because of his illness, but also because of his internalized guilt. His treatment, therefore, included involvement both with the chaplain whose presence Larry had requested and a clergyperson from his own tradition. His mother and siblings were also an integral part of the therapy because of Larry's issues of shame and punishment and his feeling that suicide was the only solution.

Though still struggling with reconciliation at the time of his death, Larry caught a glimpse of the merciful side of God and the compassionate aspect of the church. One of the last things he said to the chaplain was, "At least I can pray now and know my words are heard."

### Walter's Case

The guilt emerging from spiritual conflict was also articulated by Walter, a hospital patient, who greeted the chaplain* with the words, "Please don't judge me; I'm living under my own judgment." Despite a rational acknowl-

---

*Chaplain Rev. Alexander Tartaglia, D.Min.

edgment to the contrary, Walter could not see his AIDS outside the context of punishment for his drug abuse.

### Emily's Case

Emily attributed much of her coping ability not only to the commitment and love she has for her son but also to the much needed acceptance she received from family and friends. Emily, like other persons with AIDS, wanted to retain a meaningful place in her social settings. She longed to remain intimate, to retain the ability to reach out and care in an environment where she could be well received. In turn, like all of us, Emily wanted to experience the compassionate care of others. Her father, a social worker nearing retirement, in response to Emily's experience, changed his focus for later years to "doing more for others by moving into AIDS work."

For people like these, a religious figure's symbolic intervention of confession, forgiveness, and penance might be appropriate. For clients who do not draw upon religious resources, other alternatives might be more appropriate. For example, referral could be made to a 12-step fellowship program. This requires the individual's own responsibility for his or her actions and for making appropriate amends. Alternatively, referral for family therapy might incorporate the principles of repentance and reparation, as suggested by Madanes.[1] Involving the natural support system allows this process to occur while the client or patient is supported by his or her resources, as discussed in Chapter 8.

### Spiritual Diagnosis and HIV Disease

We have found that retaining a working distinction between the "spiritual" (finding meaning in existence) and the "religious" (communal creeds and practices)[2] has enabled us to acknowledge the limitations of religion as faced by HIV+ persons, without dismissing the spiritual concerns as either irrelevant or oppressive.[3,4] Rev. Tartaglia's tool for spiritual diagnosis (Table 9-A)* has been designed to enhance the repertoire of diagnostic and treatment options available to the practitioner with minimal training in pastoral care or theology.

This table works with four existential questions that are universal in appeal and application: "Am I Safe?,"[5,6,7] "Do I Belong?"[8] "Am I Worthy?" "Am I Valued?" The following Table 9-B is a model of how health care professionals can use the diagnostic Table 9-A in working with HIV patients or clients.

---

*Acknowledgement to Rev. James Evinger, former staff chaplain, and to the Clinical Pastoral Education students of the fall of 1989.

## TABLE 9-A

| Spiritual Diagnosis | Image of God | Experience | Existential Question | Experience | Image of God | Spiritual Diagnosis |
|---|---|---|---|---|---|---|
| Fear | Unpredictable, Capricious, Chaotic | Mistrust, Victimization, Helplessness, Passivity | "Am I safe?" "Is my world a threat, or an opportunity?" | Hope, Courage, Active agency, Opportunity | Trustworthy, Reliable | Faith |
| Alienation | Vengeful, Divisive | Social stigma, External judgment, Rejection, Estrangement | "Do I belong?" | Social acceptance, Communion, Embracement | Loving, Inclusive | Community |
| Guilt | Punishing, Judgmental | Internalized stigma, Personal responsibility for illness | "Am I worthy?" | Grace, Repentance | Merciful, Compassionate | Reconciliation |
| Despair | Withholding, Silent, Absent | Meaninglessness, Death anxiety, Non-being | "Am I valued?" "Do I leave a legacy?" "Did my life make a difference?" "Am I content? regretful?" | Vocation, Purpose, Creativity, Meaning | Blessing, Affirming, Revealing | Providence |

Table 9-B shows how spiritual themes flow throughout Tom's story and offers us a way to frame his experience, without separating the bio-psychosocial components.

### Tom's Case

Bright and articulate, Tom had always seen himself as physically, intellectually, and emotionally in control of his life—*safe*. By the time we met him, however, he felt physically vulnerable and was having difficulty with speaking and with feeding himself. "I just like to know what I'm dealing with," Tom said, almost as if knowing would make a difference.

Tom faced a dilemma shared by many HIV positive persons, a struggle with the sense of *belonging*. Tom's illness had reunited him with his family; now he grieved their imminent loss. "I'm most afraid of losing my parents now that we finally are a family. After all these years, I finally know they love me." Tom's sister and brother had also welcomed him back.

Equally powerful was the family's willingness and ability to share their private agony with the church community. Much to the family's surprise and relief, revealing the secret of Tom's sexual orientation did not result in rejection, nor did it in any way diminish the care and compassion the religious community afforded its members during times of family crisis.

Tom was discharged from the hospital and his therapist continued to include the family's pastor in his management. The congregation was invited to share in the ongoing care of Tom and his family. After Tom's death, a memorial service was held, attended by the families of Tom and his deceased partner and the congregation. This ritualized the reconciliation.

Not all stories are as hopeful as Tom's. Some experience only the isolation that accompanies this disease, rather than being welcomed by families, surrogate families, congregations, and other community groups. Nonetheless, most individuals who appear to be totally cut off from the communal support systems discover a level of acceptance from them that is inclusive and loving.

Tom's reconciliation with his family and religion of origin may serve as a metaphor for spiritual reconciliation. However he had difficulty believing that he was *worthy.* "What have I done to deserve this?" He continued to assume personal culpability for his illness.

In the face of pain and suffering, the health care provider should acknowl-

**TABLE 9-B***

| Biological (Medical) | Psychological | Spiritual (Tom's words) | Themes and Feelings | Spiritual Issues |
|---|---|---|---|---|
| Tom is 30 years old; Tom and partner diagnosed with AIDS three years ago. Partner dies. Tom treated for depression. | Grief from partner's death, close contact with partner's family. | "I still wonder why this is happening to me. What have I done to deserve this?" | Self-punitive. Looking for answers. Seeking forgiveness. Fear that this is all that his life will come to. | What would it take for Tom to feel valued? worthy? forgiven? What is the meaning of his life? What is fair and just? |
| Tom admitted to hospital. At admission, is taking AZT, Doxaprin, Percodan, Vitamins, Sinequan, Nazoral, Idometharin | Reconciliation with family after 10 years estrangement; relationship with older brother very important. Parents shocked by the rapidity, gravity and adjustment to events, but supportive. Parents not yet drawing on community support. Parents church supportive (home communion, pastoral care). | "I'm most afraid of losing my parents now that we are a family. After all these years, I finally know they love me." | Relieved, glad at family reconciliation. Not resentful, bitter over past estrangement. Unfinished emotional/ relational grief over lost opportunities. | Gratitude, thankfulness. Sense of belonging. Parable of Prodigal Son. Familial reconciliation as a metaphor for spiritual reconciliation. |

| | | | | |
|---|---|---|---|---|
| Difficulty eating and swallowing. Speech slurred. Facial droop on left side; MRI shows bilateral parietal lobe lesions. Cannot read or write. Left arm tremor makes feeding himself difficult. History of seizures. Ambulates with aid of a cane. Stereotactic biopsy shows PML. | Career as successful scientist ended. Prior to hospital admission, asked to come home to family, and family learns he has AIDS. Parents unable to provide home care. | "I'd just like to know what I'm dealing with." | Diminished control and ability, dependency, anxious, frustrated, suppressing anger, fear of unknown. | Physical vulnerability as a metaphor for spiritual vulnerability. What does it mean to Tom to hope? |
| Tom diagnosed with terminal, untreatable PML | Family perceives him as terminal with little time. | "I've made my peace with God, but I'm not sure what happens to us after death. What do you think heaven is like?" | Seeks reassurance: his cognitive belief does not resolve his existential anxiety. | Providence: worthiness, acceptance, validation of his life, hope. What does peace mean for Tom? What would it mean for him to have faith amidst fear, uncertainty, suffering and death? |

*This diagnostic chart was developed by Rev. Alexander Tartaglia, D.Min., in working with HIV patients and clients.

edge the patient's or client's need to ask "why," and then help him or her gain perspective.

Tom also asked the fundamental spiritual question of what happens to us at death. He had made his peace, convinced that life has purpose, that his life had been affirmed, and that he was *valued*.

Questions about eternal life should not be met with resistance, avoidance, or countertransference. Tom's therapist could not give Tom an absolute answer since no one is in a position to do so. However, it was important to facilitate Tom's exploration of the question. Interestingly enough, Tom's description of being at peace with God parallels the way many dying patients view life after death, as a secure, peaceful, and restful state. Including Tom's pastor in these conversations also relieved the anxiety of the therapist.

This systems framework for spiritual assessment is one that the practitioner can employ regardless of his or her own perspective on these matters. It attempts to frame both secular and religious language in the common denominator of spiritual terminology.

## The Role of Spiritual Heritage and Tradition

Spiritual issues that are universally applicable find their expression in specific faith traditions and religious institutions. Often viewed as voluntary associations around which groups organize for a common purpose, religious institutions retain historical, familial, cultural, ethnic, and personal meaning with a power of their own. This power can be harnessed creatively as the transformer of cultural values toward a just and compassionate treatment of others. They can also serve as a mirror of the normative values of a given culture, controlling individual behavior through a system of social taboos.

The role of religious institutions in the lives of individuals and family systems requires careful consideration and open negotiation.[9] The hurtful, destructive elements that reflect cultural judgmentalism require a process of healing. The creative opportunities for that healing need to draw upon the redemptive quality of religious institutions.

The therapist's or health care professional's role may be seen as threefold in attending to the faith tradition of HIV-positive clients and families: 1) negotiating the religious history of the family of origin as a way of facilitating healing; 2) taking seriously the blending of religion and culture within ethnic groups; and 3) including the resources of faith communities in addressing the multitude of physical, social, and emotional needs experienced by clients and families.[10-15]

Religious history, not unlike family history, is multigenerational. It brings to bear on an individual not only the belief system, but the moral framework of past religious traditions, which weave within the fabric of one's family system. Thus, negotiating the impact of religious history requires attending not only to the tradition of choice but also to the tradition of family origin and tradition of birth. The lives of many HIV-positive persons crystalize the need to take an extensive religious history when exploring family history.

## Paul's Case

Paul's journey toward becoming spiritual has been described in Chapter 8. The religion of Paul's family of origin would not give us an insight into what drove Paul in his spiritual quest, which had become more intense as his illness progressed. Paul's parents were self-proclaimed agnostics; his siblings were uninvolved in religious activity. There was no "apparent" formal religious training, yet from his multigenerational family, Paul was the inheritor of a deep-rooted eclectic religious heritage of which Anglicanism was a part.

One day, Paul stopped in the chaplain's office and said, "I've only a minute . . . I'm late for an appointment in the clinic but I saw your door open and wanted to share the good news . . . I know where I belong." At age 30, he was halfway through his adult membership classes in a reservedly liberal (the chaplain's term) upper middle class Episcopal church. That Easter Sunday he was baptized and publicly received into full fellowship. Not unlike the myth of being cut off from his family of origin (described in chapter 8), Paul was anything but emotionally cut off from his religious history.

## Congregational Interventions

A systems approach to care maintains the inherent value of drawing upon the strength of an individual's group and the natural resources within it. Religious and ethnic groups have long experienced the religious community or body of the church as the network through which they discover the coping mechanisms to face crisis situations. The questions are: How is this done? What helps? Our experience has taught us that creative and proactive steps that contribute to spiritual and emotional well-being can be taken by religious congregations. Research has suggested that the value of social support depends not on volume, but on the quality and properties of the support network(s).[16] Therefore, accurate assessment and appropriate referral to agencies, congregations, and groups are crucial. Table 9-C highlights some approaches and interventions that a religious community group can provide.

**TABLE 9-C**

| Congregational Interventions | Techniques and Issues |
|---|---|
| Openness to educational programs on sexuality, risk reduction, health and AIDS | First close dichotomy between body and spirit. Focus programs on health and wholeness. Focus on relationship and safety topics in sex education. Provide quality AIDS education that targets attitude change leading to behavior change. |
| Openness to non-traditional families | Consider how to include single-parent, same-gender, childless, blended, or unmarried family structures. Broaden concept of family and provide activities relevant to the diversity of family units. Provide resource list of congregations which have such programs. |
| Development of liturgy that affirms non-traditional families | Provide blessing of relational commitments. Support the internal struggles of young adults and adolescents around questions of sexual orientation and identity. |
| Support and compassion for HIV-positive individuals and their families (blood and surrogate) who seek re-entry into church | Recognize fear of rejection by those who feel cut off by religious group. Understand the individual's urge to "come home" and make home a haven by inviting full participation by the congregation. |
| Support for the worried-well | The most well-intentioned person who interacts with HIV positive people may experience anxiety, fear and then guilt. Create support groups that will accept AIDS fears and reduce guilt, to eliminate the withdrawal of potentially supportive congregants. Maintain dialogue to keep fear from festering. Dialogue will provide an environment of support to prevent persons engaged in risky behavior from withdrawing into isolation. |

| | |
|---|---|
| Support for families in the face of isolation | Recognize the burden of families and loved ones who carry the secret of a person's sexual orientation, high risk behaviors, or drug abuse.<br><br>Connect congregants who share the problem and help facilitate self-help groups.<br><br>Encourage support through community systems.<br><br>Do not be (clergy or congregant) the sole or primary support system. |
| Support for grieving persons and their families | Celebrate and remember the lives of those persons who have died.<br><br>Remember that grief comes in battalions, and deal with anticipatory grief and grief that lingers after the physical death.<br><br>Recognize that families, lovers, friends, other HIV-positive persons, colleagues, health care workers and therapists are all impacted.<br><br>Grief is collective and demands a communal response; encourage individuals to seek communal expressions of public grief and to participate at a level appropriate to their needs.<br><br>Create an interfaith network to sponsor quarterly services and yearly candlelight vigils.<br><br>Hold services on a rotating basis at diverse religious sanctuaries and in various ethnic communities. |
| Invitation/Openness for 12-Step fellowship programs to use congregational facilities | Provide a home in congregational facilities.<br><br>Be sensitive to the need for support groups for teenagers and adults to deal with alcohol abuse, drug abuse.<br><br>Do not deny entry to programs based on prejudice.<br><br>Avoid a moral message of judgment, and provide a nonblaming welcome. |
| Religious organizations as prophetic witnesses for a response to AIDS | Assume the scriptural role of witness on behalf of those who lack power: the poor, the elderly, the disabled, the disenfranchised, persons with AIDS.<br><br>Engender collective support for political and legislative action which requires the just and humane treatment of HIV-positive persons: access to health care, health insurance, jobs, personal compassion. |

Religious institutions as mediators among family members and between alienated persons and their traditions.

Actively pursue reconciliation. Initiate and mediate discussion among family members and between alienated persons and their traditions.
Use an intentional and persistent approach to reconciliation.
Promote listening and forgiveness by sensitivity to alienation.

Visitation of the sick and attendance at funerals and memorial services.

Since illness is an isolating experience, visiting the sick is a fundamental task for religious leaders, congregants, and pastoral counselors.
AIDS should not be an exception to this task.

Assistance in meeting daily needs

Maintain independent living through assistance with meals, housekeeping, and transportation.
Help HIV-positive people be cared for and die in their homes if they wish.
Enhance dignity and self-esteem by helping persons and families maintain control and choices about the routines of daily living.
See this as a unique opportunity for the local religious congregation to help this happen for members of its faith community.

Advocacy in the development of housing and/or hospice care

Understand housing for people with AIDS can be a community controversy.
Advocate community residences for AIDS individuals, as the congregation has advocated for developmental disability and mental health.
Help empower persons with AIDS by advocating semi-independent living.
Open hospice centers through cooperative efforts of individual churches.
Facilitate financial and volunteer support by members of the congregation.

Providing respite nursing care for families caring for the ill

Be sensitive to the burden of caring for terminally ill loved ones and how this interrupts routine living. Assist caretakers in meeting basic needs such as sleep and social interaction. Recognize caretaker ambivalence and guilt. Recognize the absence of "permission" to enjoy life.
Organize volunteer efforts by congregants to provide respite care on a regular basis.

| | |
|---|---|
| Providing temporary housing for out-of-town families | Since AIDS patients may be treated in medical centers far from family, the economic burden of extended stays away from home needs to be alleviated. |
| | The AIDS patients at state and federal prisons are a special problem. |
| | Recognize that such families may have no natural support system within the community. Congregations can provide such support and services and can create an interfaith network. |
| Support for congregants in health-related fields | Hospital chaplains should spend time consulting with and supporting staff as well as ministering to patients and families. |
| | Be sensitive to health care workers who may have emotional turmoil relating to work. |
| | Provide an environment where professionals who work with illness and death can cope with frustration and pain. |
| | Sponsor remembrance services for health care workers whose patients have died. |
| | Provide ritual remembrance services in the local congregation for health care workers. |

The key to effective inclusion of these congregational interventions in the treatment of HIV-positive patients and their families is the understanding and development of religious and spiritual resources by health-care professionals and the commitment to a systems approach. Professionals will want to establish a multiracial, multiethnic, multifaith resource list of congregations to which patients and families can be referred and who are available for consultation when needed. A religious community that meets some of the criteria outlined above will generally be an effective resource. Finally, professionals who are connected with such resources may invite religious and community leaders into dialogue around the care of their clients and families to allow for collaboration and to reduce mistrust and competition between secular and religious disciplines.

## THE CONCEPT OF FAMILY AMIDST CULTURAL DIVERSITY

The health-care professional needs not only to identify the spiritual and religious traditions of the particular groups that he or she serves, but also to develop an understanding of their broader cultural norms and their needs. Although it is important to know the cultural norms of the group at large, it is also necessary to map each individual family to avoid broad generalization and stereotyping. As we discussed in Chapter 8, the transitional pathway and experiences of each family need to be seen in the light of the experiences of the group.[17] We have selected two examples of communities particularly at risk for HIV to briefly illustrate the need for awareness of and sensitivity to cultural diversity.

### The African-American Family

Sensitivity to African-American extended family patterns is imperative in a multisystems approach to treatment. This sensitivity should include an awareness of the immigration and migration patterns of each family, since the term African-American is extremely broad, ranging from those who settled in the colonies to the recent wave of Eritrean refugees. The strength of kinship networks has been documented in an effort to increase understanding and empower resources in work with these families.[18,19,20] Appreciating the natural function of these kinship systems allows us to view the existing family structures as normal, thereby reducing culture bias, which can lead to a disparaging view of these families.[21,]

Hill viewed the strong or healthy African-American family as having well-defined but flexible boundaries, with balance between a high degree of organization and self-differentiation, with tolerance of difference, and the capacity for both cooperation and negotiation.[23] He viewed their strong kinship bonds and religious orientation, as well as their use of strong support systems such as the extended family, as major strengths. Pinderhughes stresses that recognition and development of these characteristics form a central goal in empowering African-American families, since "these mechanisms are in constant jeopardy of being undermined as their existence is dependent upon the very forces that they must struggle against."[24]

Nancy Boyd-Franklin, in her book *Black Families in Therapy*, describes some of the key features and different models of the kinship system.[22] She is also quick to warn against generalized assumptions that ignore the widespread existence of a nuclear family system. One of the primary strengths she describes within the extended family system is "reciprocity"—the "process of helping each other . . . exchanging and sharing support as well as goods and services . . ." (p. 43). Knowing that another can be counted on engenders family stability. She views one of the potential problems within the kinship system as the imbalance that can result and the tendency of individuals to become overly burdened (p. 44). Thus, the role of the health care professional includes clarification for the family of how the system works and the implications for individual members.

African-American extended family systems are neither homogeneous nor static. They vary in form and structure. Boyd-Franklin draws upon the contributions of previous efforts,[18,25] in describing four major extended family types:

(1) subfamilies . . . two or more related individuals within the same household or close proximity, often drawn together due to economic factors; (2) secondary members . . . which include families who take in related children (informal adoptions) or adults in transition; (3) augmented families . . . children raised in households with nonrelated members; (4) "nonblood" relatives . . . individuals who are related by function and involvement, thus experienced as "family" despite not having blood ties.[22] (pp. 45–49)

Many African-American families share the same traditions and culture of origin. However, as with other cultural groups, this does not imply uniformity and health-care providers should guard against stereotyping. There is a large African-American middle class that, while sharing many of the strengths and resources of the African-American community and family structure, does not belong to the inner city lower socioeconomic underclass. It does, however, feel a common bond and share some of the same concerns, problems, and risks of that population.[26] When one is dealing with prevention and management of HIV disease, an understanding of the context and fabric of these communities is essential to the health care provider.

As mentioned previously, the role of the health-care professional is not merely to identify how the family system is structured but to clarify how it works. The sensitive professional must begin with the assumption that the existing family structure, whatever its form, is value neutral. Imposing other cultural structural models or assessing nontraditional nuclear models as pathological would be a grave error. The family structure typically emerges in response to perceived needs and the role of the professional is to work with the family to explore and assess how these needs are functionally addressed. A systemic view of the family includes, but is not limited to, clarifying boundaries, allowing for role flexibility, and discussing family "secrets."[22] (pp. 51–63)

Appreciating the role of religion in the life of African-Americans begins with the recognition that the church has been historically the only institution "owned" by the African-American community. Not only has it served as the focus of shared experience, but also as the source of redemptive possibility. The church has been a key component of this group's extended family concept. It has served as the arena where education is valued, respect for the integrity of the individual is nurtured, and impetus for political change is sparked.

## The Puerto Rican-American Family

Although the Puerto Rican family is an example of Hispanic culture, it is important to recognize that the term Hispanic loosely links people who share the roots of a common language, but come from very different cultures. These include Mexican, Argentinean, Chilean, Bolivian, Spanish, Dominican, Puerto Rican, Cuban, and Colombian. The language and historical roots may be similar, but there is a wide variety of spoken language and cultural traditions across this group. For example, while the Puerto Rican and Spanish family systems are patriarchal, the Colombian tradition is strictly matriarchal.

The Puerto Rican family is typically viewed as the heartbeat of the culture among Puerto Rican-Americans.[27] The components that contribute to one's individual identity—sense of belonging, worthiness, and value—emerge from one's connection to the family system. As in many other traditional extended family cultures, the family is relied on to solve problems internally.[21] Common characteristics include an extended family system in which the male members hold the major decision-making power. The Puerto Rican patriarchy is based on a "godfather" system similar to the Italian one; the health care provider must attend to this internal network of authority.

Clients with traditional extended family structure generally turn first to their family system for support in addressing social, ethical, or emotional concerns. Only in the face of a new cultural context in which traditional prescriptions no longer apply, or in which they fail, is agency assistance sought.[21] The internal support system includes, first, the extended network of family members, friends, and neighbors, followed by teachers, clergy, or others believed to have expertise in the problem area. Assessing the natural support network and the client's attempts to enlist it is critical. To what extent have the internal support networks been explored by the client? What about this situation requires going beyond them? Is the family local? Have they "failed" the person seeking help? How can they be approached or mobilized as resources for treatment? What are the family lines of authority? What are the individual's expectations regarding the treatment process? What are the family's expectations?

These are a few of the early questions health care professionals will want to explore. HIV disease represents a problem for which there is no traditional extended family prescription; therefore, outsiders are invited in. It is, however, crucial to include the family in all planning and administration of treatment, since their exclusion will diminish the efficacy of the professional.[15]

Approaching the client requires sensitivity to the internal struggle prior to seeking external intervention. The professional must not undervalue the courage of the patient and family in taking this step. Respect for both the individual's integrity and the cohesion of the extended system should be underscored. Maintaining close physical proximity, assuming intimacy on a first-name basis, direct confrontation, or delving into highly personal matters too readily are among the common mistakes made by professionals. Closing emotional distance and establishing trust require patience and recognition of the importance of the family context. Movement from indirect to direct eye contact, closing the gap of physical proximity, verbal jesting, elaborated responses, and shift from avoidance of to exploration of intimate feelings are signs that the professional is gaining the trust of the client and family.

The power of persons in authority that exists in the patient's family system is carried into the clinical relationship. As an authority figure, the practitioner is apt to be viewed as the expert who will direct the process and supply answers. Clarifying the expectations and an understanding of roles in the clinical relationship will reduce misunderstanding.

The traditional family plays a key factor within Puerto Rican family systems. Males tend to hold a dominant place, while females are submissive within the family. To be "macho" or virile is valued for men, while faithfulness and obedience are valued for women. Vigilance to preserve manhood, dignity, and respect is central. Discussion of personal problems that might compromise these attributes will be avoided. Male expression of emotional vulnerability will be interpreted as a sign of personal weakness.

Women may not feel as free to speak openly when experiencing the influence of a male counterpart. Discussion of intimate matters such as sexual behavior is considered taboo even with one's own husband. The reticence to do so will be carried into clinical treatment. Loyalty to traditional norms and role expectations, even for those who rebel against them, contributes to emotional conflict when women encounter the Americanized social system. Any discussion where the potential loss of one's children or the right to reproduce is at stake will be met with resistance since it threatens traditional roles and duties.

For both men and women, a health care professional of the opposite sex can be particularly threatening. A woman can threaten traditional hierarchical norms for the male client; a man may threaten openness to discussion of intimate issues for the female client. Establishing trust and gaining confidence can be accelerated by the inclusion of professionals of the same gender and same ethnic group and by the inclusion of same-sex family members. This becomes particularly critical when one is discussing HIV disease and high-risk sexual behavior.

Therapists need to avoid formality and rigidity, and accommodate ethnic, racial, and cultural diversity. Resistance should not be viewed as negative nor lead to clients and their families being judged as noncompliant. If resistance is present, the therapist needs to be sensitive to its origins. Resistance is the responsibility of the therapist, not of the client or family. Often the use of team counseling, the inclusion of key family members (when extended family is not available), allowing the client to bring a confidant or close friend, neighbor, clergy, or other support demonstrate an understanding of, and respect for, the particular needs of the individual.

The purpose of this section is to offer some guidance to the reader in his or her work with persons of different ethnic and cultural backgrounds. No generalizations should be drawn from these insights, nor assumptions made about any individual or family. The purpose is to motivate the reader to invite clients and families into exploration of their understanding of the concerns brought to treatment. Allow them to be teachers in the process and to identify their coping mechanisms and strengths that can be mobilized toward realizing more satisfying social interaction and healing.

We have only briefly discussed African-American and Puerto Rican-American families and their cultures. Other African, Hispanic, or Latin-American cultures will require the same sensitivity to kinships, traditions, family and network structures, and rules of behavior. Other cultures (e.g. Asian, Native American, European, Aboriginal) also need to be understood in terms of such structures and behavioral rules.

## BUILDING A COMMUNITY NETWORK FOR PREVENTION AND INTERVENTION

The power of the community as illustrated throughout the book is of central importance in both the prevention and management of HIV disease. Communities are made up of complex networks that can be mobilized and strengthened to ensure that problems do not arise.[28,29,30] They can also be integral to the prevention and management of specific problems that have emerged, and may be threatening the welfare of the community.[31] Even when, as in the case of HIV disease, one's purpose is the prevention and management of the disease, other factors such as poverty, disenfranchisement, substance abuse, hemophilia, and discrimination should be included in one's purview.[32,33,34]

As was presented in Chapter 8, involving people who are not intimately connected with the issues can result in greater efficacy than including only those people at the nexus of the problem.[35-38] Also, when the larger system is involved, the energy for change is far greater and there may be resources available of which one is unaware but which could prove helpful to one's mission.[39,40,41] Those dealing with the central problem are generally the ones who are overburdened and whose vision tends to narrow to an immediate focus. They are frequently so busy that they cannot be aware of the broader implications of the problems or take time to establish contact with resources that do not appear to be directly relevant.

One first needs to establish where and who the resources are. The principle of determining what is out there at every level of the community, building on what is already there, expanding where needed, and creating only what needs creating is central to community work. In dealing with HIV disease, HIV services and programs are clearly central; however, there are many other services in communities that may be effectively involved. It is important in identifying community resources not to narrow the initial search, so that should the nature of the problems change, the support and intervention system can be adapted. For example, involvement of only gay activists, agencies, and organizations would limit response to the needs of the minority populations, substance abusers, and adolescents who are now at risk.

Community organization in this endeavor may be formal or informal. It can aim at creating networks of an entire community towards general health and welfare. Or it can be specifically directed towards one community or problem area, and take the form of the establishment of community-based agencies and organizations directed toward that problem. It can also take the form of case management or home/community-based services.[42,43] Examples of community networking directed towards dealing with HIV disease are the impressive number of community-based agencies that have sprung up around the world for this purpose. Some are general community agencies serving populations with broad needs and integrating HIV programs into their mission. Others are aimed specifically at informing the community about the disease and its prevention, while providing services for clients and families dealing with HIV.

## Community-Based Agencies

In our community, a member of our AIDS Training Program, Jackie Nudd, was one of the early organizers of what eventually became the major community-based AIDS agency, AIDS Rochester, Incorporated (ARI). Her experience was similar to those of others initiating community efforts.

*The Example of AIDS Rochester, Inc. (ARI)\** "In the winter of 1982–1983, a group of concerned people from the gay community began meeting to discuss the threat of AIDS in the larger Rochester community. We met in restaurants and in homes to try and develop a strategy for the care and edu-

---

*Jackie Nudd, former Executive Director of AIDS Rochester, Inc. and chief trainer for the community section of our University of Rochester AIDS Training Program, contributed this section of the chapter.

cation of those at high risk or with AIDS. At that time, gay men were the primary focus. By late spring, the meetings were more formal and directive. The people attending were assigned areas of expertise. Serious discussions were held, dealing with how the organization would be structured. One of the first serious decisions we made was whether the word "gay" would appear in the title of the agency. Some groups in New York State, such as the Gay Men's Health Crisis in New York City, had opted to include the word; others had not. This led to a long and difficult exchange about whom we would serve. Ultimately, the decision was made that we would not include the word gay in the name and that the philosophy of the organization would be to provide service to any and all people affected by the disease.

"In July of 1983, the group formally applied to form a not-for-profit organization under the name of AIDS Rochester, Inc. A formal board of directors was elected and committees formed. In the fall of 1983, the New York State Department of Health (NYSDOH) sent representatives to the seven major regions of the state to meet with grassroots organizations in an attempt to formalize a system for the delivery of services and educational programs. In November, 1983, ARI applied for its first grant with the NYSDOH. The first contract was awarded in January, 1984 and approved in March. In March, 1984 an executive director was hired and office space established over a cocktail lounge (the rent was free).

"The first identified Person With AIDS (PWA) contacted ARI in July of 1983; others followed rapidly. It was immediately apparent that we could not meet all the needs of our clients and their families. One of our first priorities was to do outreach to the community and identify other agencies that could assist in meeting the needs of our clients. Then, we had to educate the staff of these other agencies, so that they would be willing to provide appropriate services.

"This early recognition of our limitations and the need for community networking led to the development of our other primary philosophy: to empower the clients to take control of their own lives by providing them with information on where and how to access the community system to make it work for them. On those occasions when the system did not respond, it was our role to work within the system to meet the client's needs. We did this through education and patient advocacy at the highest administrative level.

"The agency grew from one employee in 1984 to 17 in 1989; from one client in 1983 to over 830 in 1989; and from 11 volunteers meeting in living rooms to over 800 highly trained volunteers in 1989. ARI was instrumental in helping to establish effective policies dealing with HIV infection in the Rochester community. At the state level, ARI was involved with several successful service and educational pilot programs. ARI was a leader in the field of community response to the AIDS epidemic. Those involved can be proud of the standards set forth by the agency, but more importantly of the love and caring, both given and received."

Jackie's story reflects the development and struggles of what became an extremely effective community-based AIDS agency. Its mission was not specific to any one population, but recognized the potential need of the community at large. However, its mission was specific to HIV disease. The example of Elisabet Espaillat's experience at the Puerto Rican Youth Development organization was similar in many ways and different in others. The agency was already in operation when she joined it and its mission was to meet the broad needs of a specific community—the Hispanic community. She was hired to work in their AIDS program as a community AIDS educator. Elisabet's struggles with her new role reflect the difficulties that many community workers experience when first called upon to network with others around a specific issue. They also reflect the benefits of being in an organization that considers the larger needs of the community that it serves.

*The Example of Elisabet Espaillat at Puerto Rican Youth Development and Resource Center, Inc. (PRYD)\** The PRYD center was strategically located in the heart of the largest at-risk Hispanic community in Rochester—the community they most wanted to serve. PRYD's mission was to facilitate community participation in reaching at-risk minority individuals, including substance abusers, adolescents, women, migrant workers, and immigrants from Haiti, Puerto Rico, South and Central America. The original mission of the agency was far broader than AIDS, but, with the advent of the epidemic, services had to be added. Community involvement was seen as fundamental in providing effective services to these people and their families. In fact, the agency's programs were designed to meet such specific and primary needs as high dropout rates, drug use, child abuse and neglect, teen pregnancy, living below the poverty level, and related medical, emotional, and economic problems.

Minority communities often have limited access to services and distrust a system that may be fragmented and unresponsive to their needs. In order to reach them, PRYD needed to utilize nontraditional methods and minority staff to provide culturally appropriate outreach, advocacy, health-risk assessment, and basic preventive health education, case management, support, referrals, and follow-up for individuals and families.

It became apparent to the staff that the cultural taboos of discussing sex-

*Elisabet Espaillat is on the staff at the Puerto Rican Youth Development organization. She joined our University of Rochester AIDS Training Program team as a community expert with particular knowledge of the Hispanic population.

uality in mixed gender groups and outside of the intimacy of close family and friends made broad HIV education extremely difficult. In order to resolve this problem, PRYD instituted a family outreach program. Educators visited individual families in order to provide home-based preventive education in a setting where it could be heard and appreciated. They subsequently found that they could include a few families in an educational session, provided that the families were closely acquainted or related. Close friends and neighbors were often included, the principle remaining that the families were in charge of the invitations.

Elisabet joined this HIV program and described her experience as follows:

"Being a member of the Hispanic community, I had thought that it would be easy to teach them about AIDS. However, I discovered that there were topics, such as sexuality, that were culturally sensitive. For example, the use of condoms is a generally acceptable behavior in the Anglo community. But in the Hispanic community it is not easily accepted, whether for birth control or for prevention of HIV infection. My knowledge and understanding of the community helped in my mission, but were not enough alone."

Jackie and Elisabet's experiences are examples of working in community agencies, one created specifically to work with AIDS and the other designing an AIDS program as part of its broader mission of serving its community. Community networking can also be achieved without designing formal agencies and organizations, but utilizing whatever resources are present in the community.

## A MODEL FOR COMMUNITY NETWORKING

Our model for community intervention follows the same principles presented in earlier chapters and uses the same practical outline as the initial therapy session described in Part I of Chapter 8. However, the content and order of the tasks, as well as the process, may vary depending on (a) what role the health care provider will play, (b) how the project is initiated, and (c) at whose request. The provider should never maintain a central role, since we represent only a portion of the targeted community. If the provider has been called upon to initiate and design a preventive effort, his or her leadership role should be time-limited. If the provider lives within that community, his or her role may be limited to representing his or her own personal and family needs. If one works in the target community, one's role may be limited to representing only the specific component of one's health care profession and work setting.

A clear distinction must also be made as to whether one plans to function as a temporary consultant or to remain an integral part of the endeavor. The short-term consultant should remain on the periphery of the organization, recognizing the inherent strengths of the community and helping with mobilization towards action. The health care provider who intends to remain active should help initiate the project but, once it is underway, not assume a greater role than others in the community. The withdrawal is, therefore, more a matter of timing than of principle. The primary responsibility of the provider is to ensure that equal representation of the components of the community occurs in order to avoid skewing. Once this is achieved and community members are working effectively together, the provider should hand over to them.

Initiation of a community prevention effort may come from concerned parents, teachers, government officials, health-care providers, the police, the people most impacted by the problem, those concerned that they might be impacted, or, in fact, from any facet of the community. The incentive may also come from outside the community through the agent of government, public or private organizations, individuals with a mission, or the efforts of other communities that have initiated their own projects. For example, in the case of trade unionism, initially a grass roots organization, Sol Alinsky became a brief part of many communities in order to help them organize their own efforts. The organization of public health services and widespread immunization is an example of community organization by governmental authorities for the protection of the community and the country at large. In the case of HIV disease, the initiation of community prevention efforts may come from any of these sources.

Once the incentive for community action is present, the intervention described below may be used. As mentioned above, this intervention is based on the tasks listed in Chapter 8. However, the tasks may need to be repeated at times or consolidated at others. For example, the initial joining phase often needs to include not only joining but mapping the system in order to identify its strengths and resources and to initiate the formation of a collaborative relationship. In other words, the first three tasks of the therapeutic intervention may need to be consolidated prior to the first community meeting, and subsequently repeated at it. We will, therefore, present the tasks in the order that one most often needs to perform them:

1. Joining—identifying resources and building collaborative relationships;
2. Mapping—mapping community players and their connections and contexts, creating a transitional map;
3. Establishing strengths and resources—continuing to explore what is

out there, involving them in the mission, and assisting them in recognizing their own and others' areas of competence;
4. Establishing goals—coordinating and prioritizing common community needs and plans;
5. In-meeting (session) enactment—building of collaborative networks and task forces and recognition of the intrinsic power of the individual and the system;
6. Homework—putting plans into effect;
7. Session closure and formalized greeting—planning further meetings and formalizing network connections.

The process of community networking and completing the tasks listed above may occur in two or three stages:

(1) Since the initiation of a community-wide intervention is always started by a few specific people, the initial process is best completed with this group. (2) Once the larger group has been involved, the initial process is repeated with them. Wherever possible this stage should include representatives of the entire community. (3) In some instances, however, when representatives of the whole system were not present for stage two, a third expansion is needed that once again follows the same format.

## 1. Joining, or Setting Up the Intervention

In planning to undertake a community intervention the first step, as mentioned above, is to consider the entry point. Unlike therapy, the people who present the initial request may not be at the heart of the problem. They may be a concerned group of parents, teachers, or health professionals, or they may be members of government, law enforcement, or the judicial system. At times, the mission may be one that we, as health care providers or community members, choose to undertake without a specific request. Our previous example of Jackie Nudd is one in which she and a group of her friends decided to do something about AIDS. She chose to start an agency, since there were no other community facilities. Also, since AIDS was primarily a gay disease at that time, she knew that her best change agents were likely to come from that community.

One of the first tasks in joining, regardless of who has or has not invited one into the community, is to get to know the membership of the community, how it is organized, and where the best entry points may be found. In order to do this effectively, one may have to do some initial work on identifying resources. Once this has been achieved, the decision about whom to invite follows the same principles as therapy. If one has been invited in by a group (which can range from a few individuals to 50 or more), it is necessary to ensure that one has developed a collaborative relationship with them prior to setting up a larger community meeting. If one is initiating the effort oneself, it is critical to involve a group of concerned and representative community members for the initial phase.

This group should be representative, not only of the larger system (as determined by the large systems map), but also of the hierarchical structure of the community. If all members of the group come from the top of the hierarchy, they may experience a great deal of difficulty in mobilizing members from the bottom of the pyramid. Conversely, if one starts working with people from the base of the pyramid, it may be impossible to involve managers and executives later.

We have found that the most effective mix is one that combines representation of the tip, the base, and the middle of the pyramid to ensure adequate filtering of the intervention. This is sometimes achieved by telephone or conference calls, but generally requires a meeting at which one goes through all the stages of intervention listed above. The goal of this initial phase is to reach a consensus as to the direction the group chooses to take with its community.

The health care provider with experience in running this type of intervention is generally the best chair of the initial meeting. In instances where the provider involved does not have experience in chairing meetings, an experienced community member may be asked to do so. In this event, the provider's role is that of a consultant to the process. An alternative is to request an outside consultant for the initiation of the endeavor.

To plan the maximum impact of phase two, one should ensure the widest possible representation at the first community meeting. This requires the initial group to collaborate closely in the selection of community members who will be invited. Apart from ensuring adequate representation, the group also needs to establish who the community leaders are, who should not be excluded, who has the greatest expertise or power in the community, and who has the greatest capacity to bring about change. Failure to do this initial planning may result in important segments of the community being left out. This may lead to apathy, anger at being rejected, and even opposition to the intervention by those excluded. It may also result in decreased efficacy of the network.

In addition to inclusion of every facet of the community (see Chapter 2, Figure 2-7), it is also important to view every component of the community as equally important (e.g. children, government officials, street sweepers). However, the natural hierarchy of the community should be considered as the natural leadership of the endeavor, not because they are more important, but because they have a history of "getting the job done."

Once the collaboration of the initial group is established, the initial goals designed for the larger group meeting, and the people to be invited identified, the method of invitation needs to be negotiated. It is often useful to involve members of the media in the initial meeting for the purpose of informing and inviting the larger community to the next meeting. Where this has not occurred or has not been possible, the initial group needs to identify the components of the community that each of them can access. If there is a component that apparently cannot be accessed by anyone at the meeting, members need to take responsibility for developing the necessary channels of communication to ensure that all community components will be represented at the community meeting.

After the community meeting has been convened, the chair of the initial group introduces its members to the community, summarizes the group's original reasons for meeting, and invites the community to participate in all further endeavors. The chair may then ask those present to identify what portion of the community they represent and list these on an overhead projector transparency, blackboard, or large sheet of paper. This allows those present to see the magnitude of community representation. The chair of the meeting may then congratulate those present, since a community that cares enough and is able to come together to plan already has the tools for intervention and prevention.

The process of joining and identifying resources in the larger community meeting is generally best achieved by a three-step process. First, it is helpful to join with the larger group and to map and identify its resources. This exercise is then repeated at a more specific level by smaller groups. The small groups are in a better position to start the process of networking, get to know their detailed resources, and identify specific goals and directions. The final stage of the meeting is to reconvene the larger group, receive feedback from the small groups, and design the master plan.

The technique of mapping is extremely useful both for planning future interventions and for building collaborative relationships. It also provides a framework for networking.

## 2. Mapping

While the chair of the meeting is establishing who is present in the larger group, he or she lists them, not at random, but on the larger systems diagram (Chapter 2, Figure 2-7), showing who is present in natural and ancillary support systems. It is also helpful to point out at this stage that many members represent several levels, such as personal, family, and work levels. Generally, if the meeting has been carefully convened, representatives at every level are present. If there are gaps on the map, members can be asked who has access to those categories of people to identify how they might be involved in the project.

The next task is compiling the transitional map of the community. Instead of drawing a basic genogram, components of the community are represented by a constant symbol (circles or squares may be used since gender is not critical in this diagram). The mapping process consists of establishing the community's history, how it developed, what it is facing in the present, and how it might change in the future (i.e. where it comes from, where it is now, and where it will be going). Past historical components of the community would replace the great-grandparents of the genogram. Similar to mapping families, one needs to establish: How have countrywide or world events changed the direction of the community? What about natural disasters, economics, and politics? Is the community fairly homogeneous, sharing a predominant language, culture, philosophy, religion and political preference? Does the community comprise many different groups of immigrants speaking multiple languages, eating different foods, dressing differently, and having different value systems?

What are the community connections? How do people relate or not relate? Do they use each other as resources? What are the boundaries and how are they maintained? Are there particular populations in the community that are at greater risk? Are they represented? If not, how can the existing connections of the meeting members be used to involve them?

Le Roux adds to the mapping process a geographic map demonstrating physical boundaries and transitions.[44] Are such boundaries naturally existing, for example neighborhoods divided by rivers or main roads? When did the divisions happen and did they result in the breakdown of prior neighborhoods? Is the community isolated? Is it contiguous to an area that imposes threat? During the mapping of a community in South America, it became apparent that its geographic situation placed it in the immediate path of the drug smugglers in the country at its northern boundary. This route threatened to convey not only drugs but HIV infection. This realization was important to the community as it designed its preventive plan.

Once the transitional map is drawn, a time line may be constructed, showing how contiguous events have impinged on the life of the community, while demonstrating the stresses and celebrations through recent memory. This allows the group to get a better sense of what they are actually dealing with. We have found it helpful to extend the time line into some possible future scenarios over which the community will have control if it takes definitive action.

### 3. Establishing Strengths and Resources

When the mapping process has been completed, the maps can be used to underline the strengths and resources of the community as a whole. The strength in homogeneity or diversity can be recognized and plans made to utilize that strength for the established mission. Connections both between population groups and across the levels of the larger system can be pointed out and meeting members can be asked to list the strengths of these connections. People representing resources at each level of the system can be applauded for being present and willing to participate in the endeavor.

Members can be asked to talk about the areas of competence of other members and representatives of agencies and organizations. Parents may thank teachers for their accomplishments with their children; doctors may praise parents for their success in an immunization program; families may be appreciative of self-help groups, and others of social services. This process assists greatly in the building of the community network and is best continued in a small group setting. The next stages of the intervention, establishing goals and in-meeting enactment, are also best started in the smaller groups.

The chair of the meeting asks people to divide into groups. We have found that the optimum group size is between eight and 12. The chair should stress the need for groups to be heterogeneous, comprising the different components of the community, across the large systems map, and across hierarchies. Parents should sit with other people's children or teachers; members of an office group or working team should be separated. In practice, numbering off from left to right across the room generally achieves a good mix. Members of the initial planning group are divided among the small groups to assist in the process. The group is given very clear directives. It is asked to complete the mapping process, list the strengths and resources of those present, and form an initial resource list. It is then asked to establish goals and prioritize them, ready to report back to the larger group. Each group is asked to select a recorder for this purpose.

The first task of the small group is to complete its specific mapping process, determining which components of the community it represents. It is useful at this stage for people to make lists of the members present and their special interests, competencies, addresses, and phone numbers. In this manner, they establish an initial support and resource network. We generally ask that they gain permission to be able to call upon each other for this purpose. During this process, they also familiarize themselves with the particular expertise of group members, their hopes and dreams for the community.

## 4. Establishing Goals

The group is then charged with applying the strengths and resources they have listed to the task of establishing goals for their community. Goals may be extremely varied and the process frequently becomes heated as members struggle to achieve priorities. In our experience, some groups want to design major AIDS prevention programs, others choose to collect funds for hospices, and yet others feel that their community needs better educational or health services.

It is frequently difficult for groups to prioritize goals since different components of the community may see the problems or threat very differently. Some may feel that the community is at no risk and choose to work on issues of health maintenance and education. Others may be very concerned about a situation that they regard as an emergency and will choose to prioritize immediate public health measures and expansion of treatment facilities. All perspectives should be included as equally important, but consensus needs to be reached on which to tackle first. It is helpful to design the order according to the stage of the problem. For example, in a community in which there is still a very low rate of HIV infection, preventive education in the areas of AIDS and drug abuse might be most important, whereas in a community that is facing bankruptcy because of an overloaded health care delivery system, this might need to be dealt with concurrently. In some communities, the needs might be greatest for particular risk groups; this would be important to consider in the process of prioritizing goals.

## 5. In-Meeting Enactment

Once the goals have been prioritized, the group is charged with designing specific objectives and brainstorming ways to begin to meet them. Once again, the group draws upon the strengths of its members to allocate specific members to specific goals. The network building, begun during the mapping process, is completed and resource lists are compiled. At this stage, it is important to ensure that every member of the group is in agreement with the priorities set and has specific responsibility for at least one of them. Members are then asked to make general suggestions about how the goals might be implemented.

Once this has been achieved, the large group is reconvened and the chair requests that each recorder make a brief presentation. Recorders are asked to summarize only the group's primary goals, objectives, and designs for intervention, without repeating items mentioned by previous presenters. The recorders are asked to hand in all records of maps, resource lists, addresses, and phone numbers, as well as goals and suggestions for their implementation. A volunteer is requested to compile these into a single document that can be circulated to all present. The physical network is about to be established.

The larger community group is then asked whether it chooses to continue beyond this first meeting. In our experience, the answer is invariably affirmative. Even when some members elect to drop out, they frequently volunteer to send someone in their place and ask to be kept informed of the process. They may also request permission to attend at a future date. The community group then starts to work at prioritizing the primary goals selected by the small groups. Once this has been achieved and the community is agreed upon their immediate tasks, they can proceed to design specific homework.

## 6. Homework

The homework of the volunteer compiling the network lists has already been allocated, and homework needs to be designed by and for the rest of the community group. Homework may range from writing a press release to baking cookies, or to inviting neighbors to attend the next community meeting. Educators may offer to research and design community-appropriate prevention programs; physicians may agree to expand their clinical services; clergy may offer to involve their congregations; school principals or mayors may offer the use of their schools or town halls as venues, or to convene town meetings. Others may agree to initiate and organize task forces. Wherever possible, members are assigned or choose tasks most closely related to their own field of endeavor in order to ensure success.

## 7. Session Closure and Formalized Greeting

At this stage, we have found it best for the chair (if he or she is either a consultant or the health care provider who initiated the project) to hand over to the community to elect a long-term chair who can best represent its needs and wishes. The initial chair may offer to be available for consultation or even to attend a couple of future meetings, but the leadership and responsibility must by this stage belong to the community.

Members are asked to spend time after the meeting chatting with each other, getting to know each other informally, and making arrangements to meet or talk on the telephone with at least one other person prior to the next meeting. We have found it helpful to provide refreshments for this stage to allow the meeting to end in a relaxed social process.

Although, in order to illustrate the model, we have presented this process as continuous, it is often not possible to achieve this much in a single session. We have found, as mentioned above, that the initial meeting is generally best held before the community meeting so as to ensure that adequate representation of the components of the community will be invited to the larger meeting. In either instance, the tasks that need to be completed at the first meeting are the initial four stages: joining, mapping, establishing strengths and resources, and establishing initial goals. These can be done more briefly at the initial meeting and fleshed out later (as is often done in therapy) in the larger meeting, as described above. It is important for members present at the meeting to feel that they have areas of competence, can form an initial resource network, and can share some community goals.

Future meetings may follow a similar format, with the concentration on the various tasks varying according to the stage of accomplishment. For groups who are not experienced in community organization, we have found that they progress best if the initial goals are clearly defined and well circumscribed. Success is the key ingredient, not magnitude. Once a small goal has been achieved, larger ones inevitably follow.

## REFERENCES

1. Madanes, C. (1990). Repentance and reparation in cases of sexual abuse. In C. Madanes *Sex, Love and Violence*. New York: Norton.

2. Dunphy, R. (1987). AIDS and spirituality. *Focus, A Guide to AIDS Research*, 3:1–2.

3. Fortunato, J.E. (1987). *AIDS: The Spiritual Dilemma*. (7–33). New York: Harper and Row.

4. Pruyser, P. (1976). *The Minister as Diagnostician* (pp. 60–79, 80–87). Philadelphia: Westminster Press.

5. Perelli, R.J. (1991). *Ministry to Persons with AIDS: A Family Systems Approach*. (pp. 44–55). Minneapolis: Augsburg.

6. Frankl, V. (1963). *Man's Search for Meaning*. New York: Pocket Books.

7. Sunderland, R.H., Shelp, E.E. (1987). *AIDS: A Manual for Pastoral Care*. (pp. 18–29). Philadelphia: Westminster Press.

8. Parsons, T. (1951). *The Social System*. New York: Free Press.

9. Democrat & Chronicle, Goleman, D. Psychology takes a new look at religion. Rochester: (October 12, 1991).

10. Broderick, C.B., Schrader, S.S. (1981). The history of professional marriage and family therapy. In A.S. Gurman, D.P. Kniskern (Eds.) *Handbook of Family Therapy*. New York: Brunner/Mazel.

11. Thomas, D.L., Cornwall, M. (1990). Religion and family in the 1980's: Discovery and development. *Journal of Marriage and the Family*, 52(4): 988–992.

12. Thomas, D.L., Roghaar, H.B. (1990). Postpositive theorizing: The case of religion and the family. In J. Shay (Ed.) *Fashioning Family Theory: New Approaches* (pp. 136–170). Newbury Park, CA: Sage Publications.

13. Weber, T.T., Wynn, J.C. (1986). Consultation with the clergy: A systems approach. In L.C. Wynne, S.H. McDaniel, T.T. Weber (Eds.) *Systems Consultation: A New Perspective for Family Therapy*. New York: Guilford Press.

14. Wynn, J.C. (1987). *The Family Therapist: What Pastors and Counselors Are Learning from Family Therapists*. Old Tappan, NJ: Fleming H. Revell Co.

15. Friedman, E.H. (1985). *Generation to Generation*. New York: Guilford Press.

16. Namir, S., Alumbaugh, M.J., Fawzy, F.I., Wolcott, D.L. (1989). The relationship of social support to physical and psychological aspects of AIDS. *Psychology and Health*, 3: 77–86.

17. Landau-Stanton, J. (1990). Issues and methods of treatment for families in cultural transition. In M.P. Mirkin (ED.) *The Social and Political Contexts of Family Therapy.* Needham Heights, Mass.: Allyn and Bacon.
18. Billingsley, A. (1968). *Black Families in White America.* Englewood Cliffs, NJ: Prentice Hall.
19. McAdoo, H.P. (Ed.) (1981). *Black Families.* Beverley Hills: Sage Publications.
20. White, J. (1984). *The Psychology of Blacks: An Afro-American Perspective.* Englewood Cliffs, NJ: Prentice Hall.
21. Landau, J., Griffiths, A.J., Mason, J. (1982). The extended family in transition: Clinical implications. In F. Kaslow (Ed.) *The International Book of Family Therapy.* New York: Brunner/Mazel.
22. Boyd-Franklin, N. (1989). *Black Families in Therapy: A Multisystems Approach.* New York: Guilford Press.
23. Hill, R. (1972). *The Strengths in Black Families.* New York: Emerson Hall.
24. Pinderhughes, E. (1989). *Teaching Cultural Sensitivity: Ethnicity, Race and Power at the Cross-Cultural Treatment Interface.* New York: Free Press.
25. Hill, A. (1977). *Informal Adoption Among Black Families.* Washington, DC: National Urban League Research Department.
26. Coner-Edwards, A.F., Spurlock, J. (Eds.). (1988). *Black Families in Crisis: The Middle Class.* New York: Brunner/Mazel
27. Puerto Rican Youth Development Organization, Rochester, New York.
28. Kark, S.L., Steuart, G.W. (Eds.) (1962). *A Practice of Social Medicine: A South African Team's Experiences in Different African Communities.* London: E.& S. Livingstone.
29. Gillis, L.S. (1977). Prevention of psychiatric illness. In L.S. Gillis. *Guidelines in Psychiatry* (pp. 214–222). Cape Town: David Philip.
30. Caplan, G. (1964). *Principles of Preventive Psychiatry.* New York: Basic Books.
31. Landau-Stanton, J. (1985). Competence, Impermanence and Transitional Mapping: A model for systems consultation. In L. Wynne, T. Weber, S. McDaniel (Eds.). *Systems Consultation: A New Perspective for Family Therapy.* New York: Guilford Press.
32. Mays, V.M., Albee, G.W., Schneider, S.F. (Eds.) (1989). *Primary Prevention of AIDS: Psychological Approaches.* London: Sage Publications.
33. Huber, J., Schneider, B.E. (Eds.) (1992). *The Social Context of AIDS: Sociological Contributions to Research and Policy.* Binghamton, New York: Sage Publications.
34. Duh, S.V. (1991). *Blacks and AIDS: Causes and Origins.* Binghamton, New York: Sage Publications.
35. Auerswald, E.H. (1968). Interdisciplinary versus ecological approach. *Family Process, 7* (2): 202–215.
36. Auerswald, E.H. (1983). The Gouverneur Health Services Program: An experiment in ecosystemic community care delivery. *Family Systems Medicine, 1* (3): 5–24.
37. Wynne, L., Weber, T., McDaniel, S. (Eds.) (1985). *Systems Consultation: A New Perspective for Family Therapy.* New York: Guilford Press.

38. Doherty, W.J., Burge, S.K. (1987). Attending to the context of family treatment: Pitfalls and prospects. *Journal of Marital and Family Therapy,* 13 (1): 37–47.
39. Reuveni, U. (1979). *Networking Families in Crisis.* New York: Human Sciences.
40. Schwartzman, J. (Ed.). (1985). *Families and Other Systems: The Macrosystemic Context of Family Therapy.* New York: Guilford Press.
41. Aponte, H.J. (1990). "Too many bosses:" An ecostructural intervention with a family and its community. *Journal of Strategic and Systemic Therapies,* 9 (3): 49–63.
42. Aponte, H.J., Zarski, J.J., Bixenstine, C., Cibik, P. (1991). Home/Community-based services: A two-tier approach. *American Journal of Orthopsychiatry,* 61 (3): 403–408.
43. Tavantzis, T.N., Tavantzis, M., Brown, L.G., Rohrbaugh, M. (1985). Home-based family therapy for delinquents at risk of placement. In M.P. Mirkin, Koman, S. (Eds.). *Handbook of Adolescents and Family Therapy* (pp. 69–88). New York: Gardner Press.
44. Landau-Stanton, J., Le Roux, P. *Inner City Social Systems: A Manual for Individual, Group and Family Therapists.* In Preparation.

# CHAPTER 10

# Doing the Right Thing: Systems Ethics and AIDS

There is no need to sophistically search for convoluted and irrelevant ethical issues in HIV disease. HIV disease is a test filled with realistic questions about the right thing to do. This infection touches on all levels of ethical concern and can illustrate almost any major question in medical ethics. It asks about our most basic or fundamental value choices, and about how our definition or understanding of humanness is reflected in our human values. It can be a case study of medical ethics. And because of all the intricate links between sexual values, community values, human values, and the medical value system, it is impossible to understand HIV infectious disease process without understanding ethics. It is also very difficult to fully appreciate what is the right thing to do in handling this disease.[1-4]

A sophisticated theory of ethics and of values is required to serve as a grounding for the ethical questions and the suggested answers, but a remote academic intellectualization gets in the way of helping people think about the right thing to do. Systems theory ethics is a powerful tool to help, but it is not easy to get people to see their experiences within a system theory framework. The effort is worth it, but the effort is hard. Although we talk about value systems, we're not used to seeing values or ethics from a systemic viewpoint. It's a new application to ethical theory, a needed new application, but there is always traditional resistance.[5,6,7] Still, that is what also makes this very exciting, because we can offer a new way of answering questions about what is the right thing to do.

That this is a practical task was made clear in the first specific application of systems theory to medical ethics, *Medical Genetics Casebook: A Clinical Introduction to Medical Ethics Systems Theory.*[8] Here, the framework of system theory was applied to questions in medical genetics that arose from case conferences over a three-year period. Those questions were grouped into categories and then an ethical view based on systems concepts was applied. The Chairman of the Social Issues Committee of the American Society of Human Genetics used this casebook as a basis for an essay on the types of medical problems arising in the practice of medical genetics, so it had demonstrated practical application.[9] The practicality of this ethical approach is important because an applied ethics that is impractical and fails to accurately describe the realities is not only of no use, but can be harmful.[10]

## LOOKING AT ETHICAL QUESTIONS IN HIV DISEASE FROM A SYSTEMS VIEW

### The Ethical Conflict Between Individual Good and Community Good

One of the major ethical choices, both individually and in policy planning, that HIV infectious disease process confronts us with is the choice between the needs and interests of the person and the needs and interests of the society. It is the perfect case study for the ethical tension in public health and preventive medicine. This question of what is the right thing to do occurs over and over in the history and current debate on HIV infection.

In June, 1982, the Centers for Disease Control (CDC) noted the first request for pentamidine to treat pneumocystis carinii pneumonia in a hemophiliac, and cluster studies had indicated AIDS was infectious.[11] Dr. Francis was working with the conceptual model that AIDS would resemble hepatitis in its transmission and there was already concern about the safety of blood for transfusion. But AIDS had struck in people who were already discriminated against by society, and their fear of even more severe discrimination (quarantine, gay-bashing, concentration camps) was high. From the social perspective of public health, however, insuring the safety of blood was also a very high priority.

Since there was as yet no test for the agent causing AIDS and little agreement on what might be the agent, the only way to protect the blood supply would be to screen out those high-risk groups from donating blood. That could be approached in two ways: trusting individuals who knew they were at risk to refrain from donating blood or asking screening questions before donation about sexual orientation and sexual activity. Screening would become a search for homosexuals and gay men were very concerned and angry that this would cause them considerable harm. Not screening would be allowing a lethal disease to be transmitted iatrogenically to many unknown people who received transfusions.

Although the CDC requested the Food and Drug Administration (FDA) to direct blood banks to screen donors, both the blood banks and the gay community opposed such screening. It was now early 1983, almost a year after the first warning. Consider the nurse in Chapter 4 who had a blood transfusion for open-heart surgery and was at risk for HIV. What was the right thing to do?

In San Francisco, Dr. Lorraine Day, an orthopedic surgeon, was concerned for her safety and the safety of her surgical teams. She did not refuse to operate on AIDS patients, but she wished to know her patients' HIV status. She also wanted research done on the potential for aerosolized blood to transmit the virus. By now, research had shown that HIV was the infectious agent and there was a reasonably reliable test for seropositivity (antibody to HIV). Some physicians and health care professionals wanted to see HIV testing as part of a routine work-up and the results made known to the health care team. In fact, a recent study of senior residents in internal medicine and family medicine in 10 states indicated that 74 percent supported surgeons knowing the HIV status of their patients.[12]

Related to the question of desire to know the HIV status of patients, the routine risk to health care professionals was demonstrated in a study done in a Detroit Emergency Room.[13] Three hundred and seventy Emergency Room patients were anonymously tested for both HIV-1 and HTLV-I (which can cause leukemia). Of the total, 4.1 percent were HIV-1 positive and 1.9 percent were HTLV-I positive. When this was broken down in trauma cases and medical cases, the results were similar. Of trauma cases, 4.1 percent were HIV-1 + and 1.5 percent were HTLV-I +. Of medical cases, 4.1 percent were HIV-1 + and 2.3 percent were HTLV-I +. The Emergency Room staff came into contact with 114 patients' blood and of those 114, 12 patients were positive. Staff experienced three needle-sticks, three scalpel lacerations, and four mucous membrane contacts, all potentially capable of transmitting HIV.

In our training, post-anesthesia nurses who felt they routinely treated HIV + patients had one major request—that they know the HIV status of their patients in order to be even more careful with Universal Precautions. They were double-gloving for patients they knew had Creutzfeldt-Jakob disease and they would probably double-glove for patients they knew had HIV. The nurses in Chapter 4 also discussed their experiences with Universal Precautions, and some very real practical problems. But patients feel that their medical ethics guarantee of confidentiality would be violated if such HIV status were commonly known in the hospital, and that they would be discriminated against in their medical care, either being refused care or receiving substandard care. Consider the fears about discrimination and lack of quality care described by Kevin and Emily.

People being admitted to a hospital also would be resistant to routine HIV testing on the basis of violation of Informed Consent and lack of adequate counseling. Individuals might even be resistant to HIV routine testing if one of the staff had a needle-stick from the patient or other occupational accidents that could potentially transmit HIV. Here the personal and social level needs and interests are complicated and in conflict.

There are personal needs and interests of individual health care professionals and of individual patients. There are group needs of health care professionals who might experience patient-to-physician iatrogenic transmission of HIV. Again, what is the right thing to do?

Another version of this conflict is the physician-to-patient iatrogenic transmission of HIV. Should all health care professionals, as a requirement of their employment, receive regular HIV testing, and should those who are HIV + be restricted from practicing routine invasive procedures? The tragic case in Florida in 1990 again forces this question to our attention. A young college student became a documented case of health care professional-to-patient transmission. Her dentist contracted AIDS and requested information from the CDC on the risks of continuing in practice. The guidelines at that time suggested he use gloves and mask, but that it was reasonably safe for him to continue his practice. In 1987, he extracted two molar teeth from the college student. Two years later, that college student rapidly developed AIDS. Although this was a short time between possible infection and disease progression to AIDS, it was not unknown. CDC investigators tried to eliminate other sources of infection and also did a DNA sequencing test at Los Alamos laboratories on samples of the virus from the dentist and from the student. The DNA sequencing indicated what would be expected if the dentist had been the source of infection; no other source of infection was apparent.[14]

Four other patients of this dentist, who is now deceased, tested HIV +. Although it was remotely possible that the virus profile was basically the same for the entire area where the dentist practiced and the student lived, the probabilities mounted with five infected patients and this is now considered a case of professional-to-patient transmission. We are faced with choosing between the needs of a health care professional with HIV to continue to practice, to enjoy confidentiality of status, and to enjoy his or her remaining life-span, and the general needs of the patient population not to be exposed to iatrogenic transmission of a lethal disease. What choice is the right choice and how do we go about making it?

For the gay community, the bathhouse issue represents the most striking tension between personal level values and social level values. Public health officials and homosexual physicians in San Francisco had for some time been worried about the dangerous channel for rapidly spreading infectious diseases that the bathhouses represented. Even before AIDS was known, a conference by homosexual physicians had pointed out the risk that such bathhouses entailed.[11] Venereal diseases and Hepatitis B already had been spread through bathhouses. Enteric diseases were alarmingly increasing. Diseases such as amebiasis, giardiasis, and shigellosis (up 70 percent) had risen in San Francisco, and after 1973 there had been an 8,000 percent rise of all enteric diseases. Cytomegalovirus and Epstein-Barr virus had risen to 93 percent in the gay community and were considered pandemic. Physicians were beginning to see lymph node and immune system problems and some Kaposi's sarcoma. Health officials were afraid that a new pathogen could spread very rapidly through bathhouses before anyone realized what was happening. And of course, that is exactly what happened with HIV.

However, the gay community attacked its members who carried this message and described them as homophobic, antierotic, and enemies of the new sexual freedom symbolized by the bathhouses. Gay Freedom was seen as a more important individual value than Gay Public Health or general Public Health. Larry Bye's summary of this period in San Francisco is overly positive and ignores the bitter internecine struggles and wasted opportunities for prevention that Shilts' review carefully documents.[15] By the end of 1984, when San Francisco was moving to close the bathhouses, the San Francisco AIDS Foundation still had civil rights objections to the closing. Closing the bathhouses was a choice of social level good over individual level good (civil rights). Was it the right thing to do?

There will be other examples of this primary ethical question as our experience with HIV infectious disease process grows, since it is a central question in any Public Health policy. Can ethics help us to answer the question?

Traditional ethical theories understand the conflict, but are not well-equipped to resolve it. The theories tend to fall on either side of the line, between individual good and social good, and try to remain practical by creating ad hoc exceptions. Table 10-A is oversimplified, but it allows us to see the *either/or* nature of traditional ethical theories and their attempt to use ad hoc exceptions to make the theories work.

Each column of Table 10-A views ethics from the perspective of either the individual or the group. This represents a major problem in applying such ethics to a real situation. It forces us to divide up the problem into opposing and adversarial sides, and take one of the sides almost exclusively. Rather than seeing ethics as a web, as Gilligan suggests feminine ethics does,[16] it makes us see it as a rigid hierarchical structure, with one perspective holding sway over all others. If we choose one side, we will always unbalance the real situation and rarely do the right thing. Ethics needs a more sophisticated understanding of these conflicting levels of needs and interests.

Systems theory provides just that understanding. It looks at the organization of experience and sees the growing levels of complexity as part of a large and functioning system. To severely damage one level by our choice of the right thing to do is to finally seriously harm the entire functioning system. Balance, rather than an adversarial choice, is the key.[5,7]

Consider the important ethical dilemma of personal confidentiality and freedom of choice conflicting with the health and survival of the commu-

**TABLE 10-A**

| INDIVIDUAL GOOD | SOCIAL OR COMMUNAL GOOD |
|---|---|
| *Moral Rights Theories*<br>*Legal Rights Theories* | *Utilitarian/Cost-Effective Theories* |
| Moral or civil rights ethical theories require that the right of the individual be paramount, with the exception being when that right will destroy another individual's right. It's not clear how severe the destruction must be or when this exception should be made. | Utilitarian theory and Cost-Effective modern versions assume the good of the individual is defined as the good of the greatest number of individuals, or the group. The individual is always sacrificed for the greatest good, through a calculus of the amount of happiness in the world, and there is no mechanism for making exceptions to this. |
| *Autonomy Theories* | *Natural Law Theories* |
| Autonomy theories, so common in medical ethics, assume a free individual who controls his choices, which must be protected and allowed, with the exception of those that would severely violate another person's autonomy or those that are made by an incompetent individual. | Natural Law theories hold that there is an order or design in the universe that is the purpose of human choice, and that individual human needs or interests must be secondary to that natural order. |
| *Individual Hedonism Theories* | *Altruism/Self-Sacrifice Theories* |
| Individual Hedonism (sometimes Egoism) theories concentrate on the individual's happiness, the meeting of a person's needs and interests. It is often characterized in a way that makes the consequences to the social group regrettable but acceptable. | Altruism theories are the opposite, requiring that the individual sacrifice his needs and interests for the needs and interests of others, but without specifying the limits to this altruism. |
| *Justice Theories* | *Social Contract Theories* |
| Justice theories again choose for the individual in demanding fair or just treatment for him, no matter what the social consequences. | Social Contract theories require autonomous individuals to give over freedom of ethical choice in order to achieve public safety and stability in order to safeguard life. |

nity. In Central Africa, as we have documented, that dilemma is even more serious than in the United States because the threat to the entire population is now so large that it demands a different balance between individual good and community good. Choosing for unrestrained individual rights to confidentiality and consent may now allow the spread of a deadly infectious disease to the point where it will decimate the populations of countries in Central Africa. The virus has become endemic in the national populations of Zaire and Zambia, with consequences that may rival genocide. A systems theory ethics would not find such a choice the right choice to make in such a situation, unless it were possible to argue that destroying the functioning cultural and demographic systems of Central Africa was the right thing to achieve. There could be few rational ethical arguments for choosing to unleash the Fourth Horseman of the Apocalypse and decide in favor of such destruction. That cannot be our goal.

In many cases, then, we are not aiming to produce systems collapse. Instead, we have as our goal an optimally functioning system, which implies that we must create a working balance between levels in the system. Extreme situations, such as that in Central Africa, may very well require extreme restriction of the needs of one level in order to avoid complete systems chaos. But ordinary situations, or decisions made in advance of a severe crisis, will avoid extreme sacrifices at any level of the system. There is a heavy price to pay for sacrificing the legitimate needs of either the individual level or the communal level of a system. It is tragic, therefore, to reach the crisis point where that choice must be made. Doing the right thing, then, involves the foresight to avoid such crisis points, providing the ability to set a working balance between the needs of individuals and communities, between the patient and public health.[8,17]

In the blood bank question, the potential spread of HIV through transfusions was a considerable threat not only to hemophiliacs but to the general population. The choice of initially sacrificing the needs of blood recipients in order to secure the privacy and civil rights of homosexuals who donated blood was not an ethical one. The harm to members of the homosexual community who wished to donate blood was not sufficient to balance the harm to blood recipients. Embarrassment at the office because a gay man would have to refuse to participate in a blood drive, even possible suspicion that the gay man was a homosexual, was not sufficient cause to justify the policy of taking a considerable risk with the lives of so many people as a group. Between the January, 1983, meeting of blood banks, the FDA, and the CDC, and the March, 1983, guidelines on transfusion risk, nearly one million transfusions were done in the U.S.[11] The needs of individual homosexuals could be met in other ways than placing such a large number of people at risk and the public health needs should have taken priority.

The same argument holds for the needs and interests of the blood banks. These institutions were reluctant to admit that HIV could be transmitted through transfusions and they demanded a certainty, an absolute proof that good science can never give. The blood banks were concerned about their own liability, stability, and capacity to continue operating as usual. Those organizational interests allowed them to deny the incoming evidence that blood transfusion was not safe and to resist any suggested screening solutions. In California, the for-profit organizations responded more quickly because the hemophiliac groups refused to recommend blood products that were not screened in some way for HIV. The nonprofit organizations set the balance too much in favor of their needs and interests and too little in favor of the health of the general population. That, too, was an unethical balance-setting. In both cases, the right thing to do appears clearer in retrospect: Place more weight on the public health needs and less weight on individual and organization needs.

This systems theory concept of balance, with a moveable set point for that balance, can be applied to the other questions as well. Health status information routinely appears on patients' charts, and routine work-ups are ordered with implied patient consent for many presenting complaints. The competent practice of medicine requires such medical actions, but the issue of individual discrimination complicates the decision for AIDS. The ethical problem is discrimination, not defining "confidentiality" to mean complete secrecy of health status within the medical care system. The problem can be resolved by finding ways to insure that discrimination does not occur, or it can be solved by making HIV status unknowable, the latter being a bit like "killing the messenger" because the news is bad, a response we discussed in Chapter 5. Since it is so medically important to know a patient's health status, ethically it would be more appropriate to restrict discrimination rather than to restrict medical information within the system.

Where confidentiality does become an issue is when such medical information leaves the medical system. Such information now leaves the system with far too much ease, through insurance payers' reviews, federal and state reviews, coerced patient signing of release forms, and general research on cost-effectiveness. These routine violations of privacy represent the general problem of lack of meaningful confidentiality of medical records and medical information outside the medical care system. Therefore, they represent an ongoing threat to all patients. AIDS has highlighted this issue for us, if we focus it correctly on the routine transmission of medical information from the medical care system to points outside the system.

Because of the potential for iatrogenic transmission of HIV, both from patient to physician and from physician to patient, routine HIV work-up and charting would be of considerable value *within* the medical care system. Since discrimination is a problem that can be resolved in other ways than censoring such information-gathering and use, it is not in the best interest of patients or physicians to support such censorship. For both diagnostic and treatment reasons, a routine work-up is important to the individual patient. For infection control reasons, that information is important for physicians and patients. Censoring information is a poor way to solve ethical problems and needlessly sacrificing individual interests is not an ethical solution. Physicians need to know patients' HIV status and patients should know physicians' HIV status. Mechanisms for resolving any problems that arise from that knowledge need to be put in place, because the system needs to respond to such problems, not deny them, as is currently being done by many states, countries, and professional organizations.

The bathhouse conflict represents an understandable but unfortunate choice for individual freedom over community good. The result was to seriously damage both the individual's good and the community's good. The benefit of keeping bathhouses open was questionable, but if the political and psychological benefits were seen as overriding individual and community survival, other measures could have been taken to minimize the risk to all. Mechanisms used in Europe for legal prostitution could have been employed, in addition to the ineffective educational means used in some bathhouses.

The concept of state interference in individual behavior, even for a good purpose such as health maintenance, is a dangerous one and needs careful balancing. It is too easy for a totalitarian control in the name of health to create a society that is a total institution. That would not be acceptable. But conversely, complete rejection of some collective decision to bar certain behaviors is also unworkable in the face of a severe threat to life or safety.

The level of severity is the crucial question to be debated, in order to set the balance ethically. How severe was the threat of HIV to urban gay communities? In hindsight, we know it was very severe. Should we have appreciated that severity at the time? The answer, if we look at the scientific data and the warnings of the medical experts, seems to be that we should have. There was too much distrust of experts and too much fear of discrimination to allow the affected communities to understand the HIV threat adequately. Sexual and political goals distorted the available information and the normal ambiguity of scientific probability was manipulated to spread uncertainty and rejection of scientific knowledge, even though that knowledge was more than sufficient to show the severe risk of HIV.

## Ethics and Hidden Economic, Political, and Social Agendas

Another major strength of systems theory ethics is its ability to identify hidden issues that are often framed in ethics language but require a full analysis from economic, political, legal, or social perspectives.[5,18,19] Because systems ethics has a built-in mechanism for integrating many levels and perspectives, it is well equipped to bring to light many concealed goals or agendas.

One of the most important questions in medical ethics is the utilitarian choice of cost-effectiveness and restricting access to medical care or withdrawing medical care. Traditional ethical theories can approach this question in two ways. One accepts the utilitarian or Life Boat ethics standard that the individual can be sacrificed for the efficiency or utility of the system or society.[20] Because this violates social values we would like to think we have, the economic/political first-order decision to restrict money for the medical system is usually hidden and instead the second-order decisions such as triage or rationing of scarce resources are emphasized and debated.[21,22] In other words, the resident at 2:00 a.m. who has to make a triage choice as to who gets the one available Intensive Care Unit (ICU) bed, agonizes over a choice that will result in the death of one of the two candidates for that bed, makes the choice, and goes on to practice triage another day. That is a second-order decision, given the concrete reality of only one ICU bed.

In fact, a similar AIDS case occurred at a hospital in our city. A young man suffering his second bout of pneumocystis carinii pneumonia (PCP) and with a Do Not Resuscitate (DNR) order in his chart was having difficulty breathing. He required a respirator, which at the time was available only on the ICU. There was one bed open in the ICU. A second patient, a middle-aged man who had just had a myocardial infarction (MI) but who would likely recover almost completely because there was little heart damage, also required an ICU bed. The young resident in ICU chose to admit the MI patient to the bed because of the DNR and the fact that AIDS is a terminal illness. The AIDS patient, suddenly realizing what the DNR order really meant and not accepting that meaning, wanted to change his mind because he really hadn't understood that it meant dying that evening with a PCP that could probably be treated. It was too late. The resident had seen no other medically warranted triage decision than to choose the MI patient over the AIDS patient. In the absence of a local ICU bed to transfer the AIDS patient to, and in the absence of a ventilator outside the ICU, the triage choice meant an earlier death for the AIDS patient.

That is the world of second-order decisions in economics and in medical ethics. On that level of decision-making, the resident's decision was the ethical one. Most medical ethics analysis, however, stops at that second-level decision. The resident did so, too, because he was not educated by medical ethics to go beyond that level.

But there is a first-order decision level hidden in the background, controlling the second-level options. The reason there was only one ICU bed available was not some act of God, not some natural scarcity of resources, not some inevitable fate that must be accepted. The reason for one available bed was a choice made by health economists, agency specialists, and, finally, politicians to restrict the number of hospital beds in order to cut the cost of health care. Those with the power to make such choices have decided that only "x" amount of dollars should be available for health care.[21,22]

In most countries that decision is usually not publicly debated, it is restricted to policy experts, there is no public referendum, and information about such decision is carefully controlled. In some countries, such as Zaire and Zimbabwe, it is a decision reflecting to some extent a natural shortage of resources. In other countries, although it is framed as a shortage of resources or as "saving world resources," it is much less connected to a natural shortage and more often a political prioritizing that creates an artificial shortage. Because the sick do not have high social utility, this utilitarian standard operates against the medical care system.

But this partially hidden economic agenda of utility is more open and honest than the second ethical approach, a medical ethics of Right to Die and Death with Dignity, which characterizes the euthanasia activism so prominent in medical ethics.[23,24] This activism studiously overlooks the economic pressures and frames the ethical discussion in overly cognitive models of human choice and human nature, not taking into account the full human biological system, the core family system, the fact that humans must be social beings and are defined within multiple sociocultural systems. Life and death decisions are described as civil rights or legal precedents.[25] Family messages and family dynamics are then described simply as either legal surrogate-decision-making or durable-power-of-attorney issues.[25] Emotional responses are restricted to wishes for control or to frank psychoses that indicate legal incompetence. The physical and psychosocial effects of disease (particularly chronic diseases, but even diseases that have intermittent effects such as delirium) are not considered important in the decision process. And of course, economic and social structuring of individual decisions remains unrecognized, although sociologists have long recognized that social institutions and systems structure human choice and behavior in important ways.[26] Instead, rejecting a systems model of human nature and ethical choice, the ethics of euthanasia creates a myth of the person as an independent decision process whose primary values are control and logical decision theory and whose social description or definition is as a legal-civil right.

Since ideas and frameworks do have major effects, these nonsystems models in medical ethics represent risks not only to AIDS patients but to all chronic, elderly, or terminal patients:

1. Underfunded medical systems will move to triage choices, without questioning the ethics of such socially created shortages;
2. Right-to-Die and Rational Suicide groups will structure patients to choose early death as an expression of control and autonomy, while failing to see such structuring as a means to achieve economic priorities;
3. Lack of chronic care, respite care, hospice care, experimental treatment, social services, and social valuing will be accepted without questioning; and
4. Economic pressures will continue to move patients toward physician-

assisted death and withdrawal of routine medical care, not taking into account the kind of physician this will create.

In addition to helping us identify economic agendas as one of the multilevel goals in a deep analysis of ethical issues, systems theory can also be a tool for identifying other goals. For example, there are unarticulated social goals concerning sexual mores or conventions underlying ethical questions in AIDS. A brief summary of these implicit goals follows:

1. The AIDS issue is used to advance a restrictive goal for sexual behavior. Because sexual behavior can now carry a risk of death as well as the health risk of sexually transmitted diseases (STDs), those who wish sexual behavior restricted to marriage (or permanent one-partner commitment) may use the AIDS risk to achieve that goal. Abstinence, not AIDS education and prevention, will be the goal. Required assumptions will be that all sexual behavior carries a high risk, that individuals will not and should not take high risks, and that risk can be eliminated by choosing against sex outside marriage. Or,

2. The AIDS issue is used to advance a very liberal goal for sexual behavior. Because AIDS education and prevention require sex education and education about "safer" sex, proponents of sexual behavior as pleasurable activity among adults (within or outside marriage or one-partner commitment) may use such education to attempt to liberalize social conventions about sexual behavior. Required assumptions will be that the risk of AIDS requires confronting social conventions, that education in "safer" sex is effective, and that the risk of "safer" sex is sufficiently low to satisfy public health and ethical concerns. Or,

3. Sexual behavior is seen as free rational choice in a restricted Health Belief Model of education. This reflects the same nonsystemic framework discussed above. Human sexuality is much more complicated and much more fundamental than a free-choice model assumes. It needs to be understood on multiple levels, including ethology, psychological dynamic theory, and cultural variation. Or,

4. The AIDS issue can be used to devalue homosexuality. Or,

5. The AIDS issue can be used to advance homosexual goals.

All these goals need to be identified and analyzed in a full ethical study. The most useful tool for that is systems theory, which is uniquely constructed to look at all levels before reaching an answer to an ethical question.

## Trust in Experts and Expert Obligation

Experts bear the heavy ethical burden that they should deserve the trust expected as part of the expert role. That burden is not always carried well and presents a broader question that affects all aspects of our society. Although questions have been raised about the scientific ethics of some AIDS researchers, they are minor compared to the number of incidents of scientific fraud in medical science as a whole and join a large group of issues about dishonesty or incompetence in academic and professional disciplines.[27] However, we will assume the scientific ethics of experts, because there is another important problem that systems theory ethics can more fruitfully address, that of trust.

Trust in the expert's message is a major problem in AIDS prevention and treatment. It would be unethical to either minimize or overstate AIDS risks, but that is a difficult balance to achieve. How does an expert meet his or her ethical obligation when he or she interprets the data as indicating a particular risk? How does a layperson trust the guidelines and policy recommendations based on the expert's interpretation of the data? When two experts, using the same data, come to conflicting interpretations and policy, how is the conflict to be resolved?

It is important to note that systems ethics encompasses both individual and policy decisions about what is the good. It also requires a working knowledge of ethical epistemology and philosophy of science. Practical health care professionals would prefer that such abstract analysis be abbreviated and a specific ethical protocol prescribed and applied. They prefer to assume that this protocol will be rational, accurate, and useful. This is a dangerous assumption, because ethical protocols can hide more questions than they appear to answer and are not always based on scientific probability. For example, a protocol about expert messages on risk and policy, without a foundation of the standards of scientific probability, is actually based on current wishes, political ideologies, social activism, value biases, and the expert's personal dynamics. Such a protocol appeals (fallaciously) to the authority of the expert and the often premature consensus of networking experts.[28] Protocols also don't give us the various contexts of the expert interpretation, the initial conditions within which the data are explained. Building trust in the expert message, so critical for AIDS prevention and treatment, cannot reasonably occur in such a situation.

Systems theory is very helpful here because it doesn't reduce the experts' disagreements into a raw power struggle, but has mechanisms for assisting the public in understanding the various interpretations and weighting of data. We first look at the data coming from multiple levels: animal studies, microbiology, individual cases, epidemiology, comparative public health problems. Simply assigning data to a level in the larger system allows us to include data that at first glance seemed inconsistent and also allows us to see connections between those levels. We then look at the level-perspective of the expert because there are multiple possible focuses from which to perceive a question. Some perspectives will be too biased and will need to be expanded and corrected in the larger view. A public health administrator-manager will be using a different focus than a gay political activist, and both need to appreciate the multiple focuses required to understand AIDS issues. The administrator and the activist could both give a Best-Case interpretation of the data, but for very different reasons (the blood bank donation issue, for example, where the administrator sees the risk of public panic and the activist sees the risk of individual discrimination). The patient needing a blood transfusion is focused on the Worst-Case interpretation, since *any* risk of a fatal disease is seen as highly significant.

Systems theory shows us the range of data interpretation open to an expert. In order to evaluate the expert's message, we need to know where on that range from Best-Case to Worst-Case his interpretation lies, and whether that is the most reasonable point to set. It may also be a reasonable set-point for some cases or situations and an unreasonable one for others. To further complicate the expert's message, all of this is done in the context of uncertainty because of changing knowledge and the newness of HIV infection in medical science.

The ethical obligation is to make all this clear in education and prevention. There are two obstacles to this forthrightness: the rationalization that risk-messages can cause public panic or hysteria, and the concern that some risk-messages will cause health care professionals to refuse to treat HIV + individuals (or more generally, that community members will avoid all contact with HIV + persons). The evaluation of our training of health care professionals indicated that raising death and infection anxiety is not negatively correlated with willingness-to-treat. Our training raised anxiety, but it also increased willingness-to-treat.

It is not necessarily an ethical argument, then, for always choosing the Best-Case interpretation. There is also a cost in a Best-Case bias. It erodes the trust necessary to receive and implement the risk-message, and in the long run is self-defeating. There is also the ethical question concerning the expert's obligation to each individual who hears the risk-message. A Utilitarian calculus that justifies placing a few individuals at an unacknowledged risk in order to benefit the larger group needs ethical justification much beyond the assumption that the individual must always be sacrificed.

The question of dentist-to-patient transmission of HIV mentioned earlier illustrates this well. A young college student, Kimberly Bergalis, unexpectedly developed AIDS even though available data indicated she did not engage in typical risk behaviors. Investigation indicated she was not a drug user. She claimed she had not engaged in intercourse, and HIV testing of her two boyfriends and even her father was negative for HIV. She had not had a blood transfusion. The only documented exposure appeared to be the molar extractions done by a dentist who later died of AIDS.

Dr. David J. Acer was HIV + at the time and had requested advice from the CDC. He followed their suggested infection control precautions and was wearing gloves and face mask at the time of the dental procedure. The CDC did not at that time recommend he inform his patients, and as this book was being written, New York State's Department of Health did not require that patients of HIV + professionals be informed. Kimberly Bergalis did not recall Dr. Acer's puncturing his gloves or any clear indication of blood exchange between her and the dentist. Four other patients of Dr. Acer, out of 500 tested, have tested positive for HIV, and for them, dentist-to-patient transmission was confirmed. When the CDC reported the case, however, what followed was a range of interpretation of the data.

The chair of the American Medical Association (AMA) AIDS Task Force, Dr. M. Roy Schwarz, did not think the link was "proven." By "proven," Dr. Schwarz seemed to mean in his own words: "Until science proves it unequivocally."[29] Dr. Robert T. Ferris, past chair of the Florida Board of Dentistry, wrote that "it flies in the face of everything the CDC and other governmental authorities have told us."[29] Drs. Schwarz and Ferris provide a Best-Case interpretation of the data (namely dentist-to-patient transmission had actually not occurred) based on an unscientific standard of truth: absolute proof and traditional authority. Both weighted the risk of iatrogenic transmission of HIV as very low and might have seen the disruption to the medical and dental care system as potentially high. Their set-point, however, of Best-Case cannot be justified on the basis of scientific probability.

On the other hand, the Bergalis family was convinced that dentist-to-patient transmission had occurred. They were joined by Dr. Sanford Kuvin, vice-chair of the National Foundation for Infectious Diseases, who felt that the Bergalis case was "the tip of the iceberg" and was inevitable because of the presence of blood in invasive medical procedures.[29] This is a Worst-Case interpretation, although it turned out to be the most probable interpretation based on accumulating CDC data. The real question is whether this probable transmission can justify a policy advocated by Dr. Kuvin, that the CDC advocate "testing of all health care workers and patients involved in invasive procedures."[29]

The CDC set-point is closer to Worst-Case, but the policy question depends on more than the validity of the iatrogenic transmission: "the case . . . is consistent with transmission of HIV to a patient during an invasive dental procedure, although the possibility of another source of infection cannot be entirely excluded."[14] The CDC's Kent Taylor described the case as a "*possible* transmission based on all the information we have."[29] Taylor also used epidemiological data to reduce the significance of the data, describing the case as one transmission out of 146,746 total transmissions of HIV. Both experts and the public are having difficulty sending out a risk-message on such iatrogenic transmission. For AIDS prevention and treatment purposes, the systems model, which fully describes the range of interpretation, is a necessary beginning for building trust and understanding.

This case example illustrates why common medical ethics principles will be inadequate. The principle of Informed Consent is too narrow a focus for this problem. The principle of Do No Harm makes no sense and gives no answers. The principle of Confidentiality was not meant to facilitate iatrogenic transmission of disease. These concepts are not sensitive to the interconnected levels of this case. A systems ethics has the conceptual tools needed.

### The Ethics of Accepted or Assisted Suicide and AIDS Patients

Again, this is a generic ethical question for medicine, spotlighted by HIV Infection, which is a severe and fatal disease. The multiple opportunistic diseases of AIDS are a difficult way to die. The apparently primary neurodegenerative disease (AIDS dementia) joins Huntington's, the Ataxias, Creutzfeldt-Jakob, and Amyotrophic lateral sclerosis as a tragic end to life. Various euthanasia advocacy groups have argued that such deaths can be painful and dehumanizing, and that individuals may choose a "death with dignity," either through passive refusal of treatment or active taking of their lives.[30] We once did ethics case rounds interviewing a Huntington's disease patient in her early twenties. She had made a suicide gesture, but also told us a nurse at the Huntington's clinic had given her the address of The Hemlock Society (a euthanasia group advocating the right of individuals to kill themselves and to be assisted by physicians). The patient had followed the instructions in the Society's literature and said she had a bottle in her refrigerator for when she was ready to die. She had decided to live a bit longer, but did eventually commit suicide a few years later.

In addition to the euthanasia argument, civil libertarians also argue that suicide is, or should be, a legal right, or that it is a moral decision that should not involve the State.[25] Passive suicide (the refusal to alter a lethal process) is now recognized by the legal system as a civil right of patients; a 1990 U.S. federal law requires hospitals and nursing homes receiving Medicare/Medicaid payments to inform admitted patients of their right to refuse treatment or have treatment stopped. This same legal system, of course, claims its commonwealth obligation to require helmets for motorcyclists and seat belts for car passengers.

This was graphically illustrated shortly after a hospital ethics committee meeting that had developed Do Not Resuscitate forms following passage of a New York State law giving competent patients the right to be asked about and to request Do Not Resuscitate status. The State was holding that competent adult patients could make what might be self-destructive decisions, and that the State had no compelling interest in the patients' lives that would justify intervening. We left the parking garage and within a block were stopped for a routine traffic check. The seat belt had been forgotten and the police officer promptly wrote a ticket for violation of another State law requiring motorists to wear seat belts to avoid injury or death. The State was now holding that, on the road, the lives of motorists at risk from a decision not to wear seat belts constituted a compelling State interest to intervene. But if the motorist, wearing a belt, is in an accident, is admitted to a hospital, and wishes to refuse treatment or is asked about DNR status and requests it, he or she has the right to risk life.

Finally, there is the argument raised by medical professionals, particularly physicians, that it is the right of a patient to have physician-assisted suicide and the obligation of the physician to provide it. The Kevorkian and Quill cases are the most publicized, but surveys have consistently shown a sizeable percentage of physicians who support physician-assisted suicide.[31] And on the last day of 1990, Tim Johnson, M.D., the physician commentator for the television news show, Good Morning America, cited the Netherlands experience with physician-assisted termination of life as a model for the U.S. He generally supported the concept and predicted that physician termination of life would come very shortly.

We need to add to these arguments the economic environment of cost-containment[21,22] and the Utilitarian argument of Daniel Callahan [23] that it may be necessary to ration medical care, and that the elderly will be a population whose access to care should be rationed. Health policy planners in the U.S. Health Care Finance Administration are also aware that a third of Medicare/Medicaid money goes to patients in their last three months of life. Terminal patients would also be added to this list of limited access. The Oregon experiment in a computerized cost-effective protocol for Oregon Medicaid payments resulted in the prototype-system's decision that medical care for cystic fibrosis children was not cost-effective to fund.[32] Long-term, chronic care patients would be another candidate for limited access. A systems approach to ethics requires integrating all three focuses into a full ethical analysis that may reject such sacrifices as unethical in a developed country such as the United States.

Those who are at risk for HIV, are seropositive, or are diagnosed as having AIDS should be particularly concerned with this ethical analysis because they fit into many of these populations. The current ethical framework of Rights (probably legal rights since it's not clear we're using a moral rights concept), Passive and Active Euthanasia/Suicide, Physician Obligation, and Cost-Efficiency again misses the profound systemic meaning of suicide and assisting in suicide. It describes suicide and assistance as rational and utilitarian when, in fact, it is more like a Nietzschean negation of the experienced universe, a basic emotional state.[33,34] There should also be concern because of neurodegenerative impairment and the question of competence or judgment.[35] We tend to use a legal definition of competence because medical ethics has framed suicide in civil rights terms. But a legal definition of competence is a very minimal definition, sometimes as minimal as a fluctuating awareness of person, place, and time.

Assisting in another person's death also has basic internal, emotional consequences. There are certain general patterns of dealing with these powerful effects:

1.  Physicians may distance themselves personally through routinizing or institutionalizing such killing. One of the most disturbing aspects of the Nazis' disposing of millions of persons was the impersonal, routine, and efficient manner of its execution.
2.  Physicians can deny responsibility, claiming they are facilitators of the patient's wishes or acting in compliance with legal requirements and culturally changing values.
3.  Physicians can romanticize death in a variety of ways and can "side with the aggressor (death)" as hostages begin to identify with the powerful terrorists who hold them.
4.  Physicians can be unaware of their deeper and darker psychological dynamics, including sadism, eroticizing of death, rejection of the imperfect, anger with the patient's failure to improve and their own inadequacy to cure, fear of mortality, control through killing. This should not be minimized. Dr. Kevorkian, for example, was reported to have said that the woman he was assisting with suicide rose up, at the moment of death, as if to kiss him.

Systems ethics provides a way of looking at the changes in the definition of a physician that physician-assisted suicide may make, as well as the internal effects on individual physicians. It considers the multiple levels that would be affected by, and would have input into, a decision for suicide. Messages about the worth of existence, the worth of an individual's life, the needs of the family system, the legacy of extended systems are all included in the multifocal view. From its perspective on the ethics of suicide, systems ethics would conclude:

1.  Individuals kill themselves because they *feel* like it (possibly based on factors not known to others at the time), not because it is a logical or rational conclusion.[33]
2.  If those feelings can't be realistically modified over a reasonable period of time, it would only rarely be ethical to require that the individual be a sacrifice to the needs of family, community, or society and culture, and be kept alive for the needs of others.[33,34]
3.  An honest attempt, at all levels, should be made to assure the individual of the meaning and value of life. Hidden messages from family

(overburdened), professionals (burn-out and cost-cutting pressures), community (financial cost), society (cost and denial of the person's social utility), and culture (devaluing of certain groups, few opportunities for joy in existence) may be telling the person to die. These messages need to be uncovered and dealt with.[33,34]

4. Self-suicide or assisted suicide should not be trivialized since there is serious potential for abuse in any social system.

5. It would require a major redefinition of physicians were the profession to allow and support routine physician-assisted suicides. It could easily return the profession to the negative aspects of the Shaman role, where the patient did not know whether the healer would beneficially help or maliciously destroy. Physicians delude themselves if they believe they can sanitize and institutionalize assisted death and not become agents of social agendas that are not based on the needs and interests of individual patients.

6. Certain populations of patients (including AIDS patients) are at risk of being manipulated or structured into suicide decisions that do not reflect the realistic possibilities of meaning and pleasure in life.

7. Both overtreatment and undertreatment can be causes for suicidal decisions and are capable of correction.

8. A social system that accepts and routinizes suicide creates a significant statement at all levels of the system: existence or reality is not worthwhile, the system does not care if its members destroy themselves, it is more efficient to die than to try to solve problems.

9. Only a strong intimate bond can justify requesting another person to assist in suicide.

Systems ethics does not *a priori* find suicide unethical or ethical.[33] The conclusion is a case-specific balance of the needs and interests of the multilevels of the system. For each case, the set-point for that balance will differ. But the conclusion will incorporate the dynamics of all levels of the system.

## Social Responsibility and Bonding, Self-Responsibility

A systems view of ethics requires obligation or responsibility, both to self and to extended systems, from an integrated (both/and) rather than adversarial (either/or) perspective.[5,36] It rejects a rights-perspective as based on the either-or choice of self or society. But it also rejects the communal Utilitarian perspective as based on that same forced either-or choice. Also, unlike the legalistic Rights-perspective, it can rationally base ethical obligation to self. This is important in AIDS prevention and treatment because we must assume, for the prevention and treatment to be effective, that we can show individuals that they should value their body-system and its good functioning, as well as valuing the social bonds with others, which result in ethical obligations about risk behavior.

An ethical theory that justifies a responsibility to self is essential for the Health Belief Model of education to make any sense at all.[36,37] The medical ethics Rights-model will not satisfy that requirement because it describes a claims-and-contract situation and proponents have held that the person cannot meaningfully contract with himself.[38] The libertarian civil rights version restricts only those choices that seriously limit the freedom of others, so many self-destructive choices are ethical under that theory.[39] The Autonomy Principle description in medical ethics, which is Neo-Kantian, also does not give any basis for self-responsibility, since it, too, allows any freedom of choice that is not seriously limiting to others. (Kant himself did feel that self-destruction was categorically unethical because it was a logical contradiction, he thought, to kill oneself in order to benefit oneself, a contradiction not so self-evident to others.) The Beneficence Principle also fails to capture any obligation to self.[40] The Utilitarian Principle, for all practical purposes, emphasizes the responsibility to sacrifice or deny self for the communal good.[41] That same either-or split of egoism and altruism characterizes much of religious ethics and western ethical theories which dismiss or devalue egoism (self-love, self-interest). Yet psychological studies emphasize how intimately correlative self-responsibility (self-love) and responsibility to others (altruism, empathy) actually are.[42,43]

Systems ethics provides the basic theoretical foundation for valuing the body-system and its good functioning. Since HIV infection prevention depends on this value, this is an important contribution. It indicates there is an objective ethical basis for choosing risk-reduction, but does not present that choice in a simplistic way. It gives a rational basis for the individual valuing his or her life and health, having the obligation to care for oneself validated. This is also particularly important for some at-risk groups whose members are already devalued by society and who have internalized this negative social message into feelings of self-hate, lack of worth, and sense of deserving whatever bad things happen to them. These individuals will mistakenly perceive that self-destructive behaviors and choices are appropriate for them. Systems ethics can counter this by emphasizing their truly ethical responsibility to themselves and this responsibility's value to all of us.

Some practical results can be the individual's heightened valuing of his or her sexual behavior and its constructive expressions: the reduction of high-risk sexual behavior; information-seeking about HIV risks and reasonable, self-caring choices about those risks; increased attention to infection-control; better health care decisions within the medical system; and positive advocacy for individuals.

Responsibility to others flows from adequate self-development within a larger system, the most proximate being the family system. But self-development also requires the complete cultural and social system, which supplies the very means of expression of both self-development and social bonding. Systems ethics integrates this altruism with self-development, so that ethical decisions must incorporate both in a workable balance. It shows that there will be trade-offs (costs and benefits) in any ethical choice, as a natural characteristic of ethical choice, because multiple levels are involved. A total choice for surface self-interest (egotism, selfishness) is actually a destructive barrier to fully developed self-interest (egoism). Responsibility to others develops self-interest.

With that initial understanding of responsibility to others, the issues become clearer. The individual diminishes himself or herself by not caring about the risks to others and taking this obligation too lightly. The range of possibilities here is huge and a few of these are listed below:

1. The incompetent person with HIV disease who puts others at risk because of a lack of capacity to appreciate what is involved, or because of lack of control of behavior and society's refusal to assist and take responsibility. Incompetence can be independent of HIV infection and preexisting, or caused by a prior condition and HIV disease, or caused by HIV disease alone. Risk behaviors can include throwing feces and urine, biting, cutting oneself and spraying blood, having unprotected sex, sharing drugs.

2. The marginally competent person with HIV disease who puts others at risk because of impaired capacity and judgment and society's reluctance to share responsibility. Risk behaviors can include some listed above, plus risks associated with the ability to still function marginally, such as job performance in work involving public safety or health profession fields.

3. The competent person with HIV disease who, because of rage or prior personality disorder, chooses to put others at serious risk of infection, hoping others will contract AIDS. There is sometimes expressed denial that HIV can be transmitted through the particular behavior, but there can also be full understanding that it can, along with the deliberate intention to infect others. Some states in the U.S. have made this criminal behavior with specific statutes.

4. The otherwise competent person with HIV disease who refuses to believe certain risks of infection or who does not wish to know the risks. There can be powerful internal dynamics not to accept certain transmission routes: The young mother with a baby with AIDS who becomes angry with hospital staff using universal precautions such as gloves, aprons, and mask, determined to believe that only blood and semen could contain the virus.

5. The otherwise competent person with HIV disease who uses powerful psychoactive substances (e.g., cocaine, alcohol) and as a result

engages in high-risk behaviors that he or she would not choose to do if not under the influence of the psychoactive substance.

6. The competent person with HIV disease who avoids all risk behavior but does not inform others of his or her HIV status because of privacy concerns or fear of rejection.

7. The competent person with HIV disease who avoids all risk behaviors with others and also informs relevant persons about his HIV status.

8. The competent person with HIV disease who is so fearful of spreading the infection that he or she avoids even behaviors that are low-risk and informs almost every person he interacts with about his HIV status.

9. The competent person with HIV disease who works with others to help prevent the spread of HIV and support those who are HIV +.

10. The competent person with HIV disease who volunteers for research and testing.

The ethical responsibility will vary with different individuals and situations, but some generalizations are possible. The full burden cannot be put on the individual's shoulders alone. The same social bonding that produces the ethical responsibility also means that responsibility is socially shared. Support is also an ethical obligation. On the extreme negative side of the range, society has a greater share of meeting the responsibility because the individuals are so compromised in their decision-making abilities. Civil libertarians fear society's acting on this responsibility, but it is not only reasonable, but humane. The fear is that the State will take the ethical responsibility away from all members of groups seen as at high-risk for HIV infection, but this is an extreme, or Worst-Case fear. Society can (and must) make distinctions and draw lines. Taking an extreme hands-off position may in fact so worsen situations that the possibility of balance will be lost and the pendulum *will* swing to an extreme state-intervention position. Thinking in process or systems terms allows us to appreciate this typical consequence.

With competent individuals, the accountability-share for the social system is less, but not entirely absent. Even very ethical individuals have difficulty acting ethically when the system or institution is structured to model unethical behavior. Even in these situations, then, accountability is shared at all levels. AIDS preventive education must pay special attention to the accuracy of its messages and to the dynamics that may distort or interfere in hearing the message. Gaetan Dugas (known as Patient Zero and responsible for spreading HIV infection while knowing he had "gay cancer") distorted or misunderstood that scientific knowledge is always probable rather than certain; he continued to deny that science had "proved" that his disease was spread through sexual activity.[11] Sexuality was one of the major values in his life and we can understand why he misused scientific probability. This rationalization allowed him to avoid his ethical responsibility, but at a high cost to his name and to his contacts' lives.

Prostitutes without any immediate substitute means for making a living may choose to continue prostitution even when HIV-infected. They may hear the AIDS message, with its confusing names for the disease stages and its distinction between seropositivity and AIDS, as telling them that HIV infection does not mean they have and can transmit AIDS.

Health care professionals who are HIV + (at the time of writing this book there are about 5,000 tested and reported) are aware of the potential destruction of their clinical practice if they inform their patients that they have HIV infection. They may choose to hear previous CDC summaries of the state of our knowledge about iatrogenic transmission and insist that such outdated knowledge is really permanent, absolute knowledge. This would allow them to refrain from informing patients of their HIV status, under the assumption that it is not relevant. This setting of the balance between self-interest and responsibility to others too far in the direction of self-interest is unethical. But it is unethical in a complex way that slogans about Informed Consent can't possibly describe or appreciate.

In all the ethical issues involving responsibility to self and others, systems ethics makes an important point. Aristotle was not completely correct to see the good as the Golden Mean, a middle setting between two extremes (although he was shrewd enough to understand that not all virtues were the prudent middle ground). That set-point changes in different cases and contexts and can move toward either extreme. It also is not fixed in time, but is a process that must adapt to changing data. That means that medical ethics generalizations are only rules of thumb and not universal categorical imperatives.[44,45] Questions about informing others of HIV status, restricting freedom of behavior or choice because of transmission risk, universal precautions, routine medical testing, management of preschool and elementary school HIV + students and confidentiality versus duty to warn can be answered if the initial conditions of the case are specified and the multifocal levels are incorporated. However, the answers are provisional.

## Duty to Warn/Confidentiality Conflicts

This specific question has mistakenly been turned into a legal issue. We have transmuted most of our social values and ethics questions into case law or legislative statute, at our ethical peril. This is such a pervasive American cultural response that the above statement will seem harsh. But a close look at the Duty to Warn/Confidentiality question will reveal the ethical trap in such reliance on legal resolutions.

New York State passed in 1989 an addition to its Public Health Law,

Article 27-F, specifically dealing with the handling of AIDS information.[46] It was meant to address the question of physicians informing sexual contacts of HIV+ patients. Patients could see this as a breach of confidentiality and sue the professional. Sexual contacts could use the Tarasoff precedent of the physician's duty to warn individuals about serious probable harm and sue the professional for failure to warn.[47] Information about HIV status was already being managed separately from other medical information, with implied severe legal redress for improper management. Third-party payers and regulators, however, had more or less unrestricted access to such information.

Power-brokering and the political process produced Article 27-F as a solution. It included severe legal punishment for professionals who breached patient confidentiality. It also made routine work-up for HIV problematic, created complex mechanisms for professional sharing of HIV medical information within the system, and allowed physician discretion on informing sexual contacts. It failed to limit third-party payer and regulator access to patient information (the most serious area of breach of confidentiality) and made provision for penal system and other agency sharing of information. What can we learn from the law?

1. Laws reflect the power balances in a society, not the scientific, ethical, or functional aspects. Those positions activating the most power will be reflected in the final statute. Insurance companies are extremely powerful, as are federal and state agencies. There was no real limitation on their access to patient information and violation (routinely done through coerced patient sign-off) of confidentiality.
2. Laws that are statutes rather than case precedents are inflexible and unresponsive to individual situations, and become rigidified in time. They are difficult to change even in the face of new data and changing needs. Remedicalizing HIV disease through routine HIV work-up and easy professional exchange of HIV information would now benefit patients, but that benefit (both diagnostic and treatment) is deferred by a law that codified preliminary knowledge about HIV into rigid statute.
3. Laws are passed in an activist and exaggerated atmosphere of crisis, with the real problems often overlooked or misidentified. The greatest threat to confidentiality, for example, is from insurance companies and government regulators and agencies, not from physicians. Requiring a separate counseling apparatus for HIV testing and restricting the physician's practice concerning HIV diagnosis are questionable given the thousands of physicians who routinely tell patients of diagnoses of terminal conditions (pancreatic cancer, Hurler's syndrome, Huntington's disease, Alzheimer's disease, oat-cell carcinoma, ALS, etc.).
4. Laws can create legislative overmanagement and a medical practice

based, not on science or patient need, but on possibility of lawsuit (defensive medicine). As with any overmanagement, it has negative consequences on its target profession or activity.
5. Laws push ethical questions out of consideration, making them basically irrelevant or unacceptably dangerous civil disobedience.

## SUMMARY

We haven't discussed all the ethical questions raised by this newly recognized infectious disease, but hopefully we have sketched an outline of systems ethics that can be useful in the ongoing process of identifying ethical questions and proposing answers to them. We have argued that it is superior to other theories in the history of ethics that have been applied to medical problems: Utilitarian, Mill's Civil Rights, Kantian Autonomy, Ordinary Language Intuitive Principles, Eclecticism, or Engelhardt's Negotiated Consensus.[48] We have also argued that it cannot be replaced by a Legalism.

There is more involved in systems ethics than we have described in this chapter. Its philosophic foundation requires more abstract reasoning than the health care professional might find interesting, which is one of the shortcomings of applied ethics, whether medical, business or environmental. It is, however, a naturalistic ethics, deriving (not formally deducing) ethical conclusions from scientific understanding of the human organism and its evolutionary adaptation to a universe-system in process. It can be described as an evolutionary ethics, a sociobiology within a general systems explanatory paradigm. It has an historical kinship with Aristotle, Hobbes, Hume, and Dewey. It is not incompatible with the Hippocratic tradition and it has points of contact with the natural law tradition.

This theorizing may be overly conceptual to some, as a medical colleague who is not philosophically interested continues to point out.[10] It complicates medical ethics because simple statements of guidelines, or culturally relative value systems, or committee consensus, or authoritarian value commands, or professional codes of ethics seem so much more practical and straightforward.[49] These practical modes, in fact, are how modern American medical ethics has defined itself. But it really doesn't give a valid answer to the question of what is the right thing to do.

The individual clinician may have his or her answer, as C. Everett Koop does: "I just did what I had always done as a doctor. My whole career had been dedicated to prolonging lives, especially the lives of people who were weak and powerless, the disenfranchised who needed an advocate, newborns who needed surgery, handicapped children, unborn children, people with AIDS."[50] But a firm theoretical foundation is also needed, and systems ethics can give that. If AIDS education is true education, rather than indoctrination (another large ethical issue in HIV infection), it must work to achieve valid answers. That is the ethical obligation it has to all who can potentially be affected by the HIV infectious disease process.

Despite the complexity, however, we can give a step-by-step method for applying systems ethics to a particular HIV case:[5]

1. Collect a full range of facts to determine if there really is an ethical problem or simply a misinterpretation.
2. Make a list of all the relevant levels affecting the case.
3. In any specific case, all participants should identify the level at which they have their primary role obligation.
4. The needs and interests of the levels should be described.
5. The consequences of intervention or nonintervention should be predicted fully.
6. The balance-set point that optimally meets the primary ethical obligation while maintaining reasonable systems functioning should be determined.
7. Dynamic situations should be monitored.
8. Once the ethical conclusion of a case is made, it represents typical human ethical behavior, neither saints nor sinners, nor perfection.

## REFERENCES

1. Dickens, D.M. (1988). Legal rights and duties in the AIDS epidemic. *Science* 239 (4840): 580–585.
2. Walters, L. (1988). Ethical issues in the prevention and treatment of HIV infection and AIDS. *Science*, 239 (4840): 597–603.
3. Ostrow, D.G., Traugott, M., Stryker, J. (1990). Public health policy and bioethical issues in AIDS: The case of an HIV-positive patient with neuropsychiatric impairment. In D.G. Ostrow (Ed.). *Behavioral Aspects of AIDS*. New York: Plenum.
4. Pierce, C., van de Veer, D. (1988). (Eds.) *AIDS: Ethics and Public Policy.* Belmont, CA: Wadsworth.
5. Clements, C.D. Systems ethics and the history of medical ethics. *Psychiatric Quarterly.* In Press.
6. Clements, C.D. (1989). Biology, man and culture: A unified science based on hierarchy levels. *Perspectives in Biology and Medicine, 33* (1): 70–85.
7. Clements, C.D. Systems ethics: The application of an epistemological paradigm to medical ethics. *Theoretical Medicine.* In preparation.
8. Clements, C.D. *Medical Genetics Casebook: A Clinical Introduction to Medical Ethics Systems Theory.* Clifton, NJ: Humana.
9. Rowley, P. Personal communication.
10. Pointer, N. Personal communication: "But does it mow the lawn?"

11. Shilts, R. (1987). *And the Band Played On: Politics, People, and the AIDS Epidemic.* New York: St. Martin's Press.
12. Medical resident study presented at the American Federation for Clinical Research 1989 meeting. *The Medical Post.* October 17, 1989.
13. Study presented by C. Lewandowski at the American College of Emergency Physicians 1989 meeting. *The Medical Post October 17, 1989.*
14. (June 14, 1991) Update: Transmission of HIV infection during invasive dental procedures. *MMWR 40* (23) : 377–381.
15. Bye, L. (1990). Moving beyond counseling and knowledge-enhancing interventions: A plea for community-level AIDS prevention strategies. In D.G. Ostrow (Ed.). *Behavioral Aspects of AIDS.* New York: Plenum.
16. Gilligan, C. (1982). *In a Different Voice.* Cambridge: Harvard University Press; and Clements, C.D. Gender differences in medical ethics? *The Medical Post.* November 20, 1990, p. 35.
17. Clements, C.D. (1989). "Therefore choose life": Reconciling medical and environmental bioethics. *Perspectives in Biology and Medicine, 28* (3): 407–425.
18. Clements, C.D. (1987). The silence of ethics and the economics of medicine. *The World and I,* November: 577–592.
19. Clements, C.D. (1989). Pinching pennies shortchanges medicine. *Psychiatric Times.* November.
20. Hardin, G. (1972). *Exploring New Ethics for Survival.* New York: Viking.
21. Calabresi, G., Bobbit, P. (1978). *Tragic Choices: The Conflicts Society Confronts in the Allocation of Tragically Scarce Resources.* New York: Norton.
22. Aaron, J., Schwartz, W.B. (1990). Rationing health care: The choice before us. *Science, 247:* 418–422.
23. Callahan, D. (1987). *Setting Limits: Medical Goals in an Aging Society.* New York: Simon & Schuster.
24. Veatch, R.M. (1989). *Death, Dying and the Biological Revolution: Our Last Quest for Responsibility.* New Haven: Yale University Press, Rev. Ed.
25. Weir, R.F., Gostin, L. (1990). Decisions to abate life-sustaining treatment for nonautonomous patients: Ethical standards and legal liability for physicians after *Cruzon. JAMA, 263* (14): 1845–1853.
26. Hughes, E.C. (1958). *Men and Their Work.* Glencoe, Illinois: Free Press.
27. Goodstein, D. (1991). Scientific fraud. *The American Scholar, 60:* 505–515.
28. Caton, H. (1990) *Trends in Biomedical Regulation.* Sydney: Butterworth.
29. Johnson, B., Grant, M., Sider, D. (1990). A life stolen early. *People Weekly, 34* (16): 70–78.
30. Humphrey, D., Wickett, A. (1986). *The Right to Die:Understanding Euthanasia.* New York: Harper and Row.
31. Quill, T.E. (1991). Death and dignity: A case of individualized decision making. *Medicine, 324* (10): 691–694.
32. Morell, V. (1990). Oregon puts bold health plan on ice. *New England Journal of Science, 249* (4968): 468–471.
33. Clements, C.D. (1980). The ethics of not being: Individual options for suicide.

In Mayo, Batlin (Eds.) *Suicide: The Philosophical Issues.* New York: St. Martin's Press.

34. Clements, C.D., Sider, R.C., Perlmutter, R. (1983). Suicide: Bad act or good intervention. *Journal of Suicide and Life-Threatening Behavior,* April.

35. Ciccone, J.R., Clements, C.D. (1987). The elderly and medicolegal trends in consent to treatment. In F. Rosner (Ed.) *Critical Issues in American Psychiatry and Law. III.* New York: Plenum.

36. Sider, R.C., Clements, C.D. (1984). Patients' ethical obligations for their health. *British Journal of Medical Ethics, 10:* 138–142.

37. Jeffery, R.W. (1989). Risk behaviors and health: Contrasting individual and population perspectives. *American Psychologist, 44:* 1194–1202.

38. Gorovitz, S. (1978) Health as an obligation. In W.T. Reich (Ed.) *Encyclopedia of Bioethics.* 2: 606–609.

39. Culver, C., Gert, B. (1982). *Philosophy in Medicine.* New York: Oxford University Press.

40. Beauchamp, T.L. (1979). *Principles of Biomedical Ethics.* New York: Oxford University Press.

41. Clements, C.D. (1982). Social and individual interest conflicts. In C.D. Clements *Medical Genetics Casebook: A Clinical Introduction to Medical Ethics Systems Theory* (pp. 165–169). Clifton, NJ: Humana Press.

42. Sharabony, R., Bar-Tal, D. (1982). Theories of the development of altruism: Review, comparison and integration. *International Journal of Behavioral Development, 5:* 49–80.

43. Simon, H.A. (1990). A mechanism for social selection and successful altruism. *Science, 250:* 1665–1668.

44. Clements, C.D. (1985). Bioethical essentialism and scientific population thinking. *Perspectives in Biology and Medicine, 28* (2):188–207.

45. Clements, C.D., Ciccone, J.R. (1985). Applied clinical ethics or universal principles. *Hospital and Community Psychiatry, 36* (2): 121–123.

46. New York State Public Health Law. Article 27–F HIV and AIDS-Related Information.

47. Beck, J.C. (1990). Current status of the duty to protect. In J.C. Beck (Ed.). *Confidentiality Versus the Duty to Protect: Foreseeable Harm in the Practice of Psychiatry* (pp. 9–21). Washington, D.C.: American Psychiatric Press.

48. Engelhardt, H.T. (1990). *The Foundations of Bioethics.* New York: Oxford University Press.

49. Clements, C.D. (1990). The American medical education experiment in ethics. In H. Caton (Ed.) *Trends in Biomedical Regulation* (pp. 101–112). Sydney: Butterworths.

50. Koop, C.E. (1991). *The Memoirs of America's Family Doctor.* New York: Random House.

# Name Index

329

# Subject Index

335